Essentials of Gerontological Nursing

Essentials of Gerontological Nursing

Meredith Wallace PhD, APRN-BC

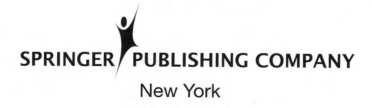

SPRINGER PUBLISHING COMPANY

New York

Copyright © 2008 Springer Publishing Company, LLC

Springer Publishing Company, LLC
11 West 42nd Street
New York, NY 10036
www.springerpub.com

Acquisitions Editor: Allan Graubard
Project Manager: Carol Cain
Cover design: Joanne E. Honigman
Composition: Apex Publishing, LLC

08 09 10/ 5 4 3 2 1

Library of Congress Cataloging-in-Publication Data

Wallace, Meredith, PhD, RN.
  Essentials of gerontological nursing / Meredith Wallace.
    p. ; cm.
  Includes bibliographical references and index.
  ISBN-13: 978-0-8261-2052-6 (alk. paper)
  ISBN-10: 0-8261-2052-0 (alk. paper)
  1. Geriatric nursing. I. Title.
  [DNLM: 1. Geriatric Nursing. WY 152 W192e 2007]
  RC954.W25 2007
  618.97'0231—dc22   2007025523

Printed in the United States of America by Bang Printing.

This book is dedicated to my loving grandfather Fiora "Bill" Metall who engendered in me a love for older adults and a passion for excellence in geriatric care.

Contents

Preface

The current standards of living, nutrition, prevention and treatment of infectious diseases, and progress in medical care have sharply increased the survival rate for people born in the United States. Once people reach adulthood, they are likely to survive to old age. In 1990, the number of Americans age 65 and older was approximately 28 million, roughly 12% of the population. By the year 2030, that percentage is projected to increase to more than 18% of the population. By the year 2020, the over-65 population in Connecticut alone is expected to increase 28% (ftp://ftp.hrsa.gov/bhpr/workforceprofiles/connecticut.pdf). In fact, the fastest-growing age group in the country is that of adults age 85 and older. According to Healthy People 2010, individuals currently aged 65 years can be expected to live an average of 18 more years than they did 100 years ago, for a total of 83 years. Those currently aged 75 years can be expected to live an average of 11 more years, for a total of 86 years (http://www.health.gov/healthypeople).

As a result of the increasing lifespan, diseases once regarded as acute in duration and imposing imminent death are now chronic diseases among older adults. The presence of disease among this population mandates quality nursing care. However, the poor perception of nursing and lack of nurses with the knowledge and experience to care for older adults clearly leaves older adults as an underserved population with a dubious quality of care. In a study of college students, negative attitudes toward the elderly were commonly found. However, intergenerational learning experiences contributed to improving these attitudes. Thus, the author recommended these experiences in order to change attitudes toward the aged (Layfield, 2004).

This evidence points clearly to the fact that a large need exists to provide quality geriatric nursing education to practicing nurses nationwide. *Essentials of Gerontological Nursing* is an effective compilation of geriatric best practices needed to effectively care for older adults. It is brief, yet comprehensive, in its approach to geriatric issues and will be a refreshing contribution to the currently existing literature that is more heavily focused on theory, and less so on clinical practice.

REFERENCES

Layfield, K. D. (2004). Impact of intergenerational service learning on students' stereotypes toward older people in an introductory agricultural computing course. *Journal of Southern Agricultural Education Research, 54,* 134–146.

Acknowledgments

The author wishes to gratefully acknowledge the many students who assisted with this book. Thanks go to Kara Diffley for her contributions on Parkinson's Disease and her editorial assistance with this book; Patricia Cino for her assistance with the sections on Alzheimer's Disease; Jay Plano for his assistance with the sections on diabetes; and George Flohr for his assistance with the sections on congestive heart failure. Also, thanks go to Paula Shevlin for her work on the Evidence-Based Practice boxes and Lindsay Neptune for assisting with the case studies. Many thanks to the Hartford Institute for Geriatric Nursing for generating so much of the knowledge evident in this book and to Dr. Mildred O. Hogstel, who provided so much inspiration for this book and for compassionate geriatric nursing care throughout her career.

Essentials of
Gerontological Nursing

CHAPTER ONE

The Graying of America

Learning Objectives

1. Discuss the concept of the Graying of America.
2. Identify special issues of aging.
3. Discuss 10 myths of aging.
4. Discuss the concept of ageism and its relevance to nursing.
5. Define ethnogeriatrics and cultural competence.
6. Describe standards of gerontological nursing and education.
7. Identify the major theoretical categories of aging.

Mrs. Molina, an 85-year-old White female, comes to the walk-in clinic with a chief complaint of dizziness and unsteady gait and states that she fell 2 weeks ago. Her vitals signs are BP 80/50, P 90, R 20, T 99.5° F, and she has no complaint of pain. She is 5'2" and weighs 90 lbs. You are the RN doing her initial assessment. You ask her why she waited so long to come in and she states "I haven't driven a car in 15 years and I don't want to be a bother to my children—they are busy enough." You then ask her what she typically eats in a day, and she tells you, "I usually don't eat anything for breakfast, just a cup of coffee. For lunch I usually have a bowl of soup, and then I make a little pasta for dinner." She then says that she has lost enjoyment in eating and cooking meals ever since her husband passed away 6 months ago.

The story of Mrs. Molina is typical of commonly occurring health care situations, and highlights the typical and complex aging older adult. Whether one is a nurse, a street sweeper, or a nuclear engineer, it is impossible to live in the United States today without hearing about the increasing elder population. According to Healthy People 2010, individuals aged 65 years can be expected to live an average of 18 more years than they did 100 years ago, for a total of 83 years. Those aged 75 years can be expected to live an average of 11 more years, for a total of 86 years (http://www.health.gov/healthypeople). Older adults are expected to represent approximately 20% of the population by the year 2030. This unprecedented increase in the number of older adults in the United States is known as the Graying of America. The Graying of America brings about multiple issues and concerns for society, including how a majority of older adults will be viewed and what resources will be available for older adults to live healthy and happy lives.

There are many reasons why people are living longer. Advances in medications to treat diseases, immunizations to prevent disease, and new diagnostic techniques to assist in the early detection and treatment of disease are among the major reasons for the increase in longevity. The development of new medications occurs daily and aids in the treatment of illnesses that once resulted in disability and death, such as heart disease and cancer. Moreover, the ability to prevent diseases such as measles, mumps, rubella, chicken pox, and polio plays a great role in allowing children and young adults to enter older adulthood. In addition, improved economic conditions and nutrition, as well as a stronger emphasis on health promotion, have undoubtedly resulted in decreases in both illness and death among the population. Many theorists have questioned the key ingredients to living a long life. In a qualitative study by Pascucci and Loving (1997), centenarians (those who have survived to the age of 100 or older) stated that clean and moral living, described as avoiding drinking and living independently, provided the rationale for their long lives. Other centenarians reported that a good attitude was essential to a long life. However, the majority of the 12 centenarians in the study had no idea why they had lived so long. This chapter will discuss the rising older population as well as special issues and myths of aging and the impact of ageism on the population. The cultural diversity of the older population will be explored with recognition of the need to develop cultural competence in order to appropriately care for older adults. Gerontological nursing education and history will be presented. The chapter will conclude with a discussion of the various theoretical explanations for aging.

ISSUES OF AGING

The great advances in science, which have created a generation of older adults that was previously nonexistent, are cause for celebration. However, the growth of the older population is not without issues that impact society and nursing practice. One of the major issues discussed frequently in society includes the need for more health care for older adults. Older adults, although living longer, tend to do so with several chronic illnesses that are in need of long-term and consistent health care. Moreover, older adults tend to have comorbid illnesses, or more than one disease at a time. The Alliance for Aging Research (2002) reports that the average older adult has three chronic medical conditions. The presence of illnesses among populations is referred to as the population's morbidity. When these illnesses result in death, this is considered the population's mortality. These acute and chronic illnesses will be discussed later in Chapter 6.

The increasing lifespan of older adults makes it possible for an individual to spend up to 40 years in older adulthood. Consequently, gerontologists have broken this stage of life into three segments: the young–old includes adults aged 65 to 75, the middle–old includes those 75–85, and those 85+ are the old–old. The division of older adults into segments allows nurses to recognize the unique differences present in each stage of older adulthood in order to provide more effective care. One of the unique issues present for the young–old is the great impact of the baby boom population on the nation's resources. The first baby boomer will turn 65 on January 1, 2011, and this population will provide the nation with the largest elderly population in history. With the great use of health promotion and health resources required by this population, society will be challenged to maintain supply with demand. The middle–old and old–old also have challenges including health and housing, as well as paying for long-term and chronic care.

Government-Funded Health Care

A major issue resulting from the increasing life span is how to pay for the many health care problems of older adults. Medicare, the current federal insurance plan for adults over the age of 65 and for those with disabilities, is experiencing great difficulty in paying for the rising medical costs consistent with the increasing population. When Medicare was originally developed, the basis for funding was a lower life span and lower medical costs. With people living longer and health care costs rising there is a growing budget deficit as payments continue to be made on behalf of Medicare recipients. Furthermore, the current Medicare coverage does not provide for long-term nursing home care or prescription drug coverage under traditional Medicare plans, although drug coverage plans may be purchased. Recently, the Medicare Prescription Drug Improvement and Modernization Act of 2003 approved prescription discount drug cards for Medicare recipients. These cards are available to over 7 million of Medicare's 41 million participants. Older adults must apply to be eligible for the discount cards, and a minimum fee may be charged depending

---

CULTURAL FOCUS

Older adults who have immigrated to the United States to live their later lives with their adult children may not have paid into the U.S. Social Security system, and, therefore, they must either buy into Medicare or become eligible for Medicaid. However, legislation passed in 1990 made it more difficult for older adults who were not citizens of the United States to access Medicaid. Nurses caring for older adults from various cultural backgrounds should question ability to pay for medication in order to decrease nonadherence to suggested health care strategies.

---

on their income. The cards provide discounts on some drugs, but not all. The *American Journal of Nursing* ("Pick a Card," 2004) reports that older adults with higher incomes may save more by using other prescription drug plans. Moreover, Social Security payments, which are a form of income for older adults who are no longer working, were designed based on a much shorter lifespan as well. Social Security payments continuing into unexpected eighth and ninth decades of life are causing the social security system to explore alternative methods. For more information on the health care delivery system implications surrounding the increasing aging population, see Chapter 2.

MEDICAL CONCERNS

Medical problems are very common among older adults. As stated earlier, it is not uncommon for older adults to have several chronic medical conditions at the same time. As a result of these medical illnesses, older adults experience a variety of problems with activities of daily living (ADLs), which include bathing, dressing, eating, toileting, continence, and transferring. These problems often impact older adult's ability to live independently, because their functional decline may prevent them from bathing on a regular basis, preparing food for themselves, or paying their bills on time, which all affect the individual's quality of life. When this occurs, older adults have several housing options. Many older adults move in with siblings or children. Others may consider subsidized or privately owned and operated housing alternatives, such as senior housing, assisted-living facilities, continuing care retirement communities, or nursing homes. Each of these environments of care provide some supervision and services to help the older adult to live as independently as possible. More information about these environments of care and the services they provide are available in Chapter 11.

AGEISM—FACTS AND MYTHS OF AGING

When nursing students enter educational programs they are often asked with which populations they would like to work. Most students answer that they wish to work with children and babies. Some students respond that they would like to work in maternity. Very few (if any) students reply that they came to nursing school to work with older adults. In fact, the society that currently exists in the United States is extremely youth-oriented. This means that older adults are not always considered and respected for their unique needs and contributions to society. Beliefs about older adulthood in the United States are perpetuated by myths of aging. The following section reports on the top 10 myths of aging and discusses why they are untrue of today's population of older adults.

Myths

Myth #1: Older adults are of little benefit to society. Older adults are often viewed as sick people in hospital units and nursing homes. As they lie in beds and consume medications and resources, it is hard to imagine what benefit they are to society, and thus they are often considered to be a burden. However, the rate of disability among older adults is continuing to decline steadily. Moreover, it is important to remember that the same older adults for whom nurses care are mothers and fathers, grandmothers and grandfathers, aunts, uncles, brothers, sisters, and friends. To those with whom they are in relationships, they are of great benefit, as they provide and receive love, care, and support. These same older adults function in professional roles as teachers, administrators, physicians, nurses, and clergy. Consequently, they are of great benefit to those they serve in these roles. Instead of viewing older adults as a burden, take the time to speak with them about their lives. Ask older adults about their favorite memories or regrets. Don't be afraid to ask for advice. When given the opportunity, it is likely that nurses as well as the rest of society will learn a lot from older adults.

Myth #2: Older adults are a drain on society's resources. As many older adults retire in their late years and collect Social Security payments and Medicare, it is assumed that they are overutilizing their resources. In fact, increasing Social Security payments over decades of life and Medicare reimbursement for rising health care costs are a significant problem for U.S. citizens. However, older adults who received Social Security and Medicare paid into the system from which they are now drawing. Moreover, while many older adults retire, many others do not. In 2002, 13.2% of older Americans were working, or actively seeking work. A Gallup poll of 986 older adults reported that, of the total sampled, only 15% of older adults wished to retire; the vast majority wanted to work as long as possible. Mandatory retirement ages and work discrimination have often forced reluctant older adults into retirement. In addition, many older adults who are retired spend a great deal of time in unpaid volunteer work, which saves employer's costs. Moreover, many retired older adults have taken on the role of custodial grandparents, relieving the states from having to pay for the full cost of foster care from a nonrelative. The 1990 Census reported that grandparents raising grandchildren had risen 44% over the previous decades. While it is true that the rising lifespan of U.S. citizens is resulting in a greater amount of expenditures on the behalf of older adults, this is not always a result of their choosing, and a great majority of the retired older adults are significantly contributing to society in ways other than traditional employment.

Myth #3: Older adults are cranky and disagreeable. When asked about initial impressions of older people, many nursing students report that older adults are cranky, disagreeable, and generally unlikable people. This myth plays an instrumental role in the lack of gerontological nurses. While it is true that there are many cranky and disagreeable older adults, it is important to note that there is an equal number of cranky and disagreeable younger adults. Moreover, the continuity theory supports that individuals move through their later years attempting to keep things much the same and using similar personality and coping strategies to maintain stability throughout life. Consequently, the coping strategies seen among older adults may be very similar to their younger characteristics. If there appears to be more difficult patients among older adults, it may be because older adults tend to approach their later years sicker than the younger population. Anyone who has ever been sick can report that being sick can make you cranky. When working with difficult older adults, remember that negative interactions with nurses may likely be a symptom of their illness, rather than a characteristic of aging. Like any other symptom, it is essential to identify the cause and treat it. In so doing, the older adult's personality will be allowed to shine through, and they will likely treat you with the respect due to a caring and concerned professional.

Myth #4: You can't teach old dogs new tricks. Patient teaching is a major component of the nursing role, regardless of which population is receiving care. This is true for older adults as well. While it is easy to think that 60 to 80 years of poor health behaviors such as drinking, smoking, or poor nutrition are impossible to break, this is simply not true. In working with the older adult population, a large amount of care will be directed toward managing pathological diseases of aging that resulted from poor health practices acquired early in life and continued into older adulthood. But, this does not mean that these diseases cannot be treated, managed, and in some cases cured. Older adults are never *too old* to improve their nutritional level, start exercising, get a better night's sleep, stop drinking and smoking, and improve their overall health and safety. The Surgeon General recently stated that the health risks of smoking may be reduced among all age groups and recommends that "geriatricians should counsel their patients who smoke, even the oldest, to quit" (U.S. Department of Health and Human Services, 2004). Moreover, older adults may still benefit from health promotion activities, even in their later years. In fact, health promotion is as important in older adulthood as it is in childhood. Further support to refute the myth that *you can't teach old dogs new tricks* may be found in the record number of older adults increasing their education. Older adults are increasingly returning to school and increasing their level of education. Many colleges and universities allow older adults to attend classes for low or no charge. In fact, 17% of older adults have a bachelor's degree or more. Keeping intellectually active is regarded as a hallmark of successful aging.

Myth #5: Older adults are all senile. The word *senile* was commonly used many years ago to describe older adults who were experiencing cognitive impairment. More recently this word has been replaced by the word *dementia,* which describes a number of illnesses that result in cognitive impairment. Becoming *senile* or *demented* as one grows older is of large concern to the aging population and their families and is the focus of a great deal of study in the older population. It is commonly believed that older adults will develop dementia as they age. However, this is always the case, as many older adults live well into their 10th decade as sharp as they were in their 20s and 30s. Memory losses are common in older adulthood, but are often falsely labeled as dementia. Dementia is not a normal change of aging, but a pathological disease process. In fact, dementia is a general term used to describe over 60 pathological cognitive disorders that develop as a result of disease, heredity, lifestyle, and perhaps environmental influences. Dementia is a chronic loss of cognitive function that progresses over a long-period of time. Alzheimer's disease (AD) is the most common cause of dementia among older adults, making up about 50% of all dementia diagnoses. There are approximately 4.5 million U.S. residents with Alzheimer's disease. Dementia is a devastating occurrence for both older adults and loved ones. Much research is being conducted on the prevention, diagnosis, early detection, and treatment of AD and related dementias.

Myth #6: Depression is a normal response to the many losses older adults experience with aging. Older adults have the highest rates of depression within the U.S. population. The frequent occurrence of loss among the older population was once used to explain the large incidence of depression among older adults. While it is true that situational life events, such as retirement, relocation, loss of spouse, financial constraints, and illness, play a role in the development or severity of depression, recent research on depression indicates that there is more to the development of depression than the experience of loss. In fact, the nature versus nurture controversy has uncovered the role of physiological factors in the development of depression among older adults. Because of the many physiological changes in older adults, this population is more susceptible to the effects of pathophysiology than any other age group. In fact, depression rates are highest among older adults with coexisting medical conditions. Moreover, 12% of older persons hospitalized for problems such as hip fracture or heart disease are diagnosed with depression. Rates of depression for older people in nursing homes range from 15% to 25%. Other factors that must be considered in assessing and managing depression are the presence of alcohol or drug abuse, past suicide attempts, and family history of depression and suicide.

Myth #7: Older adults are no longer interested in sex. It is commonly believed that older adults no longer have any interest or desire to participate in sexual relationships. Because sexuality is mainly considered a young person's activity, often associated with reproduction, society doesn't usually associate older adults with sex. In the youth-oriented society of today, many consider sexuality among older adults to be distasteful and prefer to assume sexuality among the older population doesn't exist. However, despite popular belief, sexuality continues throughout the lives of older adults. A survey of 1,709 older adults by the American Association of Retired Persons (1999) found that almost 39% had participated in sexual activity over the past week. The need to continue sexuality and sexual function should be as highly valued as other physiological needs. But for multiple reasons, most of society believes that sexuality is not part of the aging process. Consequently, nurses and other health care providers do not assess sexuality and few intervene to promote the sexuality of the older population. Reasons for nurses' lack of attention to sexuality of older adults include lack of knowledge, as well as general inexperience and discomfort.

Myth #8: Older adults smell. The age-old belief that older adults have poor personal hygiene has impacted the mind of many nursing students and health care providers of today. Moreover, the age-old recollection of nursing homes that smell of urine remains strong among those who may have visited such a home in the past. This myth plays a part in the opinion of older adults as a desirable population with whom to work. While it is true that there are older adults who have bad personal hygiene, this is definitely not the majority of the population. In fact, the number of sweat glands actually diminishes as people age, leading to less perspiration among older adults. Urinary and bowel incontinence, or the involuntary loss of urine and feces, occurs more commonly among older adults, but these are pathological changes of aging and are highly treatable. If an older adult smells of urine or feces, this is likely because they are very ill and their illnesses are not being effectively managed. Increased attention to older adult's care will likely result in improved management of hygiene, incontinence, and associated disorders.

Myth #9: The secret to successful aging is to choose your parents wisely. This comical phrase from the popular work of Rowe and Kahn on successful aging (1997) leads society to believe that little can be done to slow the aging process, because it is all set out in a nonmodifiable genetic plan dictated by lineage. This myth is dangerous, because it leads older adults and caregivers to believe that little can be done to slow or compensate for normal changes of aging or to prevent and treat pathological medical problems. While genetics certainly are responsible for some of the aging process, they become less and less important as older adults age. As life continues, the role of environment and health behaviors significantly replaces the role of genetics in determining the onset of normal and pathological aging. Rowe and Kahn (1997) report that approximately one-third of physical aging and one-half of cognitive function is a result of genetic input from parental influences. That leaves two-thirds of physical aging and one-half of cognitive function to be influenced by environmental factors and health behaviors. Consequently, there is a lot that individuals can do to prevent the onset of both normal and pathological aging processes.

Myth #10: Because older adults are closer to death, they are ready to die and don't require any special consideration at end of life. When society learns of the death of a young child or adult, the level of grief and astonishment for the loss of a young life is extraordinary and difficult to contain. This grief and astonishment often is associated with a life that was too short, or taken too suddenly. However, when individuals in society and health care workers learn of the death of an older adult, or have the opportunity to work with an older adult at the end of life, it is often assumed that the older adult is prepared for their death because of their advanced age. This myth often leads health care professionals to offer less than aggressive treatment for disease and to neglect essential components of end-of-life care for the older adult. It is important to remember that while death among older adults may occur after a long life, older adults are not necessarily ready for death. They require equal and specialized attention to physical, psychological, social, and spiritual tasks at the end of life. End of life is often a difficult time for many older adults, but it also presents the opportunity to complete important development tasks of aging, such as mending fences with loved ones, disengaging from social roles, and transcending from this life into another existence. Nurses may play an important role in helping older adults to complete these development tasks that can make the difference between experiencing a good or bad death.

Ageism

Many of the residents of the United States believe these myths of aging and allow them to be unchallenged in their perception of older adults. These myths of aging perpetuate ageism in today's society. Ageism is defined as a negative attitude or bias toward older adults, resulting in the belief that older people cannot or should not participate in societal activities or be given equal opportunities afforded to others (Holohan-Bell & Brummel-Smith, 1999).

The presence of ageism in today's society is of great concern to nurses working with older adults. Ageism affects the medical care of older adults and their access to services. It has the power to rob older adults of their dignity and respect and often forces older adults to abandon hopes of contributing to society. The danger of ageism also lies in its ability to influence policies and care decisions for older adults. Traxler (1980) proposed four reasons for the development of ageism in society, including: (a) fear of death in Western society, (b) emphasis on the youth culture, (c) poor economic potential, and (d) past research that focused attention on disability and chronicity of older adults. The following examples illustrate ageism in action.

In order to fight ageism and protect against its many harmful consequences, it is essential to re-examine the role of older adults in society. Some important facts are coming to light to dispel the myths and reframe the experience of aging. For nurses it is essential to identify ageism and mitigate its ability to influence policies and care decisions that will affect the quality of life of older adults. In so doing, nurses play an instrumental role in preventing the consequences of aging on older adults. This includes making sure that older adults are not discriminated against in selection for medical procedures or resources. Older adults as a group have taken great action to prevent the effects of ageism on health care policy. As one of the most influential and persuasive cohorts present in today's society, older adults have formed two large and influential national organizations that provide them with representation concerning legislative issues and resources for successful aging: the American Association of Retired Persons (AARP) and the National Council on Aging (NCOA). These groups are also good sources of information for students interested in exploring issues of aging.

AARP is a very important and influential organization for individuals aged 50 and older (Hogstel, 2001). The organization has substantial influence on policy making at the federal and state levels. Currently, AARP has

36 million members, which represents over 50% of older adults. The membership is growing quickly, with a new member joining AARP every 11 seconds. The name is misleading, as many of the members of AARP are not retired. The annual membership rates are reasonable, and the organization is open to all who are interested. AARP's vision is to "shape and enrich the experience of aging for each and every member of society." It is a nonprofit, nonpartisan organization whose primary goal is to help older people live with independence, dignity, and purpose. AARP offers a wide range of services, program and volunteer opportunities, and benefits to its members. Millions of people are helped each year through its free or low-cost programs, such as tax counseling and driver's training programs. The organization publishes informational bulletins and newsletters on topics of interest to older adults. An important component of the organization is its lobbying ability and influence on legislative issues of importance to older adults. With the assistance of AARP, the rights of older adults continue to be heard loudly on Capitol Hill.

The NCOA is another nonprofit organization that plays an influential role in providing information, technical assistance, and research in the field of aging. It maintains a national information clearinghouse related to aging, plans conferences on aging issues, conducts research on aging, supports demonstration programs related to aging, and keeps a comprehensive library of materials associated with every aspect of aging.

ETHNOGERIATRICS AND HEALTH CARE

Scommegna (2007) predicts an unprecedented shift in the cultural background of the U.S. population. It is reported that the White population of adults over 65 is expected to decrease from approximately 87% to 75% of all older adults in the years 1990–2030. In turn, the percentage of Black older adults is expected to rise from 8% to 9%; the percentage of Asian older adults is expected to increase from 1.4% to 5%; and the percentage of Hispanic older adults is expected to increase from 3.7% to 10.9%. These statistics are important because they predict a change in the manner in which traditional Western medicine is accepted in this country.

The United States currently functions under a health care system known popularly as the Western biomedical model. This model forms the basis of beliefs about health care in the United States. The model is based on scientific reductionism and characterized by a mechanistic model of the human body, separation of mind and body, and disrespect of spirit or soul. In practice, this model is revealed commonly through the treatment of medical problems with little respect for the impact of treatment on the older adult's life. For example, expensive medications are often prescribed for older adults with little thought as to how they could possibly be purchased on a fixed income. For many years, this model has been accepted by the older residents of the United States, and it continues to be utilized widely throughout the country. The recent increase in cultural diversity in the United States presents an unprecedented challenge to this model and the way in which health care has been practiced in the United States. However, this challenge also represents the opportunity to improve health care services to the entire population.

As each culture brings different explanations of disease origins and treatments, the traditional manner in which health is understood, maintained, or improved will likely be altered as new culture beliefs challenge traditional understanding. This has the potential to change health care practice as we know it. Improved understanding of cultures will allow a greater integration of mind, body, and spirit. This has already impacted health care as evidenced by the increased emphasis on spirituality in health care settings. O'Brien (2004) reports that the

---

EVIDENCE-BASED PRACTICE

Title of Study: Developing a Multisite Project in Geriatric and/or Gerontological Education With Emphasis in Interdisciplinary Practice and Cultural Competence

Authors: Browne, C., Braun, K., Mokuau, N., McLaughlin, L.

Purpose: A curriculum development project was designed to increase the number of professionals trained in geriatric and/or gerontological social work in Hawaii.

Methods: A 4-segment project that included: (1) developing, implementing, and testing a curriculum based on standardized learning competencies designated by project participants; (2) providing advanced training in aging, cultural competence, and interdisciplinary practice to social work professionals and masters degree students; (3) revising the curriculum to support such competencies; (4) producing a practicum handbook.

Findings: The above purposes were accomplished. This project is replicable in other communities and universities.

Implications: Although developed for the state of Hawaii, this project is replicable, and the curriculum is adaptable to other sites in need of more knowledgeable and skilled persons who work with the diverse older populations.

The Gerontologist, Vol. 42, No. 5, 698–704.

connection of mind, body, and spirit has been shown to enhance the health and spiritual well-being among older adults. In addition, alternative and complementary health care practices are more commonly seen in the clinical area.

Economically, culture also has an impact on health care. For example, there are older adults who have immigrated to the United States to live their later lives with their adult children. They may not have paid into the U.S. Social Security system, and, therefore, they must either buy into the Medicare system or become eligible for Medicaid. Medicaid, a combination federal and state program, varies from state to state and funds health care, including nursing home care for low income older adults. However, legislation passed in the 1990s made it more difficult for older adults who were not citizens of the United States to access Medicaid, which means that noncitizen older adults may not have any method with which to pay for health care.

It is imperative that health care providers become aware of the cultural diversity of the population and identify the cultural beliefs that empower health care decisions of older adults. In order to fully understand how cultural shifts in society affect the way in which health care is accessed and accepted in society, it is first necessary to understand a few terms. Increasing understanding of the great cultural shifts in society will have a substantial impact on the ability to provide health care to older adults from all cultural backgrounds. The term *culture* refers to the way of life of a population, or part of a population. Culture is usually used to discuss different societies or national origins. However, culture also reflects differences in groups according to geographic regions or other characteristics that comprise subgroups within a nation. *Acculturation* is defined as the degree to which individuals have moved from their original system of cultural values and beliefs toward a new system. The term *ethnogerontology* is the study of the causes, processes, and consequences of race, national origin, culture, minority group status, and ethnic group

---

CULTURAL FOCUS

Scommegna (2007) reports that there is an unprecedented shift in the cultural backgrounds of the U.S. population. The shift in cultural backgrounds in the United States also predicts a change in the manner in which traditional Western medicine is accepted in this country. Consequently, culturally competent care is essential among nurses caring for older adults, and improved understanding regarding complementary and alternative therapy is necessary.

status on individual and population aging in the three broad areas of biological, psychological, and social aging. The goal in providing excellent nursing care for older adults of all cultural backgrounds is cultural competence.

Cultural Competence

Cultural competence refers to the ability of nurses to understand and accept the cultural backgrounds of clients and provide care that best meets the client's needs—not the nurse's needs. Examples of cultural competence include the nurse's ability to discuss appropriate foods associated with healing with a hospitalized older adult and procure those foods to aide in the healing process. Another example is sharing in prayer with an older adult. Questioning older adults about their ability to pay for their medications or health care also shows an increased integration of mind, body, and spirit and is an example of cultural competence. Becoming culturally competent is not an easy task and requires great work. Purnell (2000) and Campinha-Bacote (2003) identify stages of cultural competence. The first stage, *unconscious incompetence,* is common to beginning nurses and is manifested by the assumption that everyone is the same. Following this stage, *conscious incompetence* occurs as the nurse begins to understand the vast differences between patients from many cultural backgrounds, but lacks the knowledge to provide competent care to culturally diverse patient populations. *Conscious competence* is the stage when knowledge regarding various cultures is actively obtained, but this knowledge is not easily integrated into practice, because the nurse is somewhat uncomfortable with culturally diverse interventions. The final stage, *unconscious competence,* occurs when nurses naturally integrate knowledge and culturally appropriate interventions into practice (Campinha-Bacote, 2003).

Developing cultural competence is increasingly challenging to nurses who were not exposed to a large variety of cultural backgrounds during childhood or early adulthood. However, with attention to several steps, cultural competence can be developed. An integral step toward cultural competence is to examine personal beliefs and the impact of these beliefs on professional behavior. This may best be accomplished by conducting a personal cultural assessment on oneself. The following questions may be helpful in guiding this assessment:

- What are your own cultural backgrounds, attitudes, and beliefs?
- Where did you get them?
- What behaviors do you have that come from your cultural background?

- Which of these behaviors are different from those of others around you or in your care?

These questions may be used individually or administered to a colleague to help uncover personal beliefs that may bias or interfere with the development of cultural competence. Once these biases are identified, they must be set aside and not allowed to interfere with the care of older adults.

Following the identification of cultural biases that may impact care, it is essential to acquire knowledge regarding population-specific, health-related cultural values, beliefs, and behaviors. These practices are often rooted in deep religious beliefs and may stand in stark contrast to the biomedical model. In addition, it is also important to explore disease incidence, prevalence, and mortality rates among cultural groups. Table 1.1 provides examples of some commonly held health care practices of the dominant cultural groups in the United States. These practices often have an influence on all aspects of health care.

It is important to remember that although older clients may be part of a specific cultural group, they may have acculturated to a certain degree during their time in the United States. Therefore, a cultural history is an essential next step in determining the basis of the client's health care beliefs and practices. Some health care facilities have begun to add cultural assessment questions to client's admission assessment. Sample questions to guide the assessment may be found in the Cultural Focus box. In conducting the assessments, approach all older adults with dignity and respect and always use a client's formal title (Mr., Mrs., Dr.). It is appropriate to ask the older adult how they would like to be addressed. If the older client speaks a language with which the nurse is not familiar, determine if the older adult client would like an interpreter or whether a family member would like to communicate the individual's needs for them. It is important to note that the fast pace in which the American culture operates may be seen as a sign of disrespect to older adults from different cultural backgrounds. A quick approach to patient care, which is often essential in busy health care climates, often is perceived as uncaring and hasty. Recognizing this allows for nurses to approach the clients more slowly and with great attention to care giving and detail. The amount of personal space, the comfort with eye contact, and the use of physical gestures, such as hand-shaking, should also be assessed to determine the older adult's comfort with these common social norms.

Two common issues in the care of older adults from various cultural backgrounds have to do with the use of complementary and alternative therapy (CAM) and end-of-life care. The Gerontological Society of America (2004) reports that one-third of older adults used alternative medicine

TABLE 1.1 Health Care Practices of Dominant Cultural Groups

Belief	Native Americans	African Americans	Asian Americans	Latin Americans
Origin of Belief	Health beliefs and views of death are older than the country and vary by tribe.	African traditions are often integrated with American Indian, Christian, and other European traditions. Many African Americans grew up with little health care.	Classical Chinese medicine influenced traditions in Japan (Kampo), Korea (Hanbang), and Southeast Asia. In parts of Asia, Taoism and Buddhism have influenced the healing traditions.	Most Latino Americans practice the biomedical model, but among some elders there may be reminiscences of other beliefs.
Focus of Health	Great emphasis on mind–body–spirit integration.	Interaction of multiple causes of health as opposed to just physical.	Characterized by need for balance between yin and yang to preserve health. Interaction of basic elements of the environment (e.g., water, fire earth, metal, and wood).	Religion is an important component of health.

View of Illness	Sometimes seen as a result of an individual's offenses.	Illness may be seen as the result of a physical cause, such as infection, weather, and other environmental factors, or from sin or great offense.	Illness is viewed as a threat to the soul.	Illness may be multidimensional in nature.
Components of Care Needed for Healing	Use of herbs from native plants, spiritual healing, harmony with environment; ritual purification ceremony may be needed to heal.	Power of religion, Christian in some cases; and use of herbs, or "root working." The use of healers is rarely seen. Home remedies may be used. Experiences of segregation and memories of the Tuskegee experiment may make older African Americans skeptical and distrustful of health care providers	The use of herbs and diet may be seen as a method of unblocking the free flow of qi (chi), or vital energy, through meridians in the body. Acupuncture, tai chi, moxibustion, and cupping are also used frequently. Illness should be addressed not only through medicine, but also through social and psychological means.	An interaction of the biomedical model with complementary and alternative therapies provides the framework for health care.

Gratefully adapted from the Stanford Geriatric Education Center's Core Curriculum in Ethnogeriatrics.

CULTURAL FOCUS

Sample Cultural History Questions

1. In what country were you born?
2. How long have you (or your ancestors) been in this country?
3. What language did you first learn to speak?
4. What language is used at home?
5. How do you identify yourself (in terms of your ethnic/racial background, heritage, or culture)?
6. What is important for others to know and understand about your background or culture?
7. How has your background or culture influenced who you are today?
8. What is the role of spirituality, faith, or religion in your life? Do you identify with any formal religion/belief system?
9. What customs or traditions are important to you/your family?
10. What does your culture/religion/heritage teach you about aging/growing older/elders or older people?
11. What has been the biggest adjustment for you/your family about life in this country?

Source: Standford Geriatric Education Center Ethnogeriatric Core Curriculum

---

in 2002. The use of CAM will be discussed in greater detail in Chapter 7. Different cultural backgrounds also show great diversity in acceptance of and discussions about death. These issues impair the appropriate use of advance directives. There are also diverse cultural rituals and traditions at the time of death that must be respected. Cultural considerations at end of life will be discussed in more detail in Chapter 12.

The final step in the acquisition of cultural competence is the development of skills for working with culturally diverse populations. This involves gaining knowledge about how to work with culturally diverse populations and consistently using those skills with older adults. The U.S. Department of Health and Human Services (DHHS) provides recommended suggestions for the integration of cultural competence into various environments of care. These recommendations are detailed in Chapter 11.

The culturally competent nurse consistently recognizes the great cultural diversity in the population and approaches care of older adults with an open and accepting attitude toward diverse health care practices. Increased respect for culture is evident during assessments, and information is gathered regarding cultural beliefs and practices. A greater integration of mind, body, and spirit as well as the use of alternative

CULTURAL FOCUS

The fast pace in which the American culture operates may be seen as a sign of disrespect to older adults from different cultural backgrounds. A quick approach to patient care, which is often essential in busy health care climates, often is perceived as uncaring and hasty. Recognizing this allows for nurses to approach the clients more slowly and with great attention to caregiving and detail.

and complementary therapies is practiced, and great respect toward the special needs of culturally diverse clients at the end of life is paid. Conducting cultural assessments, utilizing translator services in facilities, and providing culturally competent care are integral components to developing culturally competent institutions and ultimately improving care of older adults.

GERONTOLOGICAL NURSING

The increased numbers of older adults in the United States undoubtedly has a major impact on the demand of this population on the health care system. The Alliance for Aging Research (2002) reports that the average older adult has three chronic medical conditions. Consequently, more nurses are needed to care for the increasing number of older adults with chronic illness. It is commonly assumed that any nurse can take care of older adults. However, with the increasing population of older adults there has been an increase in the amount of specialized geriatric nursing knowledge needed to care for this population. Not only are more nurses needed to care for older adults, but nurses competent in the care of older adults will be needed to meet the enhanced needs of the older population. Rosenfeld, Bottrell, Fulmer, and Mezey (1999) report that "Today, a nurse's typical patient is an older adult," and "it behooves the nursing community to ensure that every nurse graduating from a baccalaureate nursing program has a defined level of competency in care of the elderly" (p. 84).

Despite the increased need, as well as the substantial growth in geriatric nursing science, the field of gerontological nursing has been slow to gain recognition as a nursing specialty. While more and more nursing programs are offering courses in geriatric nursing or integrating best geriatric nursing practices throughout programs, geriatric nursing is still not a popular specialty area among nursing students. Moreover, there is currently a nursing shortage that affects all areas of care, including older adults. The overall shortage of nurses along with the increase in older adults requiring care has resulted in a critical shortage of nurses prepared to care for older adults. A recent article in the *American Journal of Nursing* challenges whether or not nurses are prepared to meet the needs of this increased population of older adults (Stotts & Dietrich, 2004).

The terms *geriatric nursing, gerontological nursing,* and *gerontic nursing* have been used interchangeably to describe the role of nursing care of older adults. However, these terms have different meanings. Geriatric nursing refers to the nursing care of older people with health problems, or those requiring tertiary care. Gerontological nursing includes health promotion, education, and disease prevention (primary and secondary care). Gerontic nursing, although not a commonly known term, encompasses both of these aspects (Hogstel, 2001). The past several decades have seen a great increase in gerontological nursing knowledge. Rauckhorst (2003) reports that these changes began in 1966 when the American Nurses Association (ANA) first recognized geriatric nursing as a specialty. Standards to guide the practice of gerontological nursing were first published by the ANA in 1976 and later revised in 1987 and 1995.

The educational foundation in gerontological nursing has expanded greatly over the past two decades. Many more associate, baccalaureate, and certificate programs in nursing contain geriatric content than previously. The development and integration of geriatric content into nursing programs was greatly supported by the Kellogg, Robert Wood Johnson, and John A. Hartford foundations. However, despite the great progress in gerontological nursing, Kovner, Mezey, and Harrington (2002) report that 58% of baccalaureate nursing programs do not have geriatric-certified faculty. Gilje, Lacey, and Moore (2007) report that only slightly more than half of baccalaureate programs surveyed offered a stand-alone geriatric course.

The development of the first post-master's certificate and graduate programs in gerontological nursing were witnessed in the mid-1970s. These original 141 advanced programs were supported by the U.S. Public Health Service (USPHS) and cost taxpayers approximately $17 million (Hogstel, 2001). Currently, there are many graduate and post-master's certificate programs in gerontological nursing available to assist nurses in developing increased knowledge regarding the specialized needs of older adults. Graduates of these programs may practice as geriatric nurse practitioners and geriatric clinical nurse specialists to work in clinics, hospitals, home care, and nursing homes. It is important to note that the educational programs provide the education and certificate or diploma in the specialty program. However, in order to utilize these specialty titles, qualified nurses must pass an examination offered by the American Nurses Credentialing Center (ANCC). A nurse with an Associate's or Baccalaureate degree and no advanced graduate credits, 1,500 clinical practice hours

EVIDENCE-BASED PRACTICE

Title of Study: Gerontological Nursing Content in Baccalaureate Nursing Programs: Findings From a National Survey

Authors: Bottrell, M., MPH; Fulmer, T., PhD, RN, FAAN; & Mezey, M. D., EdD, RN, FAAN

Purpose: To provide a baseline of the current status of geriatric content in the baccalaureate curriculum in nursing programs.

Methods: This article is based upon a survey that was conducted in 1997 with a universe of baccalaureate nursing programs with n = 598. The findings are based on a respondent pool of 480 programs (80.3%). This survey covered curriculum, content, faculty preparation, and how programs define their needs for the future. The data analysis included the identification of baccalaureate nursing programs with exemplary offerings in gerontological care.

Findings: The survey indicates that, at present, nursing students are not being adequately prepared to care for the elderly. This study shows that the size of the full-time and part-time faculty varied dramatically in baccalaureate nursing programs, with some programs having stand-alone courses and others integrated courses. Overloaded curriculums were seen as a barrier to entering gerontology into the curriculum. Three other "barriers" were reported; these included a lack of interest among students, a lack of role models/preceptors in clinical settings, and a lack of clearly articulated gerontological curricula.

Implications: The study indicates a need for more instruction regarding the care of older adults. It calls for a concerted effort to assure that baccalaureate nursing programs offer their students the courses and clinical experiences necessary for quality care for the elderly. It suggests that the number and focus of questions on the National Council Licensure Examination-Registered Nurse reflect the knowledge base necessary for the care of the elderly. It also suggests that professional organizations should revise their standards for programs to reflect the importance of preparation for care of the elderly. It also cites the need for revised curriculum to reflect courses that will teach the skills to meet the needs of the aging society.

Journal of Professional Nursing, Vol. 21, No. 5, 268–275.

in geriatric nursing, and 30 continuing education hours may sit for Geriatric Nurse Certification through ANCC (http://www.nursingworld.org/ancc/) as well. Certification programs designed to provide the 30 continuing education hours are often available at local hospitals, colleges, and universities and on the World Wide Web.

Currently there are several organizations that specialize in geriatric nursing. The National Gerontological Nursing Organization (NGNO) was developed in 1984 to support the growth of knowledge related to gerontological nursing science (Hogstel, 2001). The Gerontological Society of America (GSA), the American Society of Aging (ASA), and the American Geriatrics Society (AGS) are multidisciplinary organizations that support aging knowledge and research. These groups have increasing numbers of nurse members with a special interest in the development and dissemination of gerontological nursing knowledge.

THEORIES OF AGING

Prior to the middle of the twentieth century, the cause of death listed on many older adults' death certificates was *old age*. It was thought that at some later point in life, the body just gave out. The growth in scientific medical and gerontological knowledge over the past century has challenged this popular view. In fact, advances in the study of older adults have made society question whether there are more appropriate physiological, social, or psychological reasons why people die. At the 55th annual meeting of the Gerontological Society of America, a presentation by Butler and Olshansky (2002) continued to debate, "Has anyone ever died of old age?"

Despite the continuing debate, the question remains: in the absence of illness, why do people die? The results of efforts to answer this question are derived from theories of aging. Biological theories explain that the reason people age and die is because of changes in the human body. Psychological theories support the idea that an older adult's life ends when they have reached all of their developmental milestones. For example, Maslow's Hierarchy of Needs states that a person's final stage is self-actualization. From a psychological viewpoint, once an older adult reaches self-actualization, they approach the end of life. Moral/spiritual theories support the idea that once an older individual finds spiritual wholeness, this transcends the need to inhabit a body, and they die. Sociological theories explain that when an older adult's usefulness in roles and relationships ends, end of life occurs.

Biological Theories

Two of the main biological categories are feature and defect theories. Feature theory is consistent with the work of Hayflick (2007) commonly known as the "Hayflick limit." The Hayflick limit essentially states that cells will divide for a finite number of times, and once they have reached this limit, the cells shrink, disperse, and eventually die, resulting in death of the body. The Hayflick limit relies heavily on the science of "programmed cell death" or "apoptosis." The manner and timeline of apoptosis is the subject of a great deal of research surrounding the aging process. Feature theory expands the work of Hayflick and focuses heavily around apoptosis. This theory purports that the aging process is contained in the design of human beings. In other words, theorists who support this theory believe that how a person ages is genetically predetermined. Consistent with this theory, little can be done to alter the aging process, despite interventions taken to promote health and prevent illness. The main purpose of aging, according to feature theory, is to improve or perfect human beings. Supporters of the feature theory look to the wide variation in lifespan among people in similar environments to support the theory. For example, two people who grow up and live their lives in the same town, performing similar jobs and having similar families may die at vastly different ages as a result of their genetic make-up. An adaptation of this theory is commonly known as programmed senescence theory. This theory states that while the aging process is dependent on genetic make-up, there is an ordered switching on and off of certain genes. The aging process, according to programmed senescence theory, begins when age-associated deficits are manifested. For example, aging could be thought to begin when an adult develops hip pain as the early sign of osteoarthritis. Further expansion of genetic theories known as longevity and senescence theory are currently being researched. Perls (2001) is studying genetic backgrounds of elderly people to differentiate between the genetics of longevity and exceptional longevity. This researcher is attempting to find differences in genetic make-up between those families that live to old age and groups of family members that live to very old age, that is, well into their nineties and hundreds.

The defect theory is a biological theory that is somewhat the opposite of feature theory. According to the defect theory, the breakdown and losses that occur with aging are accidents or mistakes. Defect theories lead researchers to believe that the cause of death of older adults generally results from a wearing out of the body, or an accumulation of mutations in DNA that can no longer be withstood. Further research is actively being conducted on this theory and the role of shortening of telomeres in the process of DNA replication during cell division. In contrast to feature theory, defect theory supports the work of health promotion and illness treatment and management as an important manner in which to prolong life. Examples of defect theory in action are seen among the large numbers of older adults who survive years after treatment for aggressive cancers or cardiac disease. Recent work related to the defect theory shows great support for the influence of caloric restriction on the aging process (http://www.azinet.com/aging/). Caloric restriction was originally conceived by Pearl (1928) as a manner in which to optimize metabolism to expand life. This theory, which has repeatedly been tested, revealed that when mice and rats were fed a calorie-restricted but nutritious diet, they lived about 50% longer than rats fed regular diets. Moreover, the study showed that the study rats were more active and youthful. This translates to about a 30% increase in longevity for human beings or 10 to 15 years of added human life.

Psychological Theories

Psychological theories support the idea that an older adult's life ends when they have reached all of their developmental psychological milestones. Theories focusing on the psychological dimension include Maslow's Hierarchy of Needs. This theory states that an individual goes through a series of developmental steps through life commencing with the need to obtain safety and fulfill biological needs such as food and water. The steps become progressively more challenging until the final stage in a person's life, known as self-actualization. According to Maslow's theory, self-actualization is obtained when a person develops an understanding of themselves within the world and accepts who they have become. From a psychological viewpoint, once an older adult reaches self-actualization, they have reached the final stage of life. Other theories within the psychological dimension include Erikson's stages of development (1997). Erikson theorizes that within each stage of life, individuals must successfully encounter and resolve a problem or crisis in order to move on to the next stage. Within the final stage, ego integrity versus despair, the older adult must successfully master changes in health, loss of loved ones, and resolution of role changes such as no longer being a parent, employee, or friend.

Moral/Spiritual Theories

Moral/spiritual theories support the idea that once an older individual finds spiritual wholeness, this transcends the need to inhabit a body, and the person approaches the end of life. Theories that fall within this category include Kohlberg's stages of moral development (Lind, Hartman, & Wakenhut, 1985) and more recently, Tornstam's (1994) theory of gerotranscendence. Kohlberg's theory of moral development states that an individual goes through a series of moral reasoning activities that become progressively more sophisticated throughout life. The most sophisticated and final step is post-conventional reasoning, which is not reached by many individuals. According to Kohlberg's theory, post-conventional reasoning is obtained when universality with the world is present and sense of higher consciousness is achieved. This stage is dependent on social interaction and is obtained when a person develops an understanding of themselves within the world and accepts who they have become. From a moral perspective, once an older adult reaches post-conventional reasoning, they have reached the final stage of life and are therefore prepared for the end of life.

Tornstam's theory of gerotranscendence supports a movement toward older adulthood throughout all stages of life, including childhood. Tornstam's theory builds upon previous work by Carl Jung. According to the theory of gerotranscendence the movement toward the aging process results in greater satisfaction with life, resulting in greater maturity and improved understanding of the world and the individual's position within it. The steps toward attaining this enhanced perspective involve self-reflection and a progression toward selflessness, as well as an interconnectedness and communication with the past and things beyond this world. Gerotranscendence often finds older adults with a decreased need to be with others, as individuals become increasingly more comfortable being alone.

Sociological Theories

Sociological theories explain that aging results as older adult's usefulness in roles and relationships changes or declines. Sociological theories to support this process include disengagement theory. This theory, which was among the first of sociological theories to explain aging, states that as relationships change or end for older adults, either through the process of retirement, disability, or death, a gradual withdrawing of the older adult is evidenced. Less involvement in activities is seen, and while new relationships may be formed these relationships are not as integral to life as previously necessary. Also within the sociological dimension is activity theory. This theory states that social activity is an essential component of successful aging. Consequently, when social activity is halted because of death of loved ones, changes in relationship, or illness and disabilities that affect relationships, aging is accelerated and death becomes nearer. The focus of activity theory is the relationship between activity and self-concept. In other words, social activity and role relationships are integral to the self-concept and harmful when disrupted or stopped. To avoid this, new roles must be developed to replace lost roles. For example, within this theory, the loss of job roles through retirement could be replaced with appropriate recreational or volunteer activities to avoid the harmful effects of the job loss on self-concept. A final theory within the sociological perspective is the continuity theory. This theory referred to earlier in the chapter supports that individuals move through their later years attempting to keep things much the same and using similar personality and coping strategies to maintain stability throughout life. Within this theory, one can look to past experiences of an older adult to predict

---

CRITICAL THINKING CASE STUDY

A 64-year-old White male had been healthy for most of his life. He was a teacher and an upstanding father who was active in the church and community. However, after experiencing signs of Coronary Artery Disease (CAD), he underwent a Coronary Artery Bypass Graft (CABG). What should have been an unremarkable recovery was tainted with many complications, and he required permanent residence in a nursing home approximately 1 hour away from his home, wife, and grown children. Within 1 month of admission, he died.

1. What theories of aging could be used to help explain why this client died when he did?
2. What factors may have contributed to this man's premature death?
3. Do you think any one theory explains the aging process and the cause of death among older adults, or do you feel a combination of theories is more useful? Why?

---

how they will encounter current and future stressors. For example, if an individual became greatly distressed after the loss of a friend in their forties, it is likely that they will experience similar distress to other losses in life. However, this theory also supports that past reflection on life and future goal setting are helpful in changing past dysfunctional strategies.

SUMMARY

Olshansky, Carnes, and Desquelles (2001) report that

> There are no lifestyle changes, surgical procedures, vitamins, antioxidants, hormones or techniques of genetic engineering available today with the capacity to repeat the gains in life expectancy that were achieved during the 20th century. The next quantum leap in life expectancy can occur only by adding decades of life to people who have already lived 70 years or more. (p. 1491)

This statement summarizes the great advances in aging that have resulted in the emergence of a population that was nonexistent a century ago. The presence of older adults in society is of great benefit to the many children and grandchildren, spouses, siblings, and friends who receive love, care, and support from their older loved one. Moreover, nurses can receive much benefit from learning about the lives of older adults. However, the emergence of this large population is not without issues that need to be addressed. The presence of multiple medical illnesses and the subsequent need for health care, the means to pay for health care, and the ability to provide housing for older adults when illness impacts their functional status are among the issues that concern nursing for older adults. Myths of aging are prevalent among society, and this chapter provided information to dispel these myths and combat ageism. Finally, the evolution of gerontological nursing education and theories of aging were discussed to complete this introduction on the Graying of America.

REFERENCES

Alliance for Aging Research. (2002). *Medical never-never land.* Retrieved August 10, 2007, from http://www.agingresearch.org/content/article/detail1698/

American Association of Retired Persons. (1999). *AARP Modern Maturity Sexuality Study.* Atlanta: NFO Research. Retrieved May 1, 2005, from http://assets.aarp.org/rgcenter/health/mmsexsurvey.pdf

Butler, R., & Olshansky, S. J. (2002). Has anybody ever died of old age? *The Gerontologist, 42*(special issue 1), 285–286.

Campinha-Bacote, J. (2003). *The process of cultural competence in the delivery of healthcare services* (3rd ed.). Cincinnati, OH: Transcultural C.A.R.E. Associates Press.

Erikson, E. H. (1997). *The life cycle completed.* New York: W.W. Norton Company.

Gerontological Society of America. (2004, July). Alternative medicine gains popularity. *Gerontology News,* 4.

Gilje, F., Lacey, L., & Moore, C. (2007). Gerontology and geriatric issues and trends in U.S. nursing programs: A national survey. *Journal of Professional Nursing, 23,* 21–29.

Hayflick, L. (2007, April). Biological aging is no longer an unsolved problem. *Annals of the New York Academy of Science,* (1100), 1–13.

Hogstel, M. O. (2001). *Gerontology: Nursing care of the older adult.* Albany, NY: Delmar Thomson Learning.

Holohan-Bell, J., & Brummel-Smith, K. (1999). Impaired mobility and deconditioning. In J. Stone, J. Wyman, & S. Salisbury (Eds.), *Clinical gerontological nursing. A guide to advanced practice* (pp. 267–287). Philadelphia, PA: W.B. Saunders.

Kovner, C. T., Mezey, M., & Harrington, C. (2002). Who cares for older adults? Workforce implications of an aging society: Geriatrics needs to join pediatrics as a required element of training the next generation of health care professionals. *Health Affairs, 21,* 78–89.

Lind, G., Hartman, G. A., & Wakenhut, R. (1985). *Moral development and the social environment: Studies in the philosophy and psychology of moral.* Edison, NJ: Transaction Publishers.

O'Brien, M. E. (2004). *A nurse's handbook of spiritual care: Standing on holy ground.* Boston: Jones & Bartlett Publishers.

Olshansky, S. J., Carnes, B. A., & Desquelles, A. (2001). Prospects for human longevity. *Science, 291*(5508), 1491–1492

Pascucci, M. A., & Loving, G. L. (1997). Ingredients of an old and healthy life: A centenarian perspective. *Journal of Holistic Nursing, 15,* 199–213.

Pearl, R. (1928). *The rate of living.* London: University of London Press.

Perls, T. (2001). Guest editorial: Genetics and phenotypic markers among centenarians. *Journal of Gerontology, 56,* M67–M70.

Pick a card—any card?: Helping patients understand the new Medicare-approved drug discount cards. (2004). *American Journal of Nursing, 104*(7), 24–26.

Purnell, L. (2000). A description of the Purnell model for cultural competence. *Journal of Transcultural Nursing, 11*(1), 40–46.

Rauckhorst, L. H. (2003). The challenge of nursing education to meet all levels of care of elders. *The Gerontologist, 43*(special issue 1), 227.

Rosenfeld, P., Bottrell, M., Fulmer, T., & Mezey, M. (1999). Gerontological nursing content in baccalaureate nursing programs: Findings from a national survey. *Journal of Professional Nursing, 15*, 84–94.

Rowe, J. W., & Kahn, R. L. (1997). Successful aging. *Aging, 10*, 142–144.

Scommegna, P. (2007). U.S. growing bigger, older and more diverse. *Population Reference Bureau*. Retrieved July 12, 2007, from http://www.prb.org/Articles/2004/USGrowing BiggerOlderandMoreDiverse.aspx

Stotts, N., & Dietrich, C. (2004). The challenge to come: The care of older adults. *American Journal of Nursing, 104*(8), 40–48.

Tornstam, L. (1994). Gerotranscendence: A theoretical and empirical exploration. In L. E. Thomas & S. A. Eisenhandler (Eds.), *Aging and the religious dimension* (pp. 203–225). Westport, CT: Greenwood.

Traxler, A. J. (1980). *Let's get gerontologized: Developing a sensitivity to aging. the multipurpose senior center concept: A training manual for practitioners working with the aging.* Springfield: Illinois Department of Aging.

U.S. Department of Health and Human Services. (2004). *The health consequences of smoking. Executive summary.* Available at http://www.cdc.gov/tobacco/sgr/sgr_2004/pdf/executivesummary.pdf

CHAPTER TWO

The Health Care Delivery System

Learning Objectives

1. Identify the impact of retirement on aging and ability to pay for health care.
2. Identify challenges for older adults within the current health care delivery system.
3. Describe the basic elements of payment for health services for older adults.
4. Identify the essential elements of Medicare as the primary payer system of older adults.
5. Discuss Medicaid, veteran's benefits, long-term care insurance, and other payment methods for older adult health care.
6. Identify resources for health care for older adults without health insurance.

Mr. Jackson is an 80-year-old man with moderate to severe dementia. He has been living with his 55-year-old daughter and her family for the past 5 years. Over the past year his cognition has declined quite rapidly, and he has required considerably more attention and supervision in order to ensure his safety. The client's daughter states that a month ago he left the house and was found walking down the middle of a busy street, and he appeared very scared and confused. Recently, the client has also become verbally abusive toward his son-in-law.

His daughter is concerned about his safety when he is left alone, but she states that financially both she and her husband need to keep their full-time jobs. The family has discussed the possibility of visiting nurse services and assisted-living facilities, but they are unsure of how they would pay for such services. They come to you for counseling on their options, as well as to obtain more information on eligibility requirements for Medicare and Medicaid.

The story of Mr. Jackson is typical of today's older adult. It is logical to assume that the highly scientific and timely interventions that are used to treat and cure disease in today's society are available to everyone. Many citizens and health care workers operate under the assumption that if something is available, it is available to all. Unfortunately, this is not the case. While the health care delivery system has improved vastly over the past century, many of the currently available interventions to detect disease early and treat disease effectively are not available to older adults because they are not able to pay for these costly interventions. A considerable amount of time is spent in nursing and medical schools on illness assessment, management, and treatment. For example, if a patient presents to the primary care provider with undiagnosed abdominal pain and rectal bleeding, they may likely be sent for a Magnetic Resonance Imaging (MRI) study to determine the cause of the symptoms. Few providers realize that this particular test costs in excess of $1,000 and may not be covered by insurance. In fact, very little time is spent on how to access and obtain care for patients in medical and nursing education programs. Little, if any, time is spent on how to assist patients without health insurance to obtain greatly needed health care.

The sad reality is that while medical science and nursing interventions have greatly increased in effectiveness over the past century, this enhanced science is not available to everyone. Consequently, many older adults are not able to access needed health care and remain part of an underserved population. The most common barrier to effective health care is the inability to pay for it. Among older adults, the inability to receive effective health care may also result from a lack of transportation to health care providers. Another barrier is the lack of primary providers of geriatric care.

There are several primary health care payment systems for older adults in the United States. The most widely used are Medicare and Medicaid. However, these two payment mechanisms are not available to all older adults. Medicare is the federally funded insurance program for older adults. Older adults who have not paid into the U.S. Social Security system, either because they were never employed or because they immigrated into the United States as older adults, must either buy into the Medicare system or become eligible for Medicaid. Medicaid, a combination federal and state payment system, varies from state to state, but it funds health care, including nursing home care for low income older adults. Legislation passed in the 1990s made it more difficult for older noncitizen immigrants to access Medicaid.

This chapter will explore the financial issues related to health care among older adults including the impact of retirement on aging and health care. The Medicare system will be explored in depth, including historical changes to this system and the effects of these changes on the delivery of health care to older adults. Other reimbursement programs for health care will also be discussed in order to prepare students to understand the basic elements of these systems and viability of these systems for older adults. The primary systems that will be discussed include: (a) Medicaid payment systems, (b) long-term care, (c) private and fee for service, and (d) veterans services for payment of health care. Finally, the chapter will conclude with an exploration of payment options for those without access to these systems.

RETIREMENT

While older adults are generally considered to be retired, many older adults are working longer and having second careers. Some older adults continue to work because of the income it provides. Others work for the social and intellectual stimulation provided by employment. Other older adults feel that working helps them to contribute to society. In 2002, 13.2% of older Americans were working, or actively seeking work.

EVIDENCE-BASED PRACTICE

Title of Study: Predictors of Perceptions of Involuntary Retirement
Authors: Szinovacz, M., Davey, A.
Purpose: To investigate situations in which retirees perceive their retirement as "forced."
Methods: Waves 1–4 on the Health and Retirement Survey were used for analyses (N = 1, 160; 572 men and 588 women). Background factors, choice and restricted choice conditions, and retirement contexts on perceptions of forced retirement were estimated using logistic regression models.
Findings: It was found that nearly one-third of workers perceive their retirement as "forced." Restricted choice through health limitations, job displacement, care obligations, marital status, race, assets, benefits, job tenure, and off-time retirement were also reflected.
Implications: Personal and policy implications are needed relating to forced retirement. Employment programs are necessary to assist persons to find alternate employment once "forced" into retirement.

The Gerontologist, Vol. 45, No. 1, 36–47.

In fact, a recent study by the Pew Research Center (2006) found that the majority of older adults plan to retire at age 61, but 77% expect to work for pay after retirement. Moreover, the traditional view of retirement at 65 to pursue a life of leisure is becoming outdated as a result of the expanding lifespan.

Some older people prefer and need to continue to work throughout their older years. Work options may be full-time or part-time. Some older adults continue to perform work similar to what they had previously done, but others change careers. Currently, there is no mandatory retirement age for U.S. residents.

Continued employment in older adulthood fills many needs. These needs are physical, psychological, social, and financial. For example, continued work helps to provide extra income and socialization. As of January 1, 2000, Social Security recipients age 65 through 69 can earn as much as they wish and still receive their full Social Security benefits. Prior to this legislation being passed, individuals age 65 through 69 had $1 deducted from their Social Security benefit for every $3 they earned (Hogstel, 2001).

For those who have chosen retirement, the continually increasing lifespan means that older adults can spend an average of 30 years not working. Rosenkoetter (2000) provides several theories to help understand retirement. For those who view it positively, retirement may be peaceful and less stressful than previous years. For these individuals, retirement can be filled with hobbies and travel. But, for others retirement can be difficult and filled with financial struggle and ill health. Older adults are not always prepared financially for retirement, and many older adults live on limited incomes.

It is important to note that when older adults retire, the health care insurance available through employers may be terminated. While some employers maintain health insurance coverage, others do not. This will force the older adult to become a Medicare recipient. Medicare provides limited benefits, as will be seen later in this chapter. These limitations often place financial demands on older individuals that when combined with lowered income post-retirement, makes paying for health care and other expenses difficult. Financial planning during the young and healthy years is the ideal way for older adults to be able to retire when desired and to live at an optimal income level. This can be facilitated through consultations with attorneys and financial planners throughout the working years. However, this is not always done. Often when older adults retire, they find themselves on fixed incomes with insufficient financial resources for the future.

Continuing to work in later years has both advantages and disadvantages. While work provides a daily structure for activities, social involvement, and the possibility of health benefits, it also prevents travel,

CRITICAL THINKING CASE STUDY

Mr. Robertson, an 80-year-old man, has worked as a mechanical engineer for the same company for 45 years. He very much enjoys his position and utilizes the company's health insurance to pay for his health care. Yet, his blood pressure is unstable requiring frequent medications and monitoring. He has recently been diagnosed with Type 2 diabetes mellitus. Because he requires frequent medical appointments, these medical conditions often interfere with his workday. While he is well over retirement age and financially stable, he does not want to leave his current position.

1. What factors should be considered in Mr. Robertson's decision to retire or not?
2. What are the pros and cons of retirement in Mr. Robertson's case?
3. How will Mr. Robertson's retirement affect his medical care?
4. What alternatives to retirement are there for Mr. Robertson?

time with family and grandchildren, as well as other opportunities for volunteering and participating in hobbies. Moreover, as adults age, the incidence of chronic illnesses increases. The average older adult has three chronic illnesses. These illnesses usually require daily management, such as the use of medication, and the presence of pain, fatigue, or side-effects of medication may negatively impact the individual's quality of work. The need to visit health care providers may interfere with a traditional work schedule. Lower quality of work and greater absences may lessen the individuals chance of promotion within competitive work environments. While some employers understand these special needs, others do not and will look to replace the older adult with a younger, healthier worker.

CHALLENGES WITHIN THE CURRENT HEALTH CARE DELIVERY SYSTEM

There have been many changes in the health care delivery system in the United States in the last 10 years. These changes include the development of new medications, treatment for early-diagnosed disease, improved surgical techniques, and enhanced diagnostic capabilities. For example, new generations of antidepressant medications, cholesterol lowering agents (statins), and blood pressure management medications have all evolved over the last decade. These improvements have played an instrumental role in preventing death and disability among adults who are fortunate enough to benefit from these new interventions.

Changes and improvements in health care treatments have been dramatic and continuous for decades. Moreover, these changes continue to evolve everyday, and progress is not likely to be slowed in the future. In other words, the vast improvements in health care will likely continue for centuries resulting in unprecedented improvements in both morbidity and mortality.

These great improvements in health care, while cause for celebration, come with a price tag. In many cases, this price tag is exceptionally high and exceeds most people's budgets. Often health care professionals do not consider the high price of new technological improvements when prescribing care or medications. However, as a result of these technological advancements, health care costs continue to increase with each passing decade (Hogstel, 2001). The Federal Interagency Forum on Age-Related Statistics (2004, p. 14) reports that most older adults are retired from work.

Changes in health care expenditures have had a great impact on the ability to access health care, because individuals must pay the rising cost of insurance and/or out of pocket health care expenditures. In the case of Medicare-eligible older adults, some of these expenses may be paid for, but many are not. Medicare reimburses health care providers and facilities for the cost of some medical expenditure, but not all older adults are eligible for Medicare, and Medicare does not pay for all health care costs. For example, most outpatient prescription medications are expensive and not covered by traditional Medicare plans. Moreover, complementary and alternative therapies (CAM), such as herbal supplements, are usually over the counter and not covered by any insurance. These herbal medications, while rising in popularity among all older cultural groups, may be the primary healing source among some Asian, Hispanic, and other cultures. Depending on the health status of the older adult, the cost of medications alone may be enough to bankrupt them. In attempts to provide increased medication coverage for Medicare recipients, a new Medicare prescription drug benefit has recently become available. This program, titled the Medicare Prescription Drug Improvement and Modernization Act of 2003, approved prescription discount drug cards for Medicare recipients. These cards are available to over 7 million of Medicare's 41 million participants. Older adults must apply to be eligible for the discount cards, and a fee of $30 may be charged depending on the individual's income. The cards provide discounts on some medications, but not all. The *American Journal of Nursing* ("Pick a Card," 2004) reports that other available prescription drug plans may benefit higher income older adults more than the Medicare plan.

CRITICAL THINKING CASE STUDY

Mrs. O'Brien is a 79-year-old immigrant from Ireland. She came to this country 1 year ago to live with her adult daughter. One week ago, her daughter found her unconscious in the bathroom of her home. She was brought to the emergency room with an elevated blood sugar level. She was diagnosed with diabetes mellitus and sent home with a prescription for insulin and a follow-up appointment in 2 weeks. Mrs. O'Brien is having great difficulty learning to fill and inject the insulin. Her daughter can prefill the syringes before she leaves for work, but she does not return in time to administer the evening dosage. As Mrs. O'Brien is an immigrant, she is not qualified for Medicare, and she has not yet applied for Medicaid assistance. Mrs. O'Brien needs help in learning about her new disease and treatment.

1. What type of insurance might Mrs. O'Brien be eligible for, given her immigrant status?
2. If Mrs. O'Brien is not eligible for Medicare, how would you suggest Mrs. O'Brien pay for her health care?
3. In your geographic area, are there services available to assist older adults such as Mrs. O'Brien to receive needed care?
4. In light of the increasingly diverse older adult population, what changes do you feel are necessary in the U.S. health care delivery system?

The lack of reimbursement for medications and treatments for illness and the inability to pay out of pocket for these expensive treatments has resulted in an increase in the rates of noncompliance or nonadherence to medication regimes. It is reported that about one-half of all patients take the medications as prescribed upon leaving the physician's office. The other half take the medications incorrectly or not at all. One-third of those who take the medications incorrectly do not take it at all, one-third take the medication sporadically, and one-third do not even fill the prescription. Compliance and adherence, while defined differently, are similar and are used interchangeably within health care professions. Compliance is defined as the degree to which a patient follows a recommended treatment regimen. For example, if the physician tells the patient to take medication to control blood pressure, it is assumed that the patient will do what the physician says they should do. Adherence is defined as the degree to which behavior corresponds to a recommended therapeutic regimen. In this case, if the physician feels a medication might help the patient to maintain blood pressure control, the physician would recommend the administration of medication, and the patient's daily intake of the medication would be considered adherent.

Noncompliance rises in correlation with the increase in chronic illness commonly seen among older adults. As the older adult is asked to commit more time and resources to maintaining health, they are less likely to adhere closely to the recommended regimen. It is also important to note that older adults from various cultural backgrounds may be nonadherent to medication and treatment regimes because such plans conflict with their cultural healing beliefs. In order to promote maximum adherence, it is essential that nurses educate the patient on the recommended treatment regimen and assess the patient's understanding, willingness, and capability to comply. In so doing, it is estimated that up to 23% of nursing home admissions, 10% of hospital admissions, and many physician visits, diagnostic tests, and unnecessary treatments could be avoided.

Reimbursement of health care has also changed as a result of increasing costs. Allowable expenses under Medicare and Medicaid plans, as well as private insurance, have diminished in many cases and have been removed altogether in other cases. For example, at a point in the early 1990s, Medicare reimbursement for home care was very flexible, allowing clients many weeks to meet their health care goals after discharge from an acute care facility. In these cases, nurses could visit clients 2 or 3 times a week to provide wound care, medication teaching, and evaluation of health status. However, changes in the Medicare allowable expenses for home care have resulted in a lack of reimbursement for home care. Currently, home care nurses are given few visits to assist older adults to meet health care goals and then are mandated to discharge them because of lack of reimbursement. Moreover, future changes are possible and will continue to affect the way older people receive health care. These changes in health care expenditures have also had a great impact on the methods of health care delivery over the past several decades. In response to the increasing costs of health care, increased amounts of the federal and state funds must be budgeted to pay for rising health care costs.

CULTURAL FOCUS

Complementary and alternative therapies (CAM), such as herbal supplements, are usually over the counter and not covered by any insurance. These herbal medications, while rising in popularity among all older cultural groups, may be the primary healing source among some Asian, Hispanic, and other cultures. Awareness of the use of CAM therapies allows nurses to assess for the interaction of these therapies with traditional medications.

Methods of health care delivery have also changed as a result of the increasing cost of health care. The dramatic changes in the health care delivery system in the past several decades have had a profound impact on the availability of health care to older adults. Consequently, Kane (2002) reports that "Geriatricians are in danger of extinction" (p. M803).

Decreased Medicare payments to hospitals, home health agencies, and nursing homes and decreased coverage of outpatient rehabilitation services have caused a reduction in the numbers of nurses available, qualified, and willing to provide care to older adults It is not clear whether or not the health care community will be prepared to manage the needs of an increasing population of older adults (Stotts & Dietrich, 2004). In addition, many physicians, nurses, nurse practitioners, and others are not aware of the specialized care needs of older adults. As noted in Chapter 1, gerontology is a fairly new science. Only recently have medical and nursing programs begun to provide specialized education on the needs of older adults. A reduction in qualified nursing staff has the potential to decrease the number of programs designed to provide geriatric health care.

Another problem with obtaining health care for older adults includes lack of transportation. Transportation to physician's offices, clinics, and other health care services is a major problem for those who can no longer drive or afford to maintain a car. While van services are available in many communities to transport older adults to medical appointments and health-related visits, they are not universally available. Moreover, these van services usually require advanced scheduling on a first-come, first-serve basis. Often, older adults must wait for extended amounts of time at the health care facility or physician's office for the van to return to bring them home, extending a short appointment to a day-long outing. Some older adults may have the option of public transportation, such as buses or subway systems, to travel to their medical appointments, and these systems have increased accessibility to accommodate chronic disabilities among older adults. However, long walks to the stations may prevent older adults from using this system, and smaller communities may not even offer public transportation. These barriers often force older adults to delay medical treatment for health-related issues.

Clearly, the many changes in the health care delivery system present challenges for older adults in receiving adequate health care. In the affluent United States, it is often assumed that anyone who needs health care can get it. But, clearly this is not the case, and there are many challenges to the current health care delivery system, including the high cost of health care and the lack of insurance of many U.S. citizens. These issues, as well as lack of providers and transportation, may lead to noncompliance or nonadherence to health care regimens and may prevent much of the population from accessing health care. Consequently, many older adults avoid health care providers and neglect health care in order to have money to eat, live in their house or apartment, and pay their bills.

FINANCING HEALTH CARE

Health care for older adults is primarily paid for by the following methods: (a) Medicare and related plans; (b) Medicaid; (c) private pay, or fee for service; (d) veteran's benefits; and (e) long-term care insurance. Each of these payment systems has specific eligibility criteria as well as inclusions and exclusions. In many cases, more than one system is used to pay for the health care service. The following section provides a discussion of each of these payment programs and their ability to pay for health care costs of older adults.

Medicare and Related Plans

Most older adults are Medicare beneficiaries and receive health care accordingly. To be eligible to receive Medicare, older adults must have contributed to Social Security and/or the Medicare system earlier in life or had a spouse who worked and contributed to these systems (Hogstel, 2001). Younger individuals may also be eligible for Medicare if they contributed to Social Security earlier in life and then developed a disability that prevents them from working. This includes individuals with end-stage renal disease (ESRD) who are receiving dialysis treatments and other younger adults with disabilities such as amyotrophic lateral sclerosis (ALS), Parkinson's disease (PD), or other adult onset neurodegenerative diseases.

Although Medicare, as a national health insurance program, was put into effect by President Johnson in July, 1965, the program was originally conceived several decades earlier by the Roosevelt administration, within the context of its vision for universal health care in the United States.

Be that as it may, Medicare was one of several programs established to improve health care for the nation's poorest, oldest, and often sickest citizens. Health insurance plans, which also became more widely available, were primarily offered to working people through their employers. Older, often retired adults were not be eligible for these plans unless they purchased them privately and paid the full premiums by themselves. However, because older adults were considered poor health risks based on their age and an increasing need for expensive health care, private insurance premiums were quite high—if older adults were eligible for this kind of insurance at all.

Medicare is highly regulated, with health care delivery provided by private physicians, hospitals nurses, nurse practitioners, and various health care facilities. Private physicians currently treating Medicare patients receive 80% of the usual customary and reasonable (UCR) fee for health care services if they accept Medicare assignment. If they do not, they can charge no more than 115% of the Medicare allowed amount, with the client required to pay the 20% remaining UCR and any other costs up to 115% (Hogstel, 2001). Needless to say, physicians are often hesitant to accept the low reimbursement for older adults available from Medicare, and patients are hesitant to receive care from physicians that do not accept Medicare assignment because of the need to finance the co-pay. There is thus a shortage of primary care physicians to treat the health care needs of older adults.

Medicare has two parts. Part A provides for hospital insurance for older adults. In the event that an older adult requires hospitalization, Medicare Part A pays for the hospital stay. In addition, Medicare Part A pays for short-term nursing home or home care visits after hospitalization. Medicare Part A also pays for hospice care, which is discussed in Chapter 12. Generally, there is no premium for this insurance. If older adults meet the eligibility for Medicare, they are automatically enrolled in Part A.

Medicare Part B pays for visits to physicians and nurse practitioners and other health care expenditures, such as X-rays, physical and occupational outpatient therapy, and laboratory tests. Monthly premiums for Part B are based on your income and, as of June 2007, range from $93.50 to $161.40. The amount is usually deducted from the recipient's monthly Social Security checks. Medicare Part B also requires recipients to pay a deductible, which is currently the first $131 yearly for Part B-covered services or items. This deductible is likely to increase annually. Coverage of Medicare for health care needs of older adults is detailed in Table 2.1.

The Medicare traditional plan, which includes Parts A and B, has undergone a great deal of scrutiny since its inception in 1965. The chief concern among older adults and providers is the limited amount

TABLE 2.1 Coverage of Medicare for Health Care Needs of Older Adults

Service or Supply	What is covered, and when?
Acupuncture	Medicare doesn't cover acupuncture.
Ambulance Services	Medicare covers limited ambulance services. If you need to go to a hospital or skilled nursing facility (SNF), ambulance services are covered only if transportation in any other vehicle would endanger your health. Medicare helps pay for necessary ambulance transportation to the closest appropriate facility that can provide the care you need. If you choose to go to another facility farther away, Medicare payment is based on how much it would cost to go to the closest appropriate facility. All ambulance suppliers must accept assignment. **Medicare generally doesn't pay for ambulance transportation to a doctor's office.** Air ambulance is paid only in the most severe situations. If you could have gone by land ambulance without serious danger to your life or health, Medicare pays only the land ambulance rate, and you are responsible for the difference.
Ambulatory Surgical Centers	Medicare covers services given in an Ambulatory Surgical Center for a covered surgical procedure.
Anesthesia	Medicare covers anesthesia services along with medical and surgical benefits. **Medicare Part A covers anesthesia you get while in an inpatient hospital.** Medicare Part B covers anesthesia you get as an outpatient.
Artificial Limbs and Eyes	Medicare helps pay for artificial limbs and eyes. For more information, see Prosthetic Devices.
Blood	Medicare doesn't cover the first three pints of blood you get under Part A and Part B combined in a calendar year. Part A covers blood you get as an inpatient, and Part B covers blood you get as an outpatient and in a freestanding Ambulatory Surgical Center.

Bone Mass Measurement	Medicare covers bone mass measurements ordered by a doctor or qualified practitioner who is treating you if you meet one or more of the following conditions: **Women** • You are being treated for low estrogen levels and are at clinical risk for osteoporosis, based on your medical history and other findings. **Men and Women** • Your X-rays show possible osteoporosis, ostcopenia, or vertebrae fractures. • You are on prednisone or steroid-type drugs or are planning to begin such treatment. • You have been diagnosed with primary hyperparathyroidism. • You are being monitored to see if your osteoporosis drug therapy is working. The test is covered once every two years for qualified individuals and more often if medically necessary.
Braces (arm, leg, back, and neck)	Medicare covers arm, leg, back, and neck braces. For more information, see Orthotics.
Breast Prostheses	Medicare covers breast prostheses (including a surgical brassiere) after a mastectomy. For more information, see Prosthetic Devices.
Canes/Crutches	Medicare covers canes and crutches. Medicare doesn't cover canes for the blind. For more information, see Durable Medical Equipment.
Cardiac Rehabilitation Programs	Medicare covers comprehensive programs that include exercise, education, and counseling for patients whose doctor referred them and who have 1) had a heart attack in the last 12 months, 2) had coronary bypass surgery, 3) stable angina pectoris, 4) had heart valve repair/replacement, 5) had angioplasty or coronary stenting, and/or 6) had a heart or heart-lung transplant. These programs may be given by the outpatient department of a hospital or in doctor-directed clinics.
Cardiovascular Screening	Medicare covers screening tests for cholesterol, lipid, and triglyceride levels every five years. Ask your doctor to test your cholesterol, lipid, and triglyceride levels so he or she can help you prevent a heart attack or stroke.

(continued)

TABLE 2.1 Coverage of Medicare for Health Care Needs of Older Adults (*Continued*)

Service or Supply	What is covered, and when?
Chemotherapy	Medicare covers chemotherapy for patients who are hospital inpatients, outpatients, or patients in a doctor's office or freestanding clinics. In the inpatient hospital setting, Part A covers chemotherapy. In a hospital outpatient setting, freestanding facility, or doctor's office, Part B covers chemotherapy.
Chiropractic Services	Medicare covers manipulation of the spine if medically necessary to correct a subluxation (when one or more of the bones of your spine moves out of position) when provided by chiropractors or other qualified providers.
Clinical Trials	Medicare covers routine costs, like doctor visits and tests, if you take part in a qualifying clinical trial. Clinical trials test new types of medical care, like how well a new cancer drug works. Clinical trials help doctors and researchers see if the new care works and if it is safe. Medicare doesn't pay for the experimental item being investigated, in most cases.
Colorectal Cancer Screening	Medicare covers several colorectal cancer screening tests. Talk with your doctor about the screening test that is right for you. All people age 50 and older with Medicare are covered. However, there is no minimum age for having a colonoscopy. **Colonoscopy:** Medicare covers this test once every 24 months if you are at high risk for colorectal cancer. If you aren't at high risk for colorectal cancer, the test is covered once every 120 months, but not sooner than 48 months after a screening sigmoidoscopy. **Fecal Occult Blood Test:** Medicare covers this lab test once every 12 months. **Flexible Sigmoidoscopy:** Medicare covers this test once every 48 months for people 50 and older. **Barium Enema:** Once every 48 months (high risk every 24 months) when used instead of a flexible sigmoidoscopy or colonoscopy.
Commode Chairs	Medicare covers commode chairs that your doctor orders for use in your home if you are confined to your bedroom. For more information, see Durable Medical Equipment on page 46.

42

Cosmetic Surgery	Medicare generally doesn't cover cosmetic surgery unless it is needed because of accidental injury or to improve the function of a malformed part of the body. Medicare covers breast reconstruction if you had a mastectomy because of breast cancer.
Custodial Care (help with activities of daily living, like bathing, dressing, using the bathroom, and eating)	Medicare doesn't cover custodial care when it's the only kind of care you need. Care is considered custodial when it's for the purpose of helping you with activities of daily living or personal needs that could be done safely and reasonably by people without professional skills or training. For example, custodial care includes help getting in and out of bed, bathing, dressing, eating, and taking medicine.
Dental Services	Medicare doesn't cover routine dental care or most dental procedures such as cleanings, fillings, tooth extractions, or dentures. Medicare doesn't pay for dental plates or other dental devices. Medicare Part A will pay for certain dental services that you get when you are in the hospital. Medicare Part A can pay for hospital stays if you need to have emergency or complicated dental procedures, even when the dental care itself isn't covered.
Diabetes Screening	Medicare covers tests to check for diabetes. These tests are available if you have any of the following risk factors: high blood pressure, dyslipidemia (history of abnormal cholesterol and triglyceride levels), obesity, or a history of high blood sugar. Medicare also covers these tests if you have two or more of the following characteristics: • age 65 or older, • overweight, • family history of diabetes (parents, brothers, sisters), • a history of gestational diabetes (diabetes during pregnancy) or delivery of a baby weighing more than 9 pounds. Based on the results of these tests, you may be eligible for up to two diabetes screenings every year.

(continued)

43

TABLE 2.1   Coverage of Medicare for Health Care Needs of Older Adults (*Continued*)

Service or Supply	What is covered, and when?
Diabetes Supplies and Services	Medicare covers some diabetes supplies, including • blood glucose test strips, • blood glucose monitor, • lancet devices and lancets, and • glucose control solutions for checking the accuracy of test strips and monitors. There may be limits on how much or how often you get these supplies. For more information, see Durable Medical Equipment on page 32. Here are some ways you can make sure your Medicare diabetes medical supplies are covered: • Only accept supplies you have ordered. Medicare won't pay for supplies you didn't order. • Make sure you request your supply refills. Medicare won't pay for supplies sent from the supplier to you automatically. • All Medicare-enrolled pharmacies and suppliers must submit claims for glucose test strips. You can't send in the claim yourself. **Medicare doesn't cover insulin (unless used with an insulin pump), insulin pens, syringes, needles, alcohol swabs, gauze, eye exams for glasses, and routine or yearly physical exams.** If you use an external insulin pump, insulin and the pump could be covered as durable medical equipment. There may be some limits on covered supplies or how often you get them. Insulin and certain medical supplies used to inject insulin are covered under Medicare prescription drug coverage. **Therapeutic Shoes or Inserts:** Medicare covers therapeutic shoes or inserts for people with diabetes who have severe diabetic foot disease. The doctor who treats your diabetes must certify your need for therapeutic shoes or inserts. The shoes and inserts must be prescribed by a podiatrist or other qualified doctor and provided by a podiatrist, orthotist, prosthetist, or pedorthist. Medicare helps pay for one pair of therapeutic shoes and inserts per calendar year. Shoe modifications may be substituted for inserts. The fitting of the shoes or inserts is covered in the Medicare payment for the shoes.

Medicare covers these diabetes services:

- **Diabetes Self-Management Training:** Diabetes outpatient self-management training is a covered program to teach you to manage your diabetes. It includes education about self-monitoring of blood glucose, diet, exercise, and insulin.

If you've been diagnosed with diabetes, Medicare may cover up to 10 hours of initial diabetes self-management training. You may also qualify for up to two hours of follow-up training each year if

- it is provided in a group of 2 to 20 people,
- it lasts for at least 30 minutes,
- it takes place in a calendar year following the year you got your initial training, and
- your doctor or a qualified non-physician practitioner ordered it as part of your plan of care.
- Some exceptions apply if no group session is available or if your doctors or qualified non-physician practitioner says you have special needs that prevent you from participating in group training.

- **Yearly Eye Exam:** Medicare covers yearly eye exams for diabetic retinopathy.
- **Foot Exam:** A foot exam is covered every 6 months for people with diabetic peripheral neuropathy and loss of protective sensations, as long as you haven't seen a foot care professional for another reason between visits.
- **Glaucoma Screening:** Medicare covers glaucoma screening every 12 months for people with diabetes or a family history of glaucoma, African Americans age 50 and older, or Hispanics age 65 and older.
- **Medical Nutrition Therapy Services:** Medical nutrition therapy services are also covered for people with diabetes or kidney disease when referred by a doctor. These services can be given by a registered dietitian or Medicare-approved nutrition professional and include a nutritional assessment and counseling to help you manage your diabetes or kidney disease.

For more information, call 1-800-MEDICARE (1-800-633-4227). TTY users should call 1-877-486-2048.

Diagnostic Tests, X-rays, and Lab Services

Medicare covers diagnostic tests like CT scans, MRIs, EKGs, and X-rays. Medicare also covers clinical diagnostic tests and lab services provided by certified laboratories enrolled in Medicare. Diagnostic tests and lab services are done to help your doctor diagnose or rule out a suspected illness or condition. Medicare doesn't cover most routine screening tests, like checking your hearing.

Some preventive tests and screenings are covered by Medicare to help prevent, find, or manage a medical problem. For more information, see Preventive Services.

(continued)

TABLE 2.1 Coverage of Medicare for Health Care Needs of Older Adults *(Continued)*

Service or Supply	What is covered, and when?
Dialysis (Kidney)	Medicare covers some kidney dialysis services and supplies, including the following: • Inpatient dialysis treatments (if you are admitted to a hospital for special care). • Outpatient maintenance dialysis treatments (when you get treatments in any Medicare-approved dialysis facility). • Certain home dialysis support services (may include visits by trained dialysis workers to check on your home dialysis, to help in dialysis emergencies when needed, and check your dialysis equipment and hemodialysis water supply). • Certain drugs for home dialysis, including heparin, the antidote for heparin when medically necessary, and topical anesthetics. • Erythropoiesis–stimulating agents (such as Epogen®, Epoetin alfa), or Darbepoetin alfa (Aranesp®) are drugs used to treat anemia if you have end-stage renal disease. For more information, see Prescription Drugs. • Self-dialysis training (includes training for you and the person helping you with your home dialysis treatments). • Home dialysis equipment and supplies (like alcohol, wipes, sterile drapes, rubber gloves, and scissors).
Doctor's Office Visits	Medicare covers medically necessary services you get from your doctor in his or her office, in a hospital, in a skilled nursing facility, in your home, or any other location. **Routine annual physicals aren't covered, except the one-time "Welcome to Medicare" physical exam. Some preventive tests and screenings are covered by Medi-care.** See Preventive Services, and Pap Test/Pelvic Exam.
Drugs	See Prescription Drugs (Outpatient).
Durable Medical Equipment (DME)	Medicare covers Durable Medical Equipment (DME) that your doctor prescribes for use in your home. Only your own doctor can prescribe medical equipment for you. Durable Medical Equipment is • (long lasting) durable, • used for a medical reason, • not usually useful to someone who isn't sick or injured, and • used in your home.

The Durable Medical Equipment that Medicare covers includes, but isn't limited to the following:

- Air-fluidized beds
- Blood glucose monitors
- Canes (canes for the blind aren't covered)
- Commode chairs
- Crutches
- Dialysis machines
- Home oxygen equipment and supplies
- Hospital beds
- Infusion pumps (and some medicines used in infusion pumps if considered reasonable and necessary)
- Nebulizers (and some medicines used in nebulizers if considered reasonable and necessary)
- Patient lifts (to lift patient from bed or wheelchair by hydraulic operation)
- Suction pumps
- Traction equipment
- Walkers
- Wheelchairs

Make sure your supplier is enrolled in Medicare and has a Medicare supplier number. Suppliers have to meet strict standards to qualify for a Medicare supplier number. Medicare won't pay your claim if your supplier doesn't have one, even if your supplier is a large chain or department store that sells more than just durable medical equipment.

Emergency Room Services

Medicare covers emergency room services. Emergency services aren't covered in foreign countries, except in some instances in Canada and Mexico. For more information, see Travel.

A medical emergency is when you believe that your health is in serious danger. You may have an injury or illness that requires immediate medical attention to prevent a severe disability or death.

When you go to an emergency room, you will pay a copayment for each hospital service, and you will also pay coinsurance for each doctor who treats you.

Note: If you are admitted to the hospital within three days of the emergency room visit for the same condition, the emergency room visit is included in the inpatient hospital care charges, not charged separately.

(continued)

TABLE 2.1 Coverage of Medicare for Health Care Needs of Older Adults (*Continued*)

Service or Supply	What is covered, and when?
Equipment	See Durable Medical Equipment.
Eye Exams	Medicare doesn't cover routine eye exams. Medicare covers some preventive eye tests and screenings: • See yearly eye exams under Diabetes Supplies and Services on page 25. • See Glaucoma Screening. • See Macular Degeneration.
Eyeglasses/Contact Lenses	Generally, Medicare doesn't cover eyeglasses or contact lenses. However, **following cataract surgery with an implanted intraocular lens**, Medicare helps pay for corrective lenses (spectacles or contact lenses) provided by a licensed and Medicare-approved opthalmologist. Services provided by a licensed and Medicare-approved opthalmologist may be covered, if they are authorized to provide this service in your state. Important: • Only standard frames are covered. • Lenses are covered even if you had the surgery before you had Medicare. • Payment may be made for lenses for both eyes even though cataract surgery involved only one eye.
Eye Refractions	Medicare doesn't cover eye refractions.
Flu Shots	Medicare covers one flu shot per flu season. You can get a flu shot in the winter and the fall flu season of the same calendar year. All people with Medicare are covered.
Foot Care	Medicare generally doesn't cover routine foot care. Medicare Part B covers the services of a podiatrist (foot doctor) for medically necessary treatment of injuries or diseases of the foot (such as hammer toe, bunion deformities, and heel spurs). See Therapeutic Shoes and Foot Exam under Diabetes Supplies and Services starting.

Glaucoma Screening	Medicare covers glaucoma screening once every 12 months for people at high risk for glaucoma. This includes people with diabetes, a family history of glaucoma, African Americans age 50 and older, or Hispanic Americans age 65 and older. The screening must be done or supervised by an eye doctor who is legally allowed to do this service in your state.
Health Education/ Wellness Programs	Medicare generally doesn't cover health education and wellness programs. However, Medicare does cover medical nutrition therapy for some people and diabetes education for people with diabetes.
Hearing Exams/ Hearing Aids	Medicare doesn't cover routine hearing exams, hearing aids, or exams for fitting hearing aids. In some cases, Medicare covers diagnostic hearing exams.
Hepatitis B Shots	Medicare covers this preventive service (three shots) for people at high or medium (intermediate) to high risk for Hepatitis B.
	Your risk for Hepatitis B increases if you have hemophilia, end-stage renal disease (permanent kidney failure requiring dialysis or a kidney transplant), or a condition that lowers your resistance to infection. Other factors may also increase your risk for Hepatitis B. Check with your doctor to see if you are at high to medium risk for Hepatitis B.
Home Health Care	Medicare covers some home health care if the following conditions are met:
	1. Your doctor decides you need medical care in your home and makes a plan for your care at home, and
	2. You need reasonable and necessary part-time or intermittent skilled nursing care and home health aide services, and physical therapy, occupational therapy, and speech-language pathology ordered by your doctor and provided by a Medicare-certified home health agency. This includes medical social services, other services, durable medical equipment (such as wheelchairs, hospital beds, oxygen, and walkers), and medical supplies for use at home.
	3. You are homebound. This means you are normally unable to leave home and that leaving home is a major effort. When you leave home, it must be infrequent, for a short time. You may attend religious services. You may leave the house to get medical treatment, including therapeutic or psychosocial care. You can also get care in an adult day care program that is licensed or certified by your state or accredited to furnish adult day care services in your state, and

(continued)

TABLE 2.1 Coverage of Medicare for Health Care Needs of Older Adults (*Continued*)

Service or Supply	What is covered, and when?
	4. The home health agency caring for you must be approved by Medicare. Medicare covers durable medical equipment (such as wheelchairs, hospital beds, oxygen, and walkers). **Note for Women with Osteoporosis:** Medicare helps pay for an injectable drug for osteoporosis in women who have Medicare Part B, meet the criteria for the Medicare home health benefit, and have a bone fracture that a doctor certifies was related to post-menopausal osteoporosis. You must also be certified by a doctor as unable to learn or unable to give yourself the drug by injection, and that family and/or caregivers are unable or unwilling to give the drug by injection. Medicare covers the visit by a home health nurse to give the drug.
Hospice Care	Medicare covers hospice care if • you are eligible for Medicare Part A, • your doctor and the hospice medical director certify that you are terminally ill and probably have less than six months to live, • you accept palliative (care to comfort) instead of care to cure your illness, • you sign a statement choosing hospice care instead of routine Medicare-covered benefits for your terminal illness, **and** • you get care from a Medicare-approved hospice program. Medicare allows a nurse practitioner to serve as an attending doctor for a patient who elects the hospice benefit. Nurse practitioners are prohibited from certifying a terminal diagnosis. **Respite Care:** Medicare also covers respite care if you are getting covered hospice care. Respite care is inpatient care given to a hospice patient so that the usual caregiver can rest. You can stay in a Medicare-approved facility, such as a hospice facility, hospital or nursing home, up to five days each time you get respite care. Medicare will still pay for covered services for any health problems that aren't related to your terminal illness.

Hospital Bed	See Durable Medical Equipment.
Hospital Care (Inpatient) for Outpatient Services.	Medicare covers inpatient hospital care when all of the following are true: • A doctor says you need inpatient hospital care to treat your illness or injury. • You need the kind of care that can be given only in a hospital. • The hospital is enrolled in Medicare. • The Utilization Review Committee of the hospital approves your stay while you are in the hospital. • A Quality Improvement Organization approves your stay after the bill is submitted. Medicare-covered hospital services include the following: a semiprivate room, meals, general nursing, and other hospital services and supplies. This includes care you get in critical access hospitals and inpatient mental health care. This doesn't include private-duty nursing, a television, or telephone in your room. It also doesn't include a private room, unless medically necessary.
Implantable Cardiac Defibrillator	Medicare covers defibrillators for many people diagnosed with congestive heart failure.
Kidney (Dialysis)	See Dialysis.
Lab Services	Medicare covers medically necessary diagnostic lab services that are ordered by your treating doctor when they are provided by a Clinical Laboratory Improvement Amendments (CLIA)–certified laboratory enrolled in Medicare. For more information, see Diagnostic Tests.
Macular Degeneration	Medicare covers certain treatments for some patients with age-related macular degeneration (AMD) like ocular photodynamic therapy with verteporfin (Visudyne®).
Mammogram (Screening)	Medicare covers a screening mammogram once every 12 months (11 full months must have gone by from the last screening) for all women with Medicare age 40 and older. You can also get one baseline mammogram between ages 35 and 39.

(continued)

51

TABLE 2.1 Coverage of Medicare for Health Care Needs of Older Adults *(Continued)*

Service or Supply	What is covered, and when?
Mental Health Care	Medicare covers mental health care given by a doctor or a qualified mental health professional. Before you get treatment, ask your doctor, psychologist, social worker, or other health professional if they accept Medicare payment. **Inpatient Mental Health Care:** Medicare covers inpatient mental health care services. These services can be given in psychiatric units of a general hospital or in a specialty psychiatric hospital that cares for people with mental health problems. Medicare helps pay for inpatient mental health services in the same way that it pays for all other inpatient hospital care. **Note:** If you are in a specialty psychiatric hospital, Medicare only helps for a total of 190 days of inpatient care during your lifetime. **Outpatient Mental Health Care:** Medicare covers mental health services on an outpatient basis by either a doctor, clinical psychologist, clinical social worker, clinical nurse specialist, or physician assistant in an office setting, clinic, or hospital outpatient department. **Partial Hospitalization:** Partial hospitalization may be available for you. It is a structured program of active psychiatric treatment that is more intense than the care you get in your doctor or therapist's office. For Medicare to cover a partial hospitalization program, a doctor must say that you would otherwise need inpatient treatment. Medicare covers the services of specially qualified non-physician practitioners such as clinical psychologists, clinical social workers, nurse practitioners, clinical nurse specialists, and physician assistants, as allowed by state and local law for medically necessary services.
Nursing Home Care	Most nursing home care is custodial care. Generally, Medicare doesn't cover custodial care. Medicare Part A only covers skilled nursing care given in a certified skilled nursing facility (SNF) or in your home (if you are homebound) if medically necessary, but not custodial care (such as helping with bathing or dressing).

52

Nutrition Therapy Services (Medical)	Medicare covers medical nutrition therapy services, when ordered by a doctor, for people with kidney disease (but who aren't on dialysis) or who have a kidney transplant, or people with diabetes. These services can be given by a registered dietitian or Medicare-approved nutrition professional and include nutritional assessment, one-on-one counseling, and therapy through an interactive telecommunications system. See Diabetes Supplies and Services.
Occupational Therapy	See Physical Therapy/Occupational Therapy/Speech-Language Pathology.
Orthotics	Medicare covers artificial limbs and eyes, and arm, leg, back and neck braces. Medicare doesn't pay for orthopedic shoes unless they are a necessary part of the leg brace. Medicare doesn't pay for dental plates or other dental devices. See Diabetes Supplies and Services (Therapeutic Shoes).
Ostomy Supplies	Medicare covers ostomy supplies for people who have had a colostomy, ileostomy, or urinary ostomy. Medicare covers the amount of supplies your doctor says you need, based on your condition.
Outpatient Hospital Services	Medicare covers medically necessary services you get as an outpatient from a Medicare-participating hospital for diagnosis or treatment of an illness or injury. Covered outpatient hospital services include
• services in an emergency room or outpatient clinic, including same-day surgery,
• laboratory tests billed by the hospital,
• mental health care in a partial hospitalization program, if a doctor certifies that inpatient treatment would be required without it,
• X-rays and other radiology services billed by the hospitals,
• medical supplies such as splints and casts,
• screenings and preventive services, and
• certain drugs and biologicals that you can't give yourself.

(continued)

53

TABLE 2.1 Coverage of Medicare for Health Care Needs of Older Adults (*Continued*)

Service or Supply	What is covered, and when?
Oxygen Therapy	Medicare covers the rental of oxygen equipment. Or, if you own your own equipment, Medicare will help pay for oxygen contents and supplies for the delivery of oxygen when all of these conditions are met: • Your doctor says you have a severe lung disease or you're not getting enough oxygen and your condition might improve with oxygen therapy. • Your arterial blood gas level falls within a certain range. • Other alternative measures have failed. Under the above conditions Medicare helps pay for • systems for furnishing oxygen, • containers that store oxygen, • tubing and related supplies for the delivery of oxygen, and • oxygen contents. If oxygen is provided only for use during sleep, portable oxygen wouldn't be covered. Portable oxygen isn't covered when provided only as a backup to a stationary oxygen system.
Pap Test/Pelvic Exam	Medicare covers Pap tests and pelvic exams (and a clinical breast exam) for all women once every 24 months. Medicare covers this test and exam once every 12 months if you are at high risk for cervical or vaginal cancer or if you are of childbearing age and have had an abnormal Pap test in the past 36 months. If you have your Pap test, pelvic exam, and clinical breast exam on the same visit as a routine physical exam, you pay for the physical exam. Routine physical exams aren't covered by Medicare, except for the one-time "Welcome to Medicare" physical exam.
Physical Exams (routine) ("One-time Welcome to Medicare" physical exam)	Routine physical exams aren't generally covered by Medicare. Medicare covers a one-time review of your health, as well as education and counseling about the preventive services you need, including certain screenings and shots. Referrals for other care, if you need them, will also be covered. **Important:** You must have the physical exam within the first six months you have Medicare Part B (deductibles and coinsurance apply).

54

Physical Therapy/ Occupational Therapy/ Speech-Language Pathology	Medicare helps pay for medically necessary outpatient physical and occupational therapy and speech-language pathology services when • your doctor or therapist sets up the plan of treatment, and • your doctor periodically reviews the plan to see how long you will need therapy. You can get outpatient services from a Medicare-approved outpatient provider such as a participating hospital or skilled nursing facility, or from a participating home health agency, rehabilitation agency, or a comprehensive outpatient rehabilitation facility. Also, you can get services from a Medicare-approved physical or occupational therapist, in private practice, in his or her office, or in your home. (Medicare doesn't pay for services given by a speech-language pathologist in private practice.) In 2007, there may be limits on physical therapy, occupational therapy, and speech-language pathology services. If so, there may be exceptions to these limits.
Pneumococcal Shot	Medicare covers the pneumococcal shot to help prevent pneumococcal infections. Most people only need this preventive shot once in their lifetime. Talk with your doctor to see if you need this shot.
Prescription Drugs (Outpatient) Very Limited Coverage	Part B covers a limited number of outpatient prescription drugs. Your pharmacy or doctor must accept assignment on Medicare-covered prescription drugs. Part B covers drugs that aren't usually self-administered when you are given them in a hospital outpatient department. You can get comprehensive drug coverage by joining a Medicare drug plan (also called "Part D"). For more information. **The following outpatient prescription drugs are covered:** • **Some Antigens:** Medicare will help pay for antigens if they are prepared by a doctor and given by a properly instructed person (who could be the patient) under doctor supervision. • **Osteoporosis Drugs:** Medicare helps pay for an injectable drug for osteoporosis for certain women with Medicare. See note for women with osteoporosis, under Home Health Care. • **Erythropoisis-stimulating agents (such as Epogen,® Epoetin alfa, or Darbepoetin alfa Aranesp®):** Medicare will help pay for erythropoietin by injection if you have end-stage renal disease (permanent kidney failure) and need this drug to treat anemia.

(continued)

55

TABLE 2.1 Coverage of Medicare for Health Care Needs of Older Adults (*Continued*)

Service or Supply	What is covered, and when?
	• **Blood Clotting Factors:** If you have hemophilia, Medicare will help pay for clotting factors you give yourself by injection.
	• **Injectable Drugs:** Medicare covers most injectable drugs given by a licensed medical practitioner, if the drug is considered reasonable and necessary for treatment.
	• **Immunosuppressive Drugs:** Medicare covers immunosuppressive drug therapy for transplant patients if the transplant was paid for by Medicare (or paid by private insurance that paid as a primary payer to your Medicare Part A coverage) in a Medicare-certified facility.
	• **Oral Cancer Drugs:** Medicare will help pay for some cancer drugs you take by mouth if the same drug is available in injectable form.
	Currently, Medicare covers the following cancer drugs you take by mouth:
	• Capecitabine (brand name Xeloda®)
	• Cyclophosphamide (brand name Cytoxan®)
	• Methotrexate
	• Temozolomide (brand name Temodar®)
	• Busulfan (brand name Myleran®)
	• Etoposide (brand name VePesid®)
	• Melphalan (brand name Alkeran®)
	As new cancer drugs become available, Medicare may cover them.
	• **Oral Anti-Nausea Drugs:** Medicare will help pay for oral anti-nausea drugs used as part of an anti-cancer chemotherapeutic regimen. The drugs must be administered within 48 hours and must be used as a full therapeutic replacement for the intravenous anti-nausea drugs that would otherwise be given. Medicare also covers some drugs used in infusion pumps and nebulizers if considered reasonable and necessary.

Preventive Services

Medicare covers the following preventive services:

- Bone Mass Measurement.
- Cardiovascular Screening Blood Tests.
- Colorectal Cancer Screening.
- Diabetes Screenings.
- Glaucoma Screening.
- Mammogram Screening.
- Nutrition Therapy Services.
- Pap Test/Pelvic Exam.
- Prostate Cancer Screening.
- Shots on page 52 including
  - flu shot,
  - pneumococcal shot, and
  - Hepatitis B shot.
- Smoking Cessation Counseling.
- One-time "Welcome to Medicare" physical exam.

Prostate Cancer Screening

Medicare covers prostate screening tests once every 12 months for all men age 50 and older with Medicare (coverage begins the day after your 50th birthday). Covered tests include the following:

- Digital Rectal Examination
- Prostate Specific Antigen (PSA) Test

Prosthetic Devices

Medicare covers prosthetic devices needed to replace an internal body part or function. These include Medicare-approved corrective lenses needed after a cataract operation (see Eyeglasses/Contact Lenses), ostomy bags and certain related supplies (see Ostomy Supplies), and breast prostheses (including a surgical brassiere) after a mastectomy (see Breast Prostheses).

Radiation Therapy

Medicare covers radiation therapy for patients who are hospital inpatients or outpatients or patients in free-standing clinics.

(*continued*)

TABLE 2.1 Coverage of Medicare for Health Care Needs of Older Adults (*Continued*)

Service or Supply	What is covered, and when?
Religious Non-medical Health Care Institution (RNHCI)	Medicare doesn't cover the religious portion of RNHCI care. Medicare covers inpatient nonmedical care when the following conditions are met: • The RNHCI has agreed and is currently certified to participate in Medicare, and the Utilization Review Committee agrees that you'd require hospital or skilled nursing facility care if it weren't for your religious beliefs. • You have a written agreement with Medicare indicating that your need for this form of care is based on your religious beliefs. The agreement must also indicate that if you decide to accept standard medical care you may have to wait longer to get RNHCI services in the future. You're always able to access medically necessary Medicare Part A services. • The care provided is reasonable and necessary.
Respite Care	Medicare covers respite care for hospice patients (see Hospice Care).
Second Surgical Opinions	Medicare covers a second opinion before surgery that isn't an emergency. A second opinion is when another doctor gives his or her view about your health problem and how it should be treated. Medicare will also help pay for a third opinion if the first and second opinions are different.
Shots (Vaccinations)	Medicare covers the following shots: Flu Shot: Once per flu season. You can get a flu shot in the fall and the winter flu seasons of the same year. Hepatitis B Shot: Certain people with Medicare at medium to high risk for Hepatitis B. Pneumococcal Shot: One shot may be all you ever need. Ask your doctor.
Skilled Nursing Facility (SNF) Care	Medicare covers skilled care in a skilled nursing facility (SNF) under certain conditions for a limited time. Skilled care is health care given when you need skilled nursing or rehabilitation staff to manage, observe, and evaluate your care. Examples of skilled care include changing sterile dressings and physical therapy. Care that can be given by non-professional staff isn't considered skilled care. Medicare covers certain skilled care services that are needed daily on a short-term basis (up to 100 days).

Medicare will cover skilled care if all these conditions are met:

1. You have Medicare Part A (Hospital Insurance) and have days left in your benefit period to use.

2. You have a qualifying hospital stay. This means an inpatient hospital stay of three consecutive days or more, including the day you're admitted to the hospital, but not including the day you leave the hospital. You must enter the SNF within a short time (generally 30 days) of leaving the hospital and require skilled services related to your hospital stay (see item 5). After you leave the SNF, if you reenter the same or another SNF within 30 days, you don't need another three-day qualifying hospital stay to get additional SNF benefits. This is also true if you stop getting skilled care while in the SNF and then start getting skilled care again within 30 days.

3. Your doctor has decided that you need daily skilled care. It must be given by, or under the direct supervision of, skilled nursing or rehabilitation staff. If you are in the SNF for skilled rehabilitation services only, your care is considered daily care even if these therapy services are offered just five or six days a week, as long as you need and get the therapy services each day they are offered.

4. You get these skilled services in a SNF that is certified by Medicare.

5. You need these skilled services for a medical condition that
   • was treated during a qualifying three-day hospital stay, or
   • started while you were getting care in the SNF for a medical condition that was treated during a qualifying three-day hospital stay. For example, if you are in the SNF because you had a stroke, and you develop an infection that requires I.V. antibiotics and you meet the conditions listed in items 1-4, Medicare will cover skilled care.

Smoking Cessation (Counseling to stop smoking)	Medicare covers minimal regular doctor's office visits, and up to 8 face-to-face visits in a 12-month period if you are diagnosed with an illness caused or complicated by tobacco use, or you take a medicine that is affected by tobacco.
Speech-Language Pathology	See Physical Therapy/Occupational Therapy/Speech-Language Pathology.
Substance-Related Disorders	Medicare covers treatment for substance-related disorders in inpatient or outpatient settings. Certain limits apply.

(continued)

59

TABLE 2.1 Coverage of Medicare for Health Care Needs of Older Adults (*Continued*)

Service or Supply	What is covered, and when?
Supplies (you use at home)	Medicare generally doesn't cover common medical supplies like bandages and gauze. Supplies furnished as part of a doctor's service are covered by Medicare, and payment is included in Medicare's doctor payment. Doctors don't bill for supplies. Medicare covers some diabetes and dialysis supplies. See Diabetes Supplies and Services on page 25 and Dialysis (Kidney). For items such as walkers, oxygen, and wheelchairs, see Durable Medical Equipment.
Surgical Dressings	Medicare covers surgical dressings when medically necessary for the treatment of a surgical or surgically treated wound.
Therapeutic Shoes	See Diabetes Supplies and Services (Therapeutic Shoes).
Transplants (Doctor Services)	Medicare covers doctor services for transplants, see Transplants (Facility Charges).
Transplants (Facility Charges)	Medicare covers transplants of the heart, lung, kidney, pancreas, intestine/multivisceral, bone marrow, cornea, and liver under certain conditions and, for some types of transplants, only at Medicare-approved facilities. Medicare only approves facilities for kidney, heart, liver, lung, intestine/multivisceral, and some pancreas transplants. Bone marrow and cornea transplants aren't limited to approved facilities. Transplant coverage includes necessary tests, labs, and exams before surgery. It also includes immunosuppressive drugs (under certain conditions), follow-up care for you, and procurement of organs and tissues. Medicare pays for the costs for a living donor for a kidney transplant.
Transportation (Routine)	Medicare generally doesn't cover transportation to get routine health care. For more information, see Ambulance Services.

Travel Outside of the United States (Health Care Coverage During Travel)	Medicare generally doesn't cover health care while you are traveling outside the United States. Puerto Rico, the U.S. Virgin Islands, Guam, American Samoa, and the Northern Mariana Islands are considered part of the United States. There are some exceptions. In some cases, Medicare may pay for services that you get while on board a ship within the territorial waters adjoining the land areas of the United States. In rare cases, Medicare can pay for inpatient hospital services that you get in a foreign country. Medicare can pay only under the following circumstances: 1. You are in the United States when a medical emergency occurs and the foreign hospital is closer than the nearest United States hospital that can treat the emergency. 2. You are traveling through Canada without unreasonable delay by the most direct route between Alaska and another state when a medical emergency occurs and the Canadian hospital is closer than the nearest United States hospital that can treat the emergency. 3. You live in the United States and the foreign hospital is closer to your home than the nearest United States hospital that can treat your medical condition, regardless of whether an emergency exists. Medicare also pays for doctor and ambulance services you get in a foreign country as part of a covered inpatient hospital stay.
Walker/Wheelchair	Medicare covers power-operated vehicles (scooters), walkers, and wheelchairs as durable medical equipment that your doctor prescribes for use in your home. For more information, see Durable Medical Equipment. **Power Wheelchair:** You must have a face-to-face examination and a written prescription from a doctor or other treating provider before Medicare helps pay for a power wheelchair.
X-rays	Medicare covers medically necessary diagnostic X-rays that are ordered by your treating doctor. For more information, see Diagnostic Tests.

Source: U.S. Department of Health & Human Services Centers for Medicare & Medicaid Services (2007). *Your Medicare benefits.* Retrieved September 2, 2007 from http://www.medicare.gov/Publications/Pubs/pdf/10116.pdf.

of reimbursement for increasingly common chronic illnesses. From a government perspective, providing increased Medicare coverage to a growing population of older adults is problematic.

In an attempt to resolve some of these issues, numerous changes and additions to the traditional Medicare plan have evolved, including Medigap: a private (nongovernmental) health insurance that Medicare recipients can purchase in order to help pay for expenditures not covered by Medicare (Hogstel, 2001). Some expenses covered by Medigap include Medicare deductibles, co-pays (the additional amount of money that the patient must pay the health care provider), health care outside the United States, and medications. Currently, within Medigap, there are 10 standard plans that cover some of the essentials here, such as deductibles. However, each Medigap plan may also have additional benefits, exclusions, premiums, and coverage (Hogstel, 2001).

Although many traditional Medicare recipients purchase a Medigap policy, older Medicare patients sometimes cannot afford the monthly premiums for these supplemental plans. Sorting through payment issues associated with traditional Medicare and Medigap plans is often troublesome for many older adults, especially those with limited education, literacy, and experience in managing administrative matters. Moreover, older adults from multiple cultures may have language barriers that make it more difficult to understand the complex Medicare and Medigap systems.

Another attempt to improve Medicare coverage and lower health care costs is Medicare Managed Care, which began as a strong movement in the early 1990s to lower the administrative costs associated with Medicare (Hogstel, 2001). Medicare recipients were asked to select a health maintenance organization (HMO) through which to receive their health care, and health care received through these HMOs would be paid for by Medicare. Unfortunately for the HMOs, older adults used considerably more health care services than Medicare reimbursements covered. As a result, HMOs lost money and, by 2000, many had withdrawn from the Medicare Managed Care business. While there are still HMOs servicing older adults in the United States, many other HMOs no longer take older adult Medicare clients.

The increase in health care costs between 1970 and 1980, resulted in changes in legislation surrounding how hospitals received reimbursement for Medicare patients. Before 1983, hospitals provided necessary care to older adults, and then, with care completed, the hospital submitted an invoice to Medicare, receiving payment for all Medicare-eligible services rendered. After this time, a prospective payment system (PPS) was implemented that calculated reimbursable costs based on the older patient's diagnosis and placed financial limits on the amount that could be reimbursed to the hospital for the older adult's stay (Hogstel, 2001). This system, known as defined diagnostic related groups (DRGs), forced hospitals to find more efficient ways to provide care to older adults. New technology has greatly assisted this effort and has played a substantial role in decreasing the hospital stays of older adults. Moreover, improvements in outpatient rehabilitation, home care, and short-term stays in skilled nursing facilities have provided alternatives to care that traditionally could only be found in the hospital setting. To illustrate this, consider an older adult patient admitted to the hospital with pneumonia. Prior to the implementation of the PPS and DRG systems, the patient would have remained in the hospital until complete healing and rehabilitation were assured, as long as two weeks if necessary. Currently, this same client may be treated at home with antibiotics or admitted for only a short period of time if intravenous therapy and intensive respiratory therapy are indicated. This change in health care delivery has some positive benefits for patients, who often meet health care goals more effectively at home and are free from the risks of hospitalization, such as nosocomial infections. However, should a problem arise, the availability of geriatric-educated nurses and physicians is much higher in the hospital setting than in these alternative locations.

As mentioned, the need for hospitals to deliver care more efficiently in response to the implementation of the PPS and DRG systems resulted in shorter hospital stays. Despite this movement, older adults continue to require care that is often delivered at home. As a result of these changes in the late 1980s and well into the 1990s, home care experienced tremendous growth. With an average of 95% of older adults living at home, and each with approximately three chronic illnesses, the need for nursing care at home is substantial. However, while the number of home care agencies grew greatly, so did the amount of fraudulent claims to the Medicare system (Hogstel, 2001). Offenders were prosecuted, but the cost to the home care system resulted in the closing

---

CULTURAL FOCUS

Sorting through payment issues associated with traditional Medicare and Medigap plans is often troublesome for many older adults, especially those with limited education, literacy, and experience in managing administrative matters. Moreover, older adults from multiple cultures may have language barriers that make it more difficult to understand the complex Medicare and Medigap systems. Awareness of these difficulties allows nurses to provide assistance in sorting out these complicated issues and ensuring access to health care.

EVIDENCE-BASED PRACTICE

Title of Study: The Impact of the 1997 Balanced Budget Amendment's Prospective Payment System on Patient Case Mix and Rehabilitation Utilization in Skilled Nursing

Authors: Yip, J., Wilber K., Myrtle, R.

Purpose: To study the impact of the 1997 Balanced Budget Amendment's prospective payment system (PPS) and whether that impact varies in the post-acute prospective payment system on Medicare-funded rehabilitation services in skilled nursing facilities (SNFs).

Methods: Interviews of 214 Medicare beneficiaries admitted to 3 SNFs in southern California. Comparisons were made between patients' admission characteristics and therapy utilization among those receiving post-acute rehabilitation before and after the implementation of PPS.

Findings: Those admitted after PPS implementations were more likely to have orthopedic problems, stroke, or poorer self-reported health. Their rehabilitation stay was shorter, and they received less therapy. Those in managed care had less reduction in treatment after SNF-PPS implementation than those in fee-for-service.

Implications: In this study, following SNF-PPS implementation, rehabilitation treatment levels were reduced. Changes in Medicare managed care were comparatively modest, whereas there were significant changes in intensity and duration of physical and occupational therapies in Medicare fee-for-service.

The Gerontologist, Vol. 42, No. 5, 653–660.

---

of almost half of the home care agencies and a more highly regulated system of reimbursement. Hogstel (2001) reports that no new home health agencies were allowed to open and those remaining continued to operate under strict regulations. The closure and merger of many home health care agencies created a shortage of services and providers for home-bound elderly.

It is important to note that this change in Medicare payment to hospitals was the impetus for private health care insurance programs to institute a PPS system as well. Consequently, it is not only the elderly who are discharged sicker and quicker, but children, new mothers and infants, and other members of the population are also discharged sooner than they would have been previously. Hospitals also made a change in staffing patterns and attempted to replace nurses with unlicensed assistive personnel (UAP) as a means to remain viable in a declining reimbursement environment. This change caused great concern about the quality of care in hospitals. While there are certainly positive aspects of this change in health care delivery, such as the ability to meet health care goals more effectively at home and the ability to remain free from the risks of hospitalization, such as nosocomial infections, should a problem arise, the need to transport to a facility with appropriate resources may be necessary, and the delay in accessing these services could increase both morbidity and mortality. This raises additional concerns for older adults who may be discharged home with no one to care for them in the immediate postoperative period.

In further attempts to repair the problems inherent in the Medicare system, three newer alternatives have evolved as alternative options in addition to the traditional Medicare plan. Medicare now offers (a) preferred provider organization plans (PPOs), (b) private fee-for-service plans, and (c) specialty plans. PPOs provide discounts to older adults who choose primary care providers and specialists who have agreed to accept Medicare assignment for patients. This saves Medicare money and provides older adults with an alternative health care provider based on costs. For example, an older adult may have had a relationship with a particular physician who chooses not to accept Medicare assignment. In this case, the older adult can still maintain the physician as their primary health care provider, but they must pay extra for visits to this physician. Medicare fee-for-service plans contract with private providers to allow older adults to go to any Medicare-approved doctor or hospital that is willing to take them. Benefits of these plans are often improved coverage, such as extra hospital days. However, providers must work with private insurance plans directly to determine coverage for the health care expenditures. Moreover, an additional premium may be involved, and there may be additional costs, such as higher co-pays. In addition, private insurance companies may choose to terminate coverage at the end of each year. Medicare is currently in the process of developing a variety of specialty plans to meet the diverse and comprehensive needs of older adults. More information on these plans will be available as they develop.

Medicaid

Medicaid is another national health insurance program to improve health care for low-income citizens of the United States, including older adults (Hogstel, 2001). However, while Medicare is regulated and administered by the federal government, Medicaid is administered by individual states. Consequently, the coverage is variable according to state regulations and coverages. Medicaid also has expanded coverage to include children and adults younger than 65 regardless of health status. Medicaid eligibility is based on specific income and asset guidelines established by individual states. Older adults who are attempting to qualify for Medicaid generally have very limited financial resources and assets (Hogstel, 2001). For older adults with limited assets and income, Medicaid may supplement current Medicare benefits and pay for health care expenses not covered by Medicare, including medications, extended hospital or nursing home stays, and durable medical equipment. For older adults with both Medicare and Medicaid coverage, Medicare is the primary payment system, and Medicaid is secondary. The Centers for Medicare and Medicaid Services (2005) estimates that approximately 6.5 million Medicare recipients also have Medicaid.

Medicaid was enacted in 1965 by the same legislation as Medicare and is also known as Title XIX of the Social Security Act. Unlike Medicare, which is funded and administered through the federal government, Medicaid is a joint partnership between federal and state governments aimed at assisting states to provide medical assistance to low income individuals. The Centers for Medicare and Medicaid Services (2005) reports that Medicaid is currently the greatest source of funding for health-related services for America's poor population.

While changes and revisions have resulted within Medicare since its inception, many changes have also occurred within the Medicaid systems. However, because Medicaid is jointly funded by each individual state, there is great variability in covered medical expenses throughout the country. Each state establishes eligibility guidelines, allowable expenses, how much will be paid for these expenses, and how the program will be run within that state. Thus, there are as many different Medicaid programs as there are states. Because of the variability in guidelines, an older adult could be eligible for Medicaid in one state and not another. In addition, an older adult may have a particular medical expense paid for under one state's Medicaid plan and find that it is not an allowable health care expense in another. To further complicate the variability in Medicaid, state governments have the authority to change Medicaid eligibility and guidelines to meet annual state budget requirements. This means that while an older adult may be eligible one year, they may be ineligible the following year; or a particular procedure or expense may be covered one year, but may not be covered the following year.

To receive the federal portion of funds within Medicaid, states are required to include in the program individuals who receive certain federal assistance programs. Generally speaking, eligibility for Medicaid is based on low income federal funds. Eligibility for Medicare does not make a person eligible for Medicaid. However, if the older adult receives Supplemental Security Income (SSI) from the federal government, they are eligible for Medicaid assistance as well. While states are not mandated to cover other low-income population groups, many cover institutionalized elderly within a certain income level set by the state and disabled older adults under the federal poverty line (FPL).

Many state Medicaid programs have also extended coverage for home- and community-based services (HCBS), if these services are keeping the older adult out of a covered nursing home stay. These services fall within a newer Medicaid program known as Program of All-inclusive Care for the Elderly (PACE). This program provides alternatives to nursing home care for persons aged 55 or older who require a nursing facility level of care. Within this program a coordinator plans medical, social service, rehabilitative, and supportive services with the specific aim of preventing costly nursing home admissions. The services within the PACE program are often received at home, but they may also consist of collaborations with adult day care and clinic providers. In addition to these groups, many state Medicaid plans also have broad language that allows coverage to medically needy (MN) individuals, although they do not fall into one of the traditionally covered groups. In these cases, older adults may have income or assets that exceed the eligibility guidelines within the state, but cannot afford costly health care.

As stated earlier in this text, legislation enacted in 1996, known as the Personal Responsibility and Work Opportunity Reconciliation Act or (Public Law 104–193) "welfare reform" bill, made legal resident aliens and other qualified aliens who entered the United States on or after that period ineligible for Medicaid for 5 years. Whether or not older adult aliens entering before 1996 or after the 5-year ban are eligible for Medicaid is decided by individual states. This means that many older adult immigrants to the United States may not have any available form of payment for health care expenses.

While allowable medical expenses within Medicaid varies by state, the federal government mandates that certain medical expenses are covered within all state Medicaid plans. Mandated covered expenses for older adults include inpatient and outpatient hospital services, physician services, nursing home services and home care services that are delivered to prevent nursing home stays, and laboratory and X-ray services. Coverage of other medical expenses, such as various diagnostic procedures, durable medical equipment, medications, eyeglasses, and hearing aides, vary by state.

CULTURAL FOCUS

Legal resident aliens and other qualified aliens who entered the United States in or after 1996 are ineligible for Medicaid for 5 years. Whether or not older adult aliens entering before 1996 or after the 5-year ban are eligible for Medicaid is decided by individual states. This means that many older adult immigrants to the United States may not have any available form of payment for health care expenses.

If an older adult is a Medicaid recipient, payment for health care expenses is provided directly to the health care provider. States have a great deal of flexibility in the amount of reimbursement for health care costs and how health care is delivered. Some states pay individual providers for services, while others require Medicaid recipients to receive care through health maintenance organizations (HMOs). Individual health care providers who accept Medicaid patients must accept Medicaid payment as payment in full. In other words, regardless of the charge, the provider may not ask the Medicaid recipient to pay any part of the medical bill. However, individual states may require some Medicaid recipients to pay deductibles or co-payments for some health care services.

While Medicaid is used by all population groups in each state, the highest expenditures are made on behalf of older adults. While children average approximately $1,200 a year in Medicaid expenditure, older adults, who make up only 9% of Medicaid recipients, average approximately $11,000 per person in annual Medicaid expenditures. Moreover, Medicaid payment for long-term care services utilized by primarily older adults was approximately $37.2 billion in 2001 (Centers for Medicare and Medicaid Services, 2005).

Medicaid has more enhanced coverage and fewer limitations than Medicare. Medicaid covers long-term care and some prescription medications, dental care, and eye care that Medicare does not cover. One of the most utilized Medicaid benefits for older adults is the coverage of long-term care in nursing facilities, which Medicare provides only for rehabilitative days (Hogstel, 2001).

Private Pay, or Fee for Service

In private pay, or fee for service, older people pay out of pocket for any health care services not covered by Medicare, Medicaid, long-term care, private insurances, or veteran's benefits. Some of the types of care not usually covered include: deductibles and co-pays for physicians, hospital visits, and prescription medication; cosmetic and/or experimental surgery and procedures; private duty nurses and home health aides; and nonmedical in-home assistance, such as home makers, companions, and chore services.

Veteran's Benefits

The Veteran's Administration (VA) is a government entity that provides health care for veterans (military personnel who fought during a war). VA health care is provided through VA medical centers and facilities located throughout the country. Eligibility for VA health care is determined through a network of VA health facilities and hospitals across the

United States. Once eligibility has been determined, qualified veterans may receive health care for low, or no, cost.

Eligibility for VA health care coverage or the amount of coverage the veteran is entitled to will depend on several factors. Most active duty military personnel who served in the Army, Navy, Air Force, Marines, or Coast Guard and were honorably discharged are eligible for VA health care coverage. In addition, military reservists and National Guard members who served on active duty on order from the federal government may also be eligible for some VA health services. Eligibility for health care coverage is not limited to those who served in combat.

The *Veterans' Health Care Eligibility Reform Act of 1996* was developed to clarify eligibility for VA health care coverage and improve health benefits for qualified beneficiaries. The legislative act resulted in the development of the current Uniform Benefits package, which is the standard enhanced health benefits plan generally available to all available veterans.

Once eligibility has been approved, VA health coverage under the Uniform Benefits package is comprehensive and provides for both inpatient and outpatient coverage at VA medical centers and facilities nationwide and abroad. Outpatient clinics provide physician services and primary and preventive care. Diagnostic testing (including laboratory tests), minor surgery, and other needed benefits, such as prescription medications, are covered for a small monetary fee for eligible patients (Hogstel, 2001). In addition, the VA will pay for hearing aides and other services after a small deductible has been met. Pharmaceutical coverage is provided even if the prescriptions were written by an outside health care provider. VA coverage improves for veterans with service-connected health problems (Hogstel, 2001).

Long-Term Care Insurance

Long-term care insurance is a more recent concept designed to meet the needs of the growing elderly population (Hogstel, 2001). Medicare pays only for acute care needs of the older adults, and Medicaid coverage is available to only those with low income and virtually no assets (such as a house). Alexander (2005) states that the possibility of older adults requiring long-term care at some point in their lives is approximately 50%. Thus, middle-income members of the older population requiring long-term care are not able to utilize Medicare or Medicaid to pay for extended nursing home stays. With an average stay of 2 to 4 years and an average cost of $70,000 per year, older adults cannot afford to pay out of pocket for nursing home stays. Consequently an illness that results in a nursing home stay has the potential to bankrupt most middle-income older adults.

Long-term care insurance was developed by private insurance companies to meet the long-term and chronic needs of older adults. Long-term care insurance was designed to pay for long-term health services when multiple chronic health problems occur that require custodial care not covered by Medicare or other insurance. There are many advantages to owning a long-term care insurance policy. But, while insurance companies that offer long-term care policies are usually very ethical, they are essentially businesses with an interest in profit. In other words, while long-term care insurance may legitimately and appropriately meet the needs of older adults who purchase it, it is often very costly. The older the adult is when the policy is purchased, the more expensive the policy. Monthly premiums vary depending on age at the time of policy purchase, the anticipated length of coverage, waiting period, and the desired amount of daily payments for health care expenses (Hogstel, 2001). Moreover, premiums are often not fixed and may increase throughout the coverage period. In some cases, the premium may rise so high that older adults are no longer able to afford to pay. This may result in policy cancellation and loss of all previous monthly premiums, just when the policy benefits are needed to cover long-term nursing home, assisted-living, or home care services.

Long-term care insurance generally provides coverage for approved care in nursing and assisted-living facilities, in addition to care in the home by health care providers and community-based services, such as care at adult day care centers. As the policies vary greatly, some services within these facilities may not be covered. Alexander (2005) reports that the coverage is needed the most when the older adult is least able to advocate for coverage, often because of illness.

Long-term care insurance is a useful insurance alternative or addition for middle-income older adults who do not qualify for Medicaid but have insufficient resources for extensive long-term care stays (Hogstel, 2001). Older individuals considering long-term care insurance should be encouraged to shop around for reputable plans that provide the anticipated policy benefits and terms. Hogstel (2001) reports that the younger an individual is when the plan is purchased, the lower the monthly premium.

The emergence of long-term care insurance is a new option for the payment of health care expenses among the elderly. Because it has only been available for the past 5 years or so, most of the current cohort of the older adult population would be charged high premiums for coverage. Thus, long-term care insurance is currently a rarely used method of paying for long-term health care needs among today's older adults. However, as baby boomers begin to consider their retirement years and plan for the future, the ability to purchase long-term care insurance and utilize it for payment of future health care expenses will increase. In the next decade, society will likely see a vast change within the health care delivery system and the reimbursement for health care as a result of the population of baby boomers reaching the age of 65.

As discussed earlier in this chapter, health care costs have risen sharply over the past several decades. When older adults have to pay out of pocket for medical expenses, they often must use funds set aside for food, rent, or other expenses of daily living. Consequently, paying privately for health care presents a great barrier to achieving health outcomes. Inability to pay out of pocket for expensive medications and treatments plays a significant role in medical noncompliance or nonadherence. As health care professionals, it is extremely important to be aware of the ability of the older adult to access the recommended diagnostic test or treatment before they are sent home from the hospital, health care office, facility, or home care agency.

Many older adults are not able to access needed health care and remain part of an underserved population.

PAYMENT OPTIONS FOR OLDER ADULTS WITHOUT RESOURCES FOR HEALTH CARE

There are many reimbursement options for older adults in the United States. However, they are not all-encompassing or available to all who need them. If older adults did not pay into the Medicare system throughout their lives, either because of their employment or immigrant status, they are not eligible for Medicare unless they specifically pay for it. Even those who receive Medicare are left with co-pays for physician, clinic, and hospital visits, and they still have medications to pay for. While Medicaid is a fairly comprehensive payment system option for low-income older adults, it is not an option available to middle or higher income older adults who may have some funds to support themselves but not enough to finance their increasingly complex and costly health care.

Regardless of the reason, there are many older adults who need financial assistance to pay for health care. Often hospitals have programs to help older adults finance their health care over a period of months, or to excuse the older adult from paying, if they legitimately cannot afford to do so. Physicians and other health care providers may offer the same payment alternatives for services received at private physicians' offices. In addition, physicians in private practice may also have samples of medications to distribute to low-income older adults. Clinics often have sliding scales to make health care within these facilities more affordable. There are also various state-run programs that have resources for financing or finding affordable health care for older adults.

As part of Title III of the Older American's Act (OAA) of 1965, increased focus was directed toward public and private health care systems to provide improved access to services and advocacy for older adults. Within this program are improved community services, such as home-delivered meals, transportation, home health care, and home-making assistance; adult day care; home repair; and legal assistance, which allows many older adults to remain functionally independent and community-dwelling. These programs are administered within local Area Agencies on Aging (AAA), which are located within each state. AAAs provide older adults and health care providers with a tremendous resource with which to access and afford health care. To locate the AAA within each state, use the "links" tab located at http://www.n4a.org/. In addition to this Web resource, the administration on aging offers a toll-free Elder-care Locator telephone number, 1-800-677-1116, designed to help older adults, families, and health care providers obtain necessary community services throughout the United States. In addition to AAAs, senior service offices within hospitals are good sources of information about hospital and community-based resources.

SUMMARY

The last several decades have seen enormous changes in the health care delivery system. As people continue to age, they tend to develop more health problems, requiring greater use of this health care system in turmoil. Medicare, the primary health insurance of older adults, has undergone a particularly large number of revisions in an attempt to lower the costs of this federally funded program. Medicaid and veteran's benefits are also available options for health care reimbursement. These programs, too, have undergone revisions that affect the care of older adults, and long-term care has assumed an important role in the health care delivery system.

As the population continues to age, it is likely to require further revisions in these systems. Nurses caring for older adults need to be aware of these revisions and advocate for the best care for older adults. However, nurses also have a duty to be respectful of the cost of this care for both clients and the larger systems that fund the care. Finally, it is the nurse's role to help older adults find assistance to access health care that is affordable so they can effectively manage health care problems.

REFERENCES

Alexander, R. (Ed). (2005). *Avoiding fraud when buying long-term care insurance: A guide for consumers and their families.* Retrieved May 14, 2005 from http://consumerlaw page.com/article/insure.shtml#intro.

Centers for Medicare and Medicaid Services. (2005). *Medicaid: A brief overview.* Retrieved May 12, 2005 from http://www.cms.hhs.gov/publications/overview-medicare-medic aid/default4.asp

Federal Interagency Forum on Age-Related Statistics. (2004). *Older Americans 2004: Key indicators of well being.* Washington, DC: U.S. Government Printing Office.

Hogstel, M. O. (2001). *Gerontology: Nursing care of the older adult.* Albany, NY: Delmar Thomson Learning.

Kane, R. L. (2002). The future history of geriatrics: Geriatrics at the crossroads. *Journal of Gerontology: Medical Sciences, 57A,* M803–M805.

Pew Research Center. (2006). *Working after retirement: The gap between expectations and reality.* Retrieved July 12, 2007, from http://pewresearch.org/assets/social/pdf/retirement.pdf

Pick a card—any card?: Helping patients understand the new Medicare-approved drug discount cards. (2004). *American Journal of Nursing, 104*(7), 24–26.

Rosenkoetter, M. (2000). Retirement. In J. Fitzpatrick, T. Fulmer, M. Wallace, & E. Flaherty (Eds.), *Geriatric nursing research digest* (pp. 34–37). New York: Springer-Vertag, Inc.

Stotts, N., & Dietrich, C. (2004). The challenge to come: The care of older adults. *American Journal of Nursing, 104*(8), 40–48.

CHAPTER THREE

Normal Changes
of Aging

Learning Objectives

1. Identify normal physiological changes common in each aging body system.
2. Discuss nursing interventions to compensate for normal aging changes.
3. Identify the prevalence, risk factors, and treatment options associated with constipation.
4. Identify the prevalence and risk factors associated with urinary incontinence.

Mr. Alexander is a 70-year-old married man who comes to your clinic requesting information on sexual dysfunction. On questioning him further he tells you that his sexual functioning has declined over the past 10 years. He states that he can no longer maintain an erection, and generally he has a hard time even achieving one. He had spoken with his doctor about Viagra, but was told that it interacted with "some heart pill" that he is already taking. When you ask him how his relationship with his wife has changed over the years he states that they are still very happy together but that they both miss being intimate. He then states, "I hate disappointing her, but I guess it's just a part of getting old. I wish there was something I could do."

The story of Mr. Alexander is typical of today's older adult. As older adults continue to age, each body system undergoes changes. The changes occur in response to exposure to environmental injury, illness, genetics, stress, and many other factors. The changes are sometimes noticeable, such as gray hair, wrinkled skin, and stooped posture. However, there are also many unnoticeable changes within the aging body that are quite undetectable to the naked eye. These changes may not become evident until the older adult undergoes a physical examination with appropriate diagnostic testing.

Normal changes of aging are sometimes considered to be inevitable and irreversible. However, there is a great deal of variability in these age-related changes. Just because an individual is advancing in years, it cannot be assumed that they will undergo specific changes. For example, while many older adults have wrinkled skin and gray hair, there are many others with unlined skin and blond, dark, or red hair; some older adults have stooped posture, others have perfect posture. Individual aging is influenced by many factors that are both preventable and reversible.

Cultural backgrounds also play an important role in how a person ages. For example, people with darker skin may possess more natural protection against the sun and, thus, may wrinkle less than those with lighter skin. It is generally agreed that biological aging changes begin to appear commonly in the third decade of life, with subsequent linear decline until death. Therefore, it is important for nurses to refrain from making assumptions about normal aging.

Differentiating normal changes of aging from pathological aging changes is an important part of health care for older adults. It is also of critical importance for nurses to understand the normal physiological changes associated with aging. In so doing, nurses will be able to differentiate these physiological changes from abnormal or pathological organ system changes. Consequently, nurses will be able to avoid misinterpreting age-related changes as those caused by disease, which can lead to costly, uncomfortable, and time-consuming therapeutic attempts to reverse normal aging. This error may then result in iatrogenesis or an untoward event while receiving care. For example, consider an 89-year-old woman newly admitted to an assisted-living facility. The admitting nurse notices a red ring around the iris of her eye and refers her to an ophthalmologist for follow-up care. She must pay for a van service to bring her to the ophthalmologist and attends the appointment only to have an adverse effect to the medication given to dilate her pupils for examination. Instead of returning to the facility, she is admitted to the hospital, where she falls out of bed and sustains a hip fracture requiring 6 weeks of rehabilitation. All of this could have been avoided if the nurse had recognized the ring around the eye as *arcus senilus*, a normal change of aging with no related visual effects.

Conversely, the incorrect assumption that changes induced by disease are age-related leads to therapeutic neglect of potentially or possibly treatable conditions. Consider a 75-year-old man who has gradually been

CULTURAL FOCUS

Cultural backgrounds also play an important role in how a person ages. For example, people with darker skin may possess more natural protection against the sun and thus may wrinkle less than older adults with lighter skin. It is generally agreed that biological aging changes begin to appear commonly in the third decade of life, with subsequent linear decline until death. Therefore, it is important for nurses to refrain from making assumptions about normal aging.

having greater problems with his memory over the past year. His wife frequently notices that he loses track of things, is unable to find the right words to express his thoughts, and forgets things that happened within an hour of their occurrence. Some may assume that it is normal for older people to experience forgetfulness as described here. However, these symptoms are not normal changes of aging, but signs and symptoms of early cognitive impairment. Failure to diagnose and treat this cognitive problem will result in heightened progression of disease as well as risk for other problems with health and functioning.

Health care may be delivered in a more efficient and effective manner if health professionals can recognize and prioritize which problems will benefit from intervention and which will not. Great variability occurs within the aging process, therefore, nurses cannot assume that older adults will exhibit specific changes of aging. While the two examples given previously may seem outrageous, the inability to differentiate normal aging changes from pathological aging changes occurs everyday and has similar complications for older adults' health. This chapter addresses the naturally occurring changes in each body system of older adults. These changes are summarized in Table 3.1. The chapter begins with changes in the cardiovascular system and the nursing interventions used to compensate for these changes.

CARDIOVASCULAR SYSTEM

As part of the normal aging process, several anatomical and functional changes occur within the geriatric cardiovascular system. One major change is that the geriatric heart becomes larger and occupies a greater amount of space within the chest. Unfortunately, this is often a symptom of pathological cardiac diseases, such as cardiomyopathy. Consequently, an individual whose heart size has increased may require a more comprehensive

TABLE 3.1 Normal Changes of Aging and Nursing Interventions

System	Normal Aging Changes	Nursing Interventions
Cardiovascular System	• Heart becomes larger and occupies a greater amount of space within the chest. • Reduction in the amount of functional muscle mass of heart. • Decreased amount of blood that is pumped throughout the circulatory system. • More adventitious S4 heart sounds. • Premature contractions and arrhythmias. • Blood flow is slower (wounds heal slower and impacts medication metabolism and distribution). • Low diastolic pressure. • Increased pulse pressure.	• Can be cardiomyopathy, so refer for diagnostic tests. • Inform patient that exercise can ultimately reduce the strain on the heart. • Heart murmurs require further tests to determine its effect. • Fatigue, SOB, DOE, dizziness, chest pain, headache, sudden weight gain, or changes in cognitive function or cognition requires full assessment. • Know that the time of effectiveness may take longer when giving meds. • Inform patient that low diastolic pressure is a risk for cerebrovascular accidents or strokes. • Inform patient that exercise lowers blood pressure.

Peripheral Vascular System	• Increase in the peripheral vascular resistance (blood has a hard time returning to the heart and lungs). • Valves in the veins don't function efficiently and form (nonpathological) edema.	• Inform patient that age, diet, genetics, and lack of exercise can transform nonpathological to pathological (atherosclerosis and arteriosclerosis), which can result in CVD. • Monitor older adults' cholesterol levels with lowering agents to prevent atherosclerosis and arteriosclerosis. • Inform patient that exercise results in lower cholesterol levels. • Discuss the right medication, exercise program, and diet for the patient as a means to slow the progression of cardiac changes.
Respiratory System	• Decreased vital respiratory capacity. • Lungs lose elasticity. • Loss of water and calcium in bones causes the thoracic cage to stiffen. • Decreased amount of cilia lining system. • Decreased cough reflex.	• Note that auscultating sounds is difficult so it must be done on all lung fields in a quiet environment. • Inform that pollution and smoking worsens the cilia (try to help stop smoking by recommending behavioral management classes, support groups/nicotine replacement therapies, antidepression medications). • Tell patients that they are at risk for choking. • Make sure patient's respiratory function is frequently assessed. • Encourage regular exercise.

(continued)

TABLE 3.1 Normal Changes of Aging and Nursing Interventions (*Continued*)

System	Normal Aging Changes	Nursing Interventions
Integumentary System	• Skin becomes thinner and more fragile. • Skin is dry and loses elasticity (wrinkles). • Sweat glands lessen, which leads to less perspiration. • Subcutaneous fat and muscular layers begin to diminish; less padding, more easily bruised. • Dryness. • Skin tears. • Fingernails and toenails become thick and brittle. • Hair becomes gray, fine, and thin. • Facial hair on women. • Decreased body hair on men and women.	• Promote the use of sun block and tell patient to avoid overexposure. • Avoid the use of soaps that dry skin and use a lotion after baths. • Protect high-risk areas such as elbows and heels with padding. • Refer to a podiatrist. • Help older adult maintain personal appearance.
Gastrointestinal System	• Inflamed gums. • Periodontal disease. • Sensitive teeth. • Tooth loss. • Decreased peristalsis of esophagus. • Decreased gut motility, gastric acid production, and absorption of nutrients. • Difficulty evaluating wastes (constipation). • Involuntary leakage of liquid stool (fecal incontinence).	• Assess older adult's ability to chew. • Refer older adult for further oral evaluation if necessary. • Assist older adults in making changes with their eating habits. • Assess nutritional health frequently. • Encourage older adult to drink water (1.5 L). • Add bulk and fiber to diet. • Promote exercise. • Enemas and laxative medications may be given in severe situations. • Diets high in fiber and bulk, adequate fluids, and exercise. • Bowel habit training (for cognitively impaired). • In severe cases, surgery may be appropriate.

Urinary System	• Kidneys experience a loss of nephrons and glomeruli. • Bladder tone and volume capacity decreases. • Incontinence (not a normal change, but occurs in response).	• Assess urinary incontinence. • Kegel exercises. • Voiding schedules (for cognitively impaired).
Musculoskeletal System	• Decrease in total muscle and bone mass. • Muscle units that combine to form muscle groups diminish.	• Encourage older adult to exercise regularly.
Sexual/Reproductive System	• Decrease in testosterone in men, and estrogen, progesterone, and androgen in women. Women: • Follicular depletion in the ovaries. • Natural breast tissue is replaced by fatty tissue. • Labia shrinks. • Decrease in vaginal lubrications and shortening and narrowing of the vagina. • Strength of orgasmic contraction diminishes, and orgasmic phase is decreased. Men: • Increased length of time needed for erections and ejaculation.	• Help older adult feel comfortable when discussing sexuality. • Give vaginal lubricants to females. • Inform men to increase the time between erections. • Discuss use of oral erective agents.

(continued)

81

TABLE 3.1 Normal Changes of Aging and Nursing Interventions (*Continued*)

System	Normal Aging Changes	Nursing Interventions
Senses	Eyes • Visual acuity declines. • Ability of pupil to constrict in response to stimuli decreases. • Peripheral vision declines. • Lens of the eye often becomes yellow. • Arcus senilus. Ears • Increased amount of hard cerumen. Taste and smell • 30% of taste buds diminish.	• Make sure older adult has a baseline eye assessment early in older adulthood and follow up eye exams yearly. • Help older adult remove cerumen. • Obtain a thorough history of taste and smell sensations and a physical examination of the nose and mouth. • Obtain a thorough diet history.
Neurological System	• Total brain weight decreases. • Shift in the proportion of gray matter to white matter. • Loss of neurons. • Increase in the number of senile plaques. • Blood flow to the cerebrum decreases.	• Help older adult maintain an active body and mind. • Encourage older adults to participate in cognitive activities.

cardiovascular assessment in order to differentiate normal from patho-logical cardiac changes.

A larger heart may lead students to equate size with function, how-ever, this is not the case. Despite the increased size of the geriatric heart, there is a total reduction in the amount of functional muscle mass within the myocardium. In addition, the force of each heart contraction dimin-ishes, which decreases the amount of blood that is pumped through the circulatory system. Moreover, the valves that control the flow of blood within the chambers of the heart and between the heart and lungs to the circulatory system become stiffer with calcification, or calcium deposits. This stiffness often prevents the full closure of these valves, resulting in both nonpathological and pathological heart murmurs. The adventitious S4 heart sound is often heard more commonly in older adults than in a younger population as a result of these anatomical heart changes. Heart murmurs among older adults often require further evaluation to deter-mine the effect of the murmur on overall cardiovascular function.

The complex system of electrical impulses that controls the beat-ing of the heart is also often affected by the normal anatomical changes in this critical organ system. Consequently, premature contractions and arrhythmias are auscultated more frequently among older adults than in the younger population. These arrhythmias are often not pathologi-cal in nature. An occasional missed heart beat or other disruption in heart rhythm that is not accompanied by fatigue, shortness of breath (SOB), dyspnea on exertion (DOE), altered circulation, or chest pain may not be cause for major concern. However, when accompanied by these symptoms, arrhythmias require immediate attention. When altered heart rates are detected among older adults, full assessment for the presence of underlying symptoms and a cardiovascular work-up are necessary to differentiate normal from pathological aging changes.

As a result of the decreased force of contraction and often the inef-fective closing of cardiovascular valves, blood flow through the body is slower. This may have several consequences for older adults. First, slower circulation often results in slower healing of wounds. For example, an older adult who sustains a skin tear to her lower leg may have the wound in various stages of healing for several weeks in comparison to a young, healthy child whose wound would be healed within a week. Slower cir-culation also impacts the length of time it takes for medications to take effect as a result of altered medication metabolism and distribution. This is important to keep in mind when administering medications to older adults and evaluating their effectiveness in treating disease symptoms.

As older adults continue to experience changes in the cardiovascular system, it is not uncommon for some to experience very low diastolic blood pressure. This occurs as the heart muscle weakens causing the pressure of the heart at rest to become greatly reduced. This may occur even in the presence of systolic hypertension and is known as isolated systolic hypertension (Hill, Tannenbaum, & Salman, 2005). Consequently, an increased pulse pressure (the distance between the diastolic and systolic blood pressure values) is frequently seen among older adults. Lower diastolic blood pressure values have recently been implicated as a risk factor for cerebrovascular accidents or strokes.

In the peripheral vascular system, older adults have an increase in the peripheral vascular resistance, which means that the blood in the peripheral parts of the body (fingers and toes) has greater difficulty returning to the heart and lungs to be reoxygenated and recirculated. The valves in the veins of the lower extremities also become incompetent, resulting in nonpathological accumulation of fluid in the lower extremities (dependent edema). These changes are often worsened by nonmodifiable and modifiable risk factors for disease. As a result of genetics, diet, and other factors, older adults also tend to have a higher risk of developing both atherosclerosis and arteriosclerosis in the cardiac and peripheral arteries, respectively.

There are several changes in the normal lab values of older adults. For example, hemoglobin (Hg) and hematocrit (Hct), and erythrocyte sedimentation rate (ESR, Sed rate), which are essential measures of oxygen carrying red blood cell production, volume, and function, are slightly decreased among older adults. Leukocytes, or white blood cells, which are essential for immune function, are also slightly decreased among older adults. Table 3.2 provides a list of laboratory values for the older adult with age-related changes described. Knowledge and awareness of the normal ranges of specific blood values for older adults will enhance effective assessment and management of disease.

While these normal changes of the aging cardiovascular system may seem to position all older adults as sick and weak, this is not the case. It is important to remember that there is great variability in the aging process, and while some may experience all these aging changes, others may experience none. Moreover, there are several interventions that nurses may recommend to older adults to slow the onset of these normal changes of aging, such as diet, exercise, and when necessary, medication. There have been many attempts to halt and reverse the aging process, however, Fisher and Morley (2002) report that "While the concept of anti-aging therapies is intriguing, there is clearly little evidence-based medicine to support most of the generally touted approaches" (p. M638).

The role of regular exercise in preventing normal changes in the cardiac system and preventing cardiac disease cannot be emphasized enough. There is overwhelming evidence that regular exercise results in lower cholesterol levels, which will reduce athero- and arteriosclerosis. Moreover, exercise has been shown to lower blood pressure and enhance weight loss, which will greatly reduce the strain on heart musculature. Despite these clearly obvious benefits of exercise, the majority of older adults do not exercise. Reasons for the lack of exercise among older adults lie in habit. Cultural beliefs surrounding exercise are important in motivating older adults to participate in exercise programs. Reijneveld, Westhoff, and Hopman-Rock (2003) report that understanding cultur-ally specific exercise choices, are critical to removing exercise barriers among culturally diverse clients. Environmental barriers (no safe place to exercise) and the presence of normal changes of aging (such as muscle aches and pains) are also significant barriers to exercise among older adults.

It is usually cautioned that older adults should take their slower cardiovascular status into consideration when exercising or engaging in heavy labor. This may mean starting new regimens slowly until it is determined how the body will react physiologically. Frequent assess-ments of cardiovascular status are also recommended to detect patholog-ical changes early, when they are more amenable to treatment. Because the cardiovascular system is one of the most vital organ systems in the body, effective functioning is critical. It is essential that nurses assess this system continually for signs and symptoms of failure. Dizziness, chest pain, SOB, DOE, headache, sudden weight gain, or changes in function or cognition should alert the nurse to conduct further assessments for pathological cardiac function.

Nurses are in an ideal role to teach the interventions necessary to help older adults to participate in exercise programs. Interventions should begin by discussing the benefits of exercise. The nurse may help older adults to choose exercise programs that they will enjoy, and encourage them to do so. Choosing the right exercises and encouragement are key factors in motivating older adults to exercise. The ideal exercise program will combine strength training, flexibility, and balance. One of the most popular forms of exercise among older adults is walking. Walking is an exercise that transcends care settings, requires little equipment (except good shoes), and is accessible 24 hours a day. Other exercises that are found to be popular among older adults include both weight-bearing and aquatic exercises. Weight-bearing and muscle-building exercises assist in maintaining functional mobility, promoting independence, and prevent-ing falls. In addition, weight-bearing exercises have been shown to be very effective in reducing bone-wasting related to osteoporosis (Swanenburg, de Bruin, Stauffacher, Mulder & Uebelhart, 2007). Aquatic exercises are a pain-free method of promoting health and increasing functional ability, especially for older adults with arthritis and osteoporosis.

The role of diet in reducing the effects of aging on cardiovascular function is substantial. Lifelong eating habits, such as a diet high in fat and cholesterol, are among many obstacles that prevent optimal nutrition and contribute to pathological cardiovascular function. Diets high in fat and cholesterol are among the leading cause of coronary artery disease. Nutritional assessment is one of the first steps toward helping older adults to meet daily nutritional requirements with a diet rich in health

TABLE 3.2   Common Laboratory Tests Used to Assess Older Adults

Test
Why Used
Cholesterol; total cholesterol (TC), high density lipoprotein (HDL), low density lipoprotein (LDL)
Normal Ranges
TC <200 mg/dl
HDL >60 mg/dl
LDL <100 mg/dl
Tests the amount of circulating cholesterol levels. Good indicator for risk of cardiovascular disease, as well as to manage medications to prevent hyperlipidemia.
Complete Blood Count (CBC); hemoglobin (Hg), Hematocrit (Hct), and white blood cells (WBC).
Normal Ranges
Males
Hg 10–17 g/dl
Hct 38–54%
Females
Hg 9–17 g/dl
Hct 35–49%
WBC 4,300–10,800 cells/mm^3
Tests for red blood cell (hg, hct, ESR) function and white blood cell function (leukocytes) to determine ability of red blood cells to carry oxygen and white blood cell role in infection.
Drug assays (e.g., digoxin, dilantin, phenytoin, theophyllin, lithium).
See individual tests for reference ranges
A collection of tests used to measure the level of certain medications within the body. Helpful in managing medication dosing.
Glucose and Hemoglobin A1C (HgA1C)
Normal Ranges
Glucose (fasting) 70–105 mg/dl
HgA1C < 8%
Used to evaluate blood sugar levels and effectiveness of glucose management medications on glucose function among older adults.
Iron (Fe)

(continued)

TABLE 3.2   *(Continued)*

Normal Ranges
Serum Iron 35–165 ug/L
Plays a role in hemoglobin and red blood cell function. Low iron is diagnostic
for iron-deficiency anemia.
International Normalized Ratio (INR)
Normal Ranges
INR 2–3
Tests bodies clotting ability. Often used to evaluate response to warfarin
therapy.
Kidney Function Tests (BUN) and Creatinine
Normal Ranges
Males
BUN 8–35 mg/dl
Serum CR 0.4–1.9 mg/dl
Females
BUN 6–30 mg/dl
Serum CR 0.4–1.9 mg/dl
Commonly used to evaluate kidney function among older adults.
Liver function tests (LFTs)
See individual tests for reference ranges
Used to evaluate normal and pathological liver functioning
Prostate Specific Antigen (PSA)
Normal Ranges
PSA < 4 ug/L
Used to detect early signs of pathological prostate activity, such as benign pros-
tatic hypertrophy (BPH), or prostate cancer.
Thyroid Function Tests (T3, T4, TSH)
Normal Ranges
T3 75–220 ng.dl
T4 4.5–11.2 ug/dl
TSH 0.4–4.2 uU/ml
As thyroid problems are prevalent among older adults, these tests are frequently
used to determine thyroid function.
Vitamin Assays
See individual tests for reference ranges
Tests for function of vitamins within the body, such as vitamin X. Vitamins play
an essential role in all bodily system functions.

food choices. Teaching appropriate food choices is essential to changing
nutritional patterns and improving poor dietary patterns among older
adults. Taking small steps toward good nutrition, by slowly replacing
unhealthy food choices with healthier alternatives, is the most appropriate nursing intervention to help achieve nutritional outcomes.

CULTURAL FOCUS

Cultural beliefs surrounding exercise are important in motivating older adults to participate in exercise programs. Lewis, Szabo, Weiner, McCall, and Piterman (1997) report that understanding culturally specific exercise choices, such as Tai Chi for the Indo-Chinese, are critical to removing exercise barriers among culturally diverse clients.

RESPIRATORY SYSTEM

In addition to the cardiac system, older adults experience changes in their respiratory system as well. Changes experienced in the respiratory system include an overall decreased vital respiratory capacity, which means less air is inspired and expired. In addition, older adults' lungs tend to lose elasticity as they age, making the lungs less flexible and further impairing the ability to effectively inhale and exhale. Loss of water and calcium in the bones also causes the thoracic cage to stiffen adding an even greater force against effective respiration.

There is often a decreased amount of cilia lining in older adults' respiratory systems. These hair-like structures play an important role in alerting the older adult to foreign items in the respiratory system, such as food. The decrease in cilia is worsened by the presence of smoking and other environmental pollutants, which flatten the cilia to the respiratory passageway, rendering it ineffective. Moreover, older adults may have a decreased cough reflex as part of the normal changes of the neurological system. The combination of loss of cilia and decreased cough reflex place the older adult at high risk for choking, aspiration of food products, and the development of pneumonia and other infectious respiratory diseases.

Despite these seemingly important anatomical changes of aging, older adults without respiratory illnesses are able to breathe effectively. However, these changes in the respiratory system place the older adult at a higher risk for the development of disease. Consequently, frequent assessment of respiratory function and efficient treatment of disease is critical to maintaining respiratory health. It is important to note that because of the changes in the thoracic cage, assessing lung sounds in this population may be challenging. Listening to all lung fields directly on the skin, in a quiet environment, is often necessary to detect minor changes in respiratory sounds that could indicate pathological processes. Frequent assessments of respiratory function are also recommended to detect pathological changes early, at a more treatable stage. Nurses should assess respiratory status regularly and be alert for SOB, DOE, or changes in function or cognition that could alert the nurse to a developing respiratory pathological process, such as infection or tumor development.

The respiratory system is a critical organ system. While changes in the respiratory system will vary among the older population, smoking cessation and exercise are two important interventions that will help to maintain respiratory health.

The benefits of exercise are numerous. Among older adults, regular exercise programs help to increase vital capacity, prevent normal and pathological changes of aging, and reverse the effects of smoking. As stated earlier, many older adults do not participate in exercise programs, despite their obvious benefits. Nurses can play an essential role in helping older adults choose the right exercise and encourage regular exercise participation. As with cardiovascular status, it is usually cautioned that older adults should progress slowly when beginning a physically demanding program.

Cigarette smoking is one of the most critical negative predictors of longevity. Smoking is well-known as a risk factor for the development of multiple respiratory diseases including chronic obstructive pulmonary diseases, such as bronchitis, asthma, emphysema, and bronchiectasis, as well as cancer of the lung (U.S. Department of Health and Human Services, 2004). Today's older adults are among the first individuals who have potentially smoked throughout their entire adult lives. The effects of smoking are silent and often occur slowly over time. Moreover, symptoms of lung disease are not often experienced until extensive damage has occurred. Despite the many years older adults may have smoked, it is possible for older adults to experience the benefits of smoking cessation. It is also important to note that older adults may be more motivated to quit smoking than their younger counterparts, because they are likely to experience some of the damage that smoking has caused.

Nurses are in an ideal position to assist older adults to quit smoking to promote health or while recovering from an acute illness or managing chronic illnesses. Interventions to stop smoking usually surround behavioral management classes and support groups, which are available to community-dwelling older adults. Nicotine-replacement therapy and anti-depression medications are also helpful in assisting the older adult to quit smoking.

INTEGUMENTARY SYSTEM

The skin of older adults generally becomes thinner and more fragile as they age. The decreased amount of subcutaneous tissue allows for less water, and the skin becomes dry and loses its elasticity. Consequently, small lines and wrinkles appear on the skin. The appearance of lines and wrinkles is closely associated with the amount of sun exposure sustained throughout older adult's lives, especially the early years. In fact, the skin that has not been exposed to the sun (i.e., skin on the underside of the arm) may be quite free of lines and wrinkles and appear very youthful.

Nurses caring for older adults know that people enjoy the sun. Moreover, some sun is healthy. The sun produces vitamin D within the body, which is necessary for calcium metabolism. However, overexposure to the harmful rays of the sun can accelerate the normal aging changes and place the older adult at high risk for the development of pathological skin problems, such as cancer. Nursing interventions to reduce the effects of sun exposure on the skin and prevent against disease onset include the use of sun protection. It is presently recommended that older adults should be counseled to use sun block and avoid over exposure to the sun.

In addition to the wrinkling of the skin, the number of sweat glands diminishes as people age, leading to less perspiration among older adults. The subcutaneous fat and muscular layers of the skin also begin to diminish. These changes have several common and noticeable effects. First, these changes result in dryness of the skin, which often is uncomfortable and can lead to skin tears. These skin tears occur under seemingly little trauma and may be very difficult to heal. In addition, the loss of subcutaneous tissue beneath the skin of older adults results in less padding and a higher rate of bruising with minimal trauma. The dryness of the skin, in combination with decreased perspiration, leads to the need to bathe less frequently. Nurses caring for older adults may recommend that older adults and caregivers avoid the use of soaps that further dry the skin and replace moisture lost during bathing with a recommended moisturizer. Moreover, great care must be taken to prevent the skin from skin tears. The use of clothing and protection of high risk areas, such as elbows and heels, with appropriate padding, may be helpful in preventing skin tears. Preventing older adults from falls and traumas is a substantial issue for nurses caring for the elderly, and this will be discussed in greater detail in Chapter 5. Changes in subcutaneous tissue, fat, and muscle among older adults result in less protection against temperature extremes. Consequently, older adults exposed to extreme heat or cold are at risk for developing hyperthermia and hypothermia, respectively. Proper environmental control and adequate hydration are essential to prevent these devastating consequences of normal aging changes.

Through the normal aging process, fingernails and toenails become thick and brittle, and thus, nail care may become more difficult for the aging adult to accomplish independently. Changes in vision and pain perception may further complicate the task of nail care. In some facilities and care agencies, nurses may assist older adults with nail care. However, it is generally recommended that older adults enter the care of a podiatrist when normal and pathological aging changes make independent nail care difficult. Nurses may play an instrumental role in detecting the need for external assistance with nail care and make an appropriate referral. This is essential in order to maintain hygiene and prevent infections.

Another change in the older adult's integumentary system occurs in the hair. This is one of the most obvious effects of aging and among the most feared. The hair of older adults may become gray, fine, and thin, but there is great variation among change in hair patterns as people age. Some older adults may experience the loss of hair, or alopecia, which may or may not be hereditary. As a result of hormone shifts, the appearance of facial hair may be seen among women, and decreased body hair generally occurs with both sexes.

Because many of the changes older adults experience in the integumentary system affect their appearance, it is important to consider the effect of these changes on the self-concept and self-esteem of older adults. As in youth, it is important to remember that older adults also take great care in their personal appearance, including personal hygiene, hair, and clothing. It is the role of nurses and other health care professionals to recognize the importance of personal appearance and to help older adults maintain and enhance their personal appearance. As older adults continue to populate society, it is likely that the appreciation of the beauty of this population will continue to grow.

GASTROINTESTINAL SYSTEM

Older adults experience a great deal of change within the important gastrointestinal system, which starts at the mouth and ends at the rectum. At the start of the system, older adults commonly experience problems chewing and swallowing food. This often results from the lack of availability of fluorinated water in the early years as well as inadequate dental care. It was not until the year 1945 that Grand Rapids, Michigan, became the first city in the United States to fluoridate its drinking water. Fluorination of drinking water, which continues to be supported by the American Dental Association, is done to prevent tooth decay by reducing the effects of harmful bacteria in the water. Because most of today's cohort of older adults was already beyond their developmental years by this time, they did not benefit from the presence of fluorination in the water. Consequently, inflamed gums or periodontal disease is common among older adults. Moreover, sensitive teeth and tooth loss is seen regularly among older adults. Tooth and gum problems often prevent older adults from being able to chew (masticate) food. This may lead to a decrease of food choices and self-denial of soft food related to its poor taste or appearance. Nurses must consistently assess client's ability to chew food and refer clients with assessed problems in this area for further oral evaluation.

Decreased peristalsis of the esophagus slows the passage of food through the next stage of the alimentary canal, which often results in the need for older adults to chew food longer and eat more slowly. In teaching older adults about the normal changes of aging, it is important to introduce these changes and encourage older adults to make changes in their daily eating habits. Midway through the gastrointestinal system, older adults may experience decreased gut motility, gastric acid production, and absorption of nutrients. While these changes may not be independently pathological, they put older adults at high risk for the development of nutritional deficiencies. Frequent assessment of nutritional health, using necessary laboratory and physical assessment instruments, is helpful for nurses to determine the effect of these normal aging changes on nutritional status.

There are several changes in the normal lab values related to gastrointestinal function. Total albumin levels, which are essential indicators of both liver function and malnutrition among older adults, lessen with aging, in direct relation to reduced liver size and function. In addition, the enzyme alkaline phosphatase (ALP), which is a measure of liver function, increases with age. A decrease in plasma calcium necessary for adequate bone production and maintenance also occurs as part of the aging process. Serum potassium, which is essential in helping nutrients cross cell membranes, and serum glucose both increase among older adults. The increase in serum glucose will be discussed in greater depth in Chapter 6 because of its role in positioning older adults at higher risk for Type 2 diabetes. Table 3.2 provides a list of laboratory values for the older adult with age-related changes described. Knowledge and awareness of the normal ranges of specific blood values for older adults will enhance effective assessment and management of disease.

On the other end of the gastrointestinal system, decreased peristalsis of the large intestine slows the passage of food through the next stage of the alimentary canal and out of the body. The increased time when the digestive mass is in the bowel allows for greater time for water absorption resulting in a higher incidence of constipation among the older population. The two major bowel elimination problems that occur in the elderly are constipation and fecal incontinence. These problems are caused in part by normal changes of aging, but also result from the use of multiple medications, the intake of foods low in dietary fiber, and the lack of physical activity among older adults.

Constipation

Constipation, defined as the abnormally delayed or infrequent passage of accumulated, often dry, feces in the lower intestines, is the most common complaint among older adults (Beers & Jones, 2000). Many nurses who care for older adults find that older adults are often preoccupied with the risk for, or presence of, constipation, which results in frequent requests for medication. Annells and Koch (2002) report that laxatives are the most commonly sought after treatment for constipation, with approximately one-third of older adults requesting weekly laxatives to reduce constipation. Constipation is a substantial problem for older adults and has extensive effects on functional health. Moreover, untreated constipation may result in life-threatening effects. Constipation also requires excessive nursing resources for effective management (Lagman, 2006).

In addition to normal aging changes, lack of physical activity is a major contributor to constipation. Environmental changes that result in less privacy also contribute to constipation. Nursing interventions to minimize the risk of constipation include encouraging adequate fluids. For older adults who are not severely ill, daily fluid intake should be between 30 and 35 ml fluid/kg (National Collaborating Center for Acute Care, 2006). Maintaining a diet with sufficient bulk, such as green leafy vegetables and grains, is also helpful in reducing constipation. Exercise has a quick and favorable effect on constipation. Moreover, dietary modifications, such as the increase of fiber and fluid, can stimulate the colon and resolve constipation. Stool softener medications, enemas, and laxative medications may be used when constipation is severe.

Bowel Incontinence

Bowel incontinence is defined as an involuntary unexpected leakage of liquid stool. It is estimated that approximately 45% of nursing home residents suffer from this condition (University of North Carolina Center for Functional Gastrointestinal and Motility Disorders, 2006). Fecal incontinence results in part from normal aging changes to the bowel. However, there are other causes of bowel incontinence as well, including: (1) history of urinary incontinence, (2) neurological disease, (3) poor mobility, (4) severe cognitive decline, and (5) age greater than 70. The University of North Carolina Center for Functional Gastrointestinal and Motility Disorders(2006) reports that fecal incontinence is associated with hemorrhoids, diarrhea, constipation, childbirth injuries, diabetes, ulcerative colitis, and dementia. As with constipation, diets high in fiber and bulk, adequate fluids, and exercise are helpful in preventing and treating bowel incontinence. In cognitive-impaired older adults, bowel habit training may be helpful. This may be accomplished by first determining times throughout the day when older adults are most often incontinent. The information for this may be gathered through examination of the bowel diary. Once the pattern of incontinent episodes is determined, the older adult may be encouraged and assisted to the toilet a half hour before the usual time of incontinence in order to prevent the incontinent episode from occurring. In severe cases of fecal incontinence, resulting from tears in the anal sphincter, surgery may be an appropriate treatment.

URINARY SYSTEM

Changes in the urinary system occur frequently as people age. The kidneys, which are responsible for concentrating urine and filtering metabolic products for elimination, experience a total loss of nephrons and glomeruli as people age. In the older adult, the bladder tone and volume capacity may decrease as well. This results in a high incidence of urinary incontinence (UI), or involuntary loss of urine among older adults. Studies have shown that between 10% and 58% of women and 6% to 28% of men experience daily incontinence (Gray, 2003).

There are several changes in the normal lab values of older adults within the genitourinary system. For example, the blood urea nitrogen (BUN) values, which are commonly used to measure kidney function, are increased as a result of decreased renal function. BUN values among older adults are heavily influenced by dietary protein intake. Because lean body mass declines with age, the total production of creatinine increases, while creatinine clearance declines by almost 10% per decade after age 40. These are essential indicators of kidney function among older adults. Normal changes in lab values are summarized in Table 3.2.

Urinary Incontinence

Urinary incontinence (UI) is not a normal change of aging, but it occurs frequently among the older population in response to normal aging changes. Because of the stigma associated with this embarrassing disorder, it is not readily diagnosed. Gray (2003) reports that UI occurs in up to 11% of community-dwelling older adults. There are many types of UI, but the two most frequent types of UI in the older population are stress and urge incontinence. Stress incontinence results when the strength of the urethral sphincter decreases and is unable to stop the flow of urine. This most commonly occurs in response to weakened pelvic muscles that support the bladder. Older patients with stress incontinence frequently report losses of small volumes of urine during laughing, sneezing, coughing, or running/jumping. This type of UI occurs very commonly with aging. The other common type of UI is urge incontinence, which results in the loss of a large volume of urine. There are many causes of urge incontinence, including neurological problems or infection. However, in many cases of older people with UI, no known causes are identified. The risk for developing UI increases with age, obesity, chronic bronchitis, asthma, and childbearing. Many older adults experience a combination of both types of incontinence, known as mixed.

Assessing UI is the first step in solving this embarrassing problem. It is important to note that Bradway (2004) and other researchers report that UI in women is a culturally bound experience. Narratives of women with long-term UI revealed that it is an individual experience and interpreted and managed according to culture, individual and shared experiences, and interactions with health care professionals, friends, and family members. Consequently, many clients, including those from diverse cultural backgrounds, may be reluctant to discuss incontinence. Nurses must understand this and be sure to ask culturally appropriate assessment questions.

After assessing the presence of UI, many interventions are available to assist with these types of incontinence. The 2003 State of the Science on Urinary Incontinence (Mason, Newman, & Palmer, 2003) reports that practice related to urinary incontinence must change. "Use of absorbent products is often the intervention applied to everyone. Individualized care for UI isn't provided" (p. 2). They further report that devices and medications should take a back seat to effective nursing interventions for UI, including behavioral interventions, such as pelvic floor exercises and bladder training.

The easiest nursing intervention for cognitively intact older adults with incontinence is to teach pelvic floor exercises, also known as Kegel exercises. These exercises strengthen pelvic muscles to aid in the retention of urine. Wyman (2003) found that pelvic floor muscle exercises combined with lifestyle modification and bladder training exercises were very effective in helping older adults with UI. While these exercises work well to help older adults improve incontinence, they are challenging to learn. Thus, nurses are instrumental in teaching older adults the correct pelvic floor muscle exercise method. Older women may be taught to place a finger in their vagina and squeeze around it. The correct technique occurs when pressure is felt on the finger. Once the correct muscle is identified, clients should be instructed to hold the squeeze for 3 to 4 seconds and then relax for 3 to 4 seconds. It is recommended that the exercises be performed 15 times, 2 or 3 times a day. Improvement in urinary incontinence will be seen in 6 to 12 weeks. Nurses may suggest that clients do the exercises to music first thing in the morning and last thing at night. Biofeedback, which provides clients with verification of the correct technique while they are practicing the exercise, may be useful and is available at many urology practices nationwide. More information on kegel exercises may be found at http://www.biolifedynamics.com/kegel_exercises.html.

CULTURAL FOCUS

Researchers report that UI in women is a culturally bound experience. Narratives of women with long-term UI revealed that it is an individual experience and interpreted and managed according to culture, individual and shared experiences, and interactions with health care professionals, friends, and family members. Consequently, many clients, including those from diverse cultural backgrounds may be reluctant to discuss incontinence. Nurses must understand this and be sure to ask culturally appropriate assessment questions.

Voiding schedules have also been shown to be effective in the treatment of UI (Wyman, 2003), especially for older adults who are cognitively impaired. Voiding schedules begin by determining times throughout the day when older adults are most often incontinent. The information for this may be gathered through examination of the bladder diary. Once the pattern of incontinent episodes is extracted, the older adult may be encouraged and assisted to void a half hour before the usual time of incontinence in order to prevent the incontinent episode from occurring. In addition, medications that act as anticholinergics or smooth muscle relaxants assist in increasing bladder capacity to decrease the urge to void.

Urinary incontinence is often a rationale for the insertion of an indwelling catheter. This procedure, however, is a nearly guaranteed method of acquiring a urinary tract infection. Indwelling urinary catheters are contraindicated to treat UI in the older population. As discussed earlier, although it is time-consuming, the nurse must initiate a record of voiding times for 24 hours and then plan to offer the opportunities to void about 30 minutes prior to usual voiding times. This bladder schedule will prevent the negative consequences of UI and afford the older adult dignity and respect.

MUSCULOSKELETAL SYSTEM

Multiple changes occur in the musculoskeletal status of older adults. These changes often have a great impact on the health and functioning of older adults. As people age, there is a decrease in total muscle and bone mass. The decrease in bone mass occurs as bones lose calcium, causing the bone structure to shrink and weaken. All of this places the older adult at a higher risk for fractures. When the bone loss becomes more severe, the older adult may be diagnosed with osteoporosis. Osteoporosis is a pathological disease of the bone and will be discussed more comprehensively in Chapter 9. Changes in the normal lab values related to musculoskeletal function include a decrease in plasma calcium necessary for adequate bone production and maintenance. Moreover, total alkaline phosphatase (ALP) may rise as a consequence of Paget's disease or minor bone trauma or fracture among clients with osteoporosis. Table 3.2 provides a list of laboratory values for the older adult with age-related changes described. Knowledge and awareness of the normal ranges of specific blood values for older adults will enhance effective assessment and management of disease.

Individual muscle units that combine to form muscle groups also diminish with age. It is important to note that both the decrease in bone and muscle mass may be counteracted with exercise. Exercise is essential to healthy aging, producing positive effects on older adults, including the ability to maintain strength and flexibility throughout older adulthood. All older adults should be encouraged to find an exercise program that they enjoy and participate in it regularly. As discussed earlier in this chapter, walking and aquatic exercises are among two of the most

---

EVIDENCE-BASED PRACTICE

Title of Study: Changes in Postural Stability in Women Aged 20 to 80 Years

Authors: Low Choy, N., Brauer, S., Nitz, J.

Purpose: To identify the relationship between vision and postural stability in order to introduce falls—prevention strategies.

Methods: Measurements of postural stability in 453 women aged 20 to 80 years using the Balance Master force-plate system, while performing the modified Clinical Test for the Sensory Interaction and Balance, and the Single-Limb Stance Test.

Findings: Aged 60- to 70-year-old women were more unsteady than younger women in bilateral stance on a firm surface with eyes closed. Initial instability was noted in 40-year-olds when single-limb stance was tested with eyes closed. Further instability was evidenced in 50-year-olds when a foam surface was introduced. A further decline in stability was demonstrated for each subsequent decade when the eyes were closed in single-limb stance.

Implications: Age, visual acuity, and support surface were significant variables influencing postural stability in women. The cause(s) of this instability and subsequent decline in stability requires further investigation and research.

Journal of Gerontology, Medical Sciences 2003, Vol. 58A, No. 6, 525–530.

common exercises enjoyed by older adults. However, there are many exercise programs to choose from. Tai chi, yoga, and pilates are among the more recent forms of exercise that have gained in popularity among older adults. Early research on these forms of exercise reveals great benefits. For older adults, consistent involvement in exercise programs assists greatly in reducing the normal changes of aging on the musculoskeletal system. For an enhanced discussion of the role and benefits of exercise in older adults, see Chapter 5.

SEXUALITY/REPRODUCTIVE SYSTEM

It is commonly believed that older adults no longer desire to participate in sexual activities and lack sexual desires. This has led to a major neglect in the consideration of normal changes in the sexuality and reproductive systems. Moreover, this myth of aging has resulted in a failure to assess the sexuality and reproductive system in older adults. Consequently, many normal changes of aging sexual and reproductive systems are unknown to older adults. In addition, many pathological diseases, such as gynecological cancers and impotence, are left undetected and untreated.

It is important to note that despite popular belief, sexuality continues throughout the lifespan of older adults. The need to continue sexuality and sexual function must be considered along with the other physiological changes of aging. In both men and women, the reduced availability of sex hormones in the older adult results in less rapid and less extreme vascular responses to sexual arousal (Masters, 1986). The overall decrease in testosterone in men and estrogen, progesterone, and androgen in women results in changes in: (a) arousal, (b) orgasm, (c) postorgasm, and (d) the extragenitals (Masters, 1986).

Aging women experience follicular depletion in the ovaries as a result of a decrease in circulating hormones. This further leads to a decrease in the secretion of estrogen and progesterone (Masters, 1986). Natural breast tissue is replaced by fatty tissue, changing the external appearance of the breast. The labia shrink and may hang in folds because of lack of subcutaneous tissue. The vulva may appear to be dry and have pale appearance without rugations, and the introitus atrophies. There is a decrease in vaginal lubrications and a shortening and narrowing of the vagina. The strength of the orgasmic contraction diminishes, and the orgasmic phase is decreased. Normal changes of aging women may result in an increased time to respond during sexual activity and dyspareunia (painful intercourse). Older women may have an inhibited sexual desire, orgasmic dysfunction, and vaginismus as a result of a decrease in the amount of circulating hormones. Interventions to counteract these changes may entail the use of vaginal lubricants to release friction during intercourse and to decrease pain for the female. Moreover, because of the change in response time, it may be necessary to increase the period of time of foreplay prior to the sexual act to allow the body enough time to physically respond to sexual feelings.

Specific changes of aging that occur among older men include an increased length of time needed for erections and ejaculation (Ferrie, 2003). Erections become more dependent on direct penile stimulation. Semen volume is decreased, and the refractory period between ejaculations increases. Older men also find that pubic hair is thinner, and the testicles may shrink in size. As with the aging female, the aging male may need to increase the time for foreplay in order for the body to respond physically to sexual feelings. In addition, a more rapid withdrawal following ejaculation may be needed to maintain the tension in condoms and prevent leakage of sperm into the partner, which could cause the spread of sexual transmitted disease (STD). Older men should also be taught the need to increase the time between erections as a result of normal aging changes. For more information on the prevention of STDs among older adults, see Chapter 5.

Impotence is more commonly seen among older men as a result of increased illness, medication usage, and surgery within this population. However, impotence is not a normal change of aging. In fact, in the absence of this pathological problem, older men are usually free to continue functioning sexually throughout their lives. A collection of symptoms that are commonly known as andropause, or "male menopause," are currently being researched. This syndrome, developing in response to the slow decline in testosterone as well as other factors, may result in behavior changes and depression among older men (Ferrie, 2003).

A nurse's reluctance to assess and plan care for older adults surrounding sexuality has a substantial impact on older adult's health and functioning. Older adults experience many physiological changes in their reproductive systems that impact their ability to function sexually. Because the topic of sexuality is not widely discussed, older adults do not always fully understand these changes. In fact, a study of 68 older adults living in the community revealed that only 67% of the sample was able to answer sexual knowledge questions correctly (Walker & Ephross, 1999). Despite, older adults' lack of knowledge regarding sexuality, teaching regarding normal and pathological aging changes is not provided, and interventions to compensate for these changes are not planned. Consequently, older adults may stop functioning sexually, because they think they are "abnormal" or ill, and no one is available to counsel them otherwise.

EVIDENCE-BASED PRACTICE

Title of Study: Andropause: Knowledge and Perceptions Among the General Public and Health Care Professionals

Authors: Anderson, J., Faulkner, S., Cranor, C., Briley, J., Gevirtz, F., Roberts, S.

Purpose: This study assesses the knowledge and perceptions of andropause, the natural age-related decline in testosterone in men, among health care providers and the general public.

Methods: Health care providers and members of the general public participated in brief surveys via a medical information telephone line. Trained clinical interviewers administered the questionnaire and documented the findings.

Findings: Of 443 general public participants, 377 (85%) agreed to participate in the survey. Of these, 77% had heard of andropause—male menopause—and 63% had taken TRT (testosterone replacement therapy). Out of 88 health care provider callers, 57 (65%) participated in the survey. Of these participants, 65% were pharmacists, 80% had patients with low testosterone symptoms, and 50% reported that patients rarely or never spoke of low testosterone. Among HCPs and the general public, respectively, 98% and 91% knew that low testosterone is treatable with medication, and 60% and 57% knew that it results in osteoporosis. Only 25% of HCPs and 14% of the general public knew that low testosterone does not cause loss of urinary control.

Implications: Some health care providers, as well as members of the general public, are knowledgeable about some aspects of low testosterone and have misconceptions about others. Therefore, it is clear that education is needed in this area.

Journal of Gerontology, Medical Sciences 2002, Vol. 57, No. 12, M793–M796.

In addition to normal aging changes, older adults experience other barriers that prevent full sexual function. These include the loss of partners in older adulthood and pathological illnesses, such as impotence or diabetes, that affect sexual function. As nurses, it is critical to perceive sexuality as equally important to other physiological systems when planning care.

CHANGES IN THE SENSES

Older adults experience changes in the five senses as a result of normal aging. Overall visual acuity declines, and the ability to discriminate colors becomes less acute. The ability of the pupil to constrict quickly in response to stimuli decreases and peripheral vision declines. The lens of the eye often becomes yellow, resulting in the development of cataracts in the older population. Because of the normal changes in the aging eye, the older adult is at higher risk for diseases such as cataracts and glaucoma. Older adults should have a baseline eye assessment early in older adulthood, with follow-up eye appointments at least annually. A nonpathological anatomical change seen frequently in older adults is known as arcus senilus, which is a ring that appears around the older adult's iris but has no impact on vision. Consequently, no nursing interventions are necessary.

As a result of decreased body water, older adults tend to accumulate an increased amount of hard cerumen in their ears, which may affect hearing. The removal of the cerumen often requires assistance of a health care professional, and this may increase hearing acuity. Hearing impairments, while not a normal change of aging, occur frequently in the older population as a result of environmental exposure to noise pollution, as well as genetics. The prevalence of presbycusis, or high-pitched hearing loss, also rises with age. The usual intervention for older adults who become hearing impaired is consultation with a hearing professional. Hearing aides, which are fitted to the ears of older adults and enhance the sounds of the environment, may be an effective method to improve hearing in the older population. Newer, more advanced methods of hearing enhancement are currently being researched.

Older adults also experience an overall decline in both the senses of taste and smell. This is due to an average decrease of approximately 30%

CRITICAL THINKING CASE STUDY

Mrs. Pinkus is a pleasant, 90-year-old woman who resides in a skilled nursing facility. She is alert and oriented but sometimes forgetful. She is near-sighted and hard of hearing in her left ear. She enjoys dessert with her dinner. She is continent of bowel and bladder and ambulates independently. Her past medical history includes frequent episodes of pneumonia, hypertension, and a right breast carcinoma.

1. What findings in Mrs. Pinkus's profile would be considered normal changes of aging?
2. Are there pathological changes present in Mrs. Pinkus's profile? If so, what are they?
3. What nursing interventions could be implemented to compensate for normal changes of aging?
4. Do you feel the role of ageism may impact the nurse's ability to differentiate between normal and pathological changes of aging?

in the number of taste buds (Malazemoff, 2004). While this decline is a normal aging change, a sudden decline in the ability to smell or taste may be a symptom of disease. For example, Malazemoff (2004) reports that the presence of gingivitis, periodontal disease, and other disorders common to older adults further reduces the ability to taste and smell food. This change is often difficult for older adults who relied heavily upon the smell of good food to maintain their nutritional level. It also explains why older adults may not recognize odors often evident to others, such as that of spoiled or burning food. The decline in taste and smell sensations may lead to attempts to enhance the taste of food with increased salt and sugar. However, depending on the presence of diseases, such as hypertension or diabetes, these food supplements may be problematic. Malazemoff (2004) recommends a thorough history of taste and smell sensations, as well as a physical examination of the nose and mouth to differentiate normal from pathological changes in aging. In addition, a thorough dietary assessment, beginning with a 24-hour recall, is essential to identify the impact of the change of taste and smell on the older adult's diet.

NEUROLOGICAL CHANGES

Many people believe that as individuals age, cognitive impairment is inevitable. While there are changes in the neurological system as people age, these changes do not result in cognitive impairment. Chronic cognitive impairment is a pathological change of aging resulting from dementia. Dementia is a general term used to describe over 60 pathological cognitive disorders that occur as a result of various disease processes, heredity, lifestyle, and perhaps, environmental influences. It is defined by the Alzheimer's Association as a "loss of mental function in two or more areas such as language, memory, visual and spatial abilities, or judgment severe enough to interfere with daily life" (1999).

Some of the normal changes of aging that occur include a reduction in total brain weight. There has been a documented shift in the proportion of gray matter to white matter, and there is a total loss of neurons and an increase in the number of senile plaques seen in the brain of older adults upon autopsy. Older adults also experience a decrease in blood flow to the cerebrum. The way these anatomical changes in the brain translate into human behavior has great variability. Some older adults are often thought of as "forgetful" and "slow." Memory losses are also common to older adulthood, but are often falsely labeled as dementia. However, dementia is a pathological illness of the cognitive system and is definitely not a normal change of aging. Many older adults live well into their 10th decade as intellectually keen as they were in their twenties and thirties.

Because of the great concern older adults have about becoming cognitively impaired in older age, nurses are often called upon to provide information on maintaining cognitive and intellectual capacity. The most appropriate interventions to prevent the effects of normal aging on cognitive functioning and reducing the risk for the development of dementia are to maintain an active mind and body. Older adults should be encouraged to participate in cognitive activities such as work, games, or a course of study. Many colleges and universities allow older adults to attend classes for low or no charge. In fact, 17% of older adults have a bachelor's degree or more. Keeping intellectually active is regarded as a hallmark of successful aging.

SUMMARY

It is clear that as people age, each body system undergoes changes. The changes are caused by many factors including exposure to environmental injury, illness, genetics, stress, and many others. Most of these changes occur over many years and are considered normal among older adults. However, these changes often place the older adult at high risk for the development of disease. It is extremely important to differentiate normal from pathological changes in order to prevent improperly treating normal changes and failing to treat those that result from illness.

Teaching regarding the normal changes of aging should be the first intervention made with all aging adults to help them understand what is going on in their bodies. In addition, many interventions are available to compensate for these changes as well as to prevent the development of disease as a consequent of these interventions. Teaching and assurance by the nurse that these changes are a normal part of aging allow older adults to understand their bodies, to feel comfortable learning how to compensate for these changes, and to discover how to prevent the development of disease.

REFERENCES

Alzheimer's Association. (1999). Alzheimer's disease and related dementias fact sheet. Retrieved from http://www.ncdhhs.gov/aging/ad/ADRD_FactSheet.pdf

Annells, M., & Koch, T. (2002). Older people seeking solutions to constipation: The laxativemire. *Journal of Clinical Nursing, 11*(5), 903.

Beers, M. H., & Jones, T. V. (Eds.). (2000). *The Merck manual of geriatrics* (3rd ed.). Rahway, NJ: Merck Research Laboratories.

Bradway, C. K. W. (2004). Narratives of women with long-term urinary incontinence. Unpublished doctoral dissertation, University of Pennsylvania, Philadelphia.

Ferrie, B. W. (2003, April 28). What is male menopause? *Advance for Nurses, 5,* 27–28.

Fisher, A., & Morley, J. E. (2002). Antiaging medicine: The good, the bad and the ugly. *The Journals of Gerontology, 57*(10), M636–M639.

Gray, M. L. (2003, March). Gender, race and culture in research on urinary incontinence. *American Journal of Nursing,* (Suppl.), 20–25.

Hill, M., Tannenbaum, S., & Salman, A. (2005). Hypertension. In J. Fitzpatrick & M. Wallace (Eds.), *Encyclopedia of nursing research* (pp. 287–290). New York: Springer Publishing Company.

Lagman, R. L. (2006). Constipation—Not a mundane symptom. *Journal of Supportive Oncology, 4*(5) 223–224.

Lewis M, Szabo R, Weiner K, McCall L, Piterman L.(1997). Cultural barriers to exercise amongst the ethnic elderly. *Internet Journal of Health Promotion.* Retrieved August 25th, 2007 from http://www.rhpeo.org/ijhp-articles/1997/4/.

Malazemoff, W. (2004). When the nose no longer knows—Smell and taste disorders in elders. *Nursing Spectrum, 8*(8), 12–14.

Mason, D. J., Newman, D. K., & Palmer, M. H. (2003). Changing UI practice. *American Journal of Nursing,* (Suppl.), 2–3.

Masters, W. H. (1986, August 15). Sex and aging—Expectations and reality. *Hospital Practice,* 175–198.

National Collaborative Centre for Acute Care. (2006). *Nutrition support in adults. Clinical guideline 32.* London: National Center for Health & Clinical Excellence.

Reijneveld, S. A., Westhoff, M. H., & Hopman-Rock, M. (2003). Promotion of health and physical activity improves the mental health of elderly immigrants: Results of a group randomised controlled trial among Turkish immigrants in the Netherlands aged 45 and over. *Journal of Epidemiology and Public Health, 57,* 405–411.

Swanenburg, J., de Bruin, E. D., Stauffacher, M., Mulder, T., & Uebelhart, D. (2007). Effects of exercise and nutrition on postural balance and risk of falling in elderly people with decreased bone mineral density: Randomized controlled trial pilot study. *Clinical Rehabilitation, 21*(6), 523–524.

University of North Carolina Center for Functional Gastrointestinal and Motility Disorders. (2006). *Understanding fecal incontinence.* Retrieved July 13, 2007, from http://www.med.unc.edu/ibs

U.S. Department of Health and Human Services. (2004). *The health consequences of smoking. Executive summary.* Available at http://www.cdc.gov/tobacco/sgr/sgr_2004/pdf/executivesummary.pdf.

Walker, B. L., & Ephross, P. H. (1999). Knowledge and attitudes toward sexuality of a group of elderly. *Journal of Gerontological Social Work, 31,* 85–107.

Wyman, J. F. (2003, March). Treatment of urinary incontinence in men and older women. *American Journal of Nursing,* (Suppl.), 26–35.

CHAPTER FOUR

Assessing Older Adults

Learning Objectives

1. List techniques necessary for the systematic assessment of older adults.
2. Discuss challenges and solutions to obtaining health histories and physical examinations on older adults.
3. Identify alterations in older adult lab values.
4. Identify critical components of comprehensive geriatric assessment.
5. State the two key components of assessing older adults.

Mr. Joseph is a 68-year-old man who has Down syndrome and is very hard of hearing. He recently had a physical exam and routine blood work done at the physician's office you work at. He is currently 30 lbs overweight, and his total cholesterol is 280. His physician asks you to do some teaching regarding lifestyle modifications that can be done to lose weight and lower his cholesterol. However, when he comes in you have a hard time communicating the information because he is so hard of hearing. In addition, you are unsure of whether or not he understands the material. He shakes his head when you ask if he has any questions, but he looks very confused. By the end of the session he looks very frustrated and upset and hurries to leave. You schedule a follow-up appointment in a week to see how he's doing and reinforce the material.

The story of Mr. Joseph happens frequently among older adults. Health assessment of older adults is a process of collecting and analyzing data. It is the first step in the nursing process. It is also essential in order to formulate effective plans of care for older adults. The assessment of older adults focuses on physiological findings, including normal changes of aging, psychosocial data, functional abilities, and cognitive dimensions of well-being. While nurses may assume that the assessment of older adults is similar to that of a younger adult, older adult assessments must pay close attention to the differentiation between normal and pathological changes, as well as the impact of these changes on functional status. Moreover, these assessments must consider potential subtle changes in function and cognition that indicate early signs of disease in this population.

This chapter provides information on health assessment techniques necessary for the assessment of older adults. Challenges to obtaining health histories and physical examinations among older adults will be discussed. Altered presentation of commonly occurring diseases among the elderly will be identified, and the reader will be provided with material on appropriate assessment of function and cognition.

SYSTEMATIC GERIATRIC ASSESSMENT

The nurses' assessment of older adults requires the ability to actively listen as well as to use all other senses to gather data. This often draws upon experience and expertise gained over time in working with the older population. An inexperienced nurse is often frustrated by the length of time needed for the geriatric assessment, and the inability of some older adults to keep focused on providing the necessary information. For example, consider an 86-year-old woman with mild cognitive impairment (MCI) who presents to a medical unit with a small bowel obstruction (SBO). This assessment will probably take a long time, and it may be necessary to consistently encourage the client to focus on answering the questions. In an effort not to be rude, the nurse may allow the patient to continue providing unessential information. Written forms and checklists can help the nurse to keep the client more focused.

The physical assessment of the older adult demands that the health care team include special considerations that are unique to the geriatric population. Environmental adaptations are usually necessary to compensate for the older adult's physiological and psychological changes of aging. Modifications to the physical environment start with a room that is comfortably warm to the client and not exposing the client any more than is necessary. Changes in subcutaneous tissue, fat, and muscle among older adults provide less protection against temperature extremes, consequently, older adults are more sensitive to temperature changes. Amella (2004) states that the "key to providing appropriate treatment to older adults is going beyond the usual history and physical parameters to examine mental, functional, nutritional and social-support status" (p. 43).

The room should be adequately bright but with indirect lighting to compensate for diminished visual acuity. Fluorescent lighting and window glare should be avoided. Straight-backed chairs with arms that are cushioned for comfort should be utilized, making sure that the client's height allows for ease in rising from them. The examination table should be low and well padded to protect from discomfort. The head of the examination table should rise up, as some older adults may have difficulty lying flat for any amount of time. There should be adequate space in the examination room to accommodate mobility aides. The room should be free from distraction and background noises. It is important to take into consideration the energy level of the older adult and conduct the physical examination at the individual's own pace. Minimize skin exposure of the older adult to prevent chilling. These factors may indicate the need to conduct the examination over more than one session. It is helpful to organize the examination to reduce the changes in body positions and conserve the client's energy.

Because the older adult may become disoriented in a different environment and/or have sensory impairments, various techniques need to be utilized to assess each individual adequately. At the start of the examination, it may be worthwhile for the examiner to spend some extra time establishing a nonthreatening relationship. As a sign of respect, older adults should be addressed by their last name and title. The first name should be used only if invited to do so. The nurse must allow the older client enough time to respond to questions. The nurse should speak facing the client and use commonly accepted wording. Allowing hearing-impaired clients to see the nurse's entire face and body so that they may detect lip reading and body language may be helpful. If the client wears hearing aids, make sure they are on and working properly. For clients with visual deficits, nurses must make sure that the clients have their glasses on and plan to use visual cues as needed. Family members can provide important information, but the examiner needs to focus on the client.

Older adult health assessment, which requires a substantial amount of nursing time and resources, often conflicts with the hurried and short-staffed health care environment in which older adults receive care (Hogstel, 2001). Geriatric interdisciplinary teams (GITs)—made up of physicians, nurses, physical therapists, occupational therapists, recreational therapists, social workers, psychologists, and nursing assistants—make assessment more efficient by assigning components of the assessment to the most qualified member of the team. After completing assigned components of the assessment, GIT members gather together to plan care for the older adult, which is generally more comprehensive and effective than when individual team members work alone (Fulmer et al., 2005). Geriatric interdisciplinary team care has been effective in managing the complex syndromes experienced by chronically ill and frail older adults with multiple co-morbidities, because such care requires skills that are not possessed by any one professional. Positive outcomes of geriatric teams have been revealed in multiple studies,

---

EVIDENCE-BASED PRACTICE

Title of Study: Pain Perceptions of the Oldest Old: A Longitudinal Study
Authors: Zarit, S., Griffiths, P., Berg, S.
Purpose: To assess self-reported pain in the elderly and examine its changes over time relative to other changes in health and functioning.
Methods: This was a population-based sampling of the oldest-old (86–92 years of age) in Sweden. Interviews were administered regarding their pain, and other areas of health function.
Findings: At baseline, pain was prevalent in 34% and rose to 40% at follow-up. Incidents of new pain cases were 16% during that time period. Pain was significantly related to the following: sleep disturbances, medication usage, global subjective health, depressive symptoms, and mobility, though the magnitude was relatively small.
Implications: There is an increase in the number of persons reporting pain over a period of time after the age of 85. The relatively small association of pain with other areas of functioning suggests adaptation among the oldest-old.

The Gerontologist, Vol. 44, No. 4, 459–468.

---

including one by Li, Porter, Lam, and Jassal (2007). These researchers found that a team approach to care delivery resulted in quicker hospital discharge and improved functional status. The Institute of Medicine (IOM) of the National Academy (2001), in attempts to reduce medical errors and improve patient outcomes, challenges all health care professionals to recognize the need for effective interdisciplinary team care for multiple patient populations.

As discussed in Chapter 1, the older adult population is becoming increasingly culturally diverse. Consequently, during the assessment, close attention must be paid to culturally appropriate behaviors. It is important to determine how the older adult would like to be addressed and the language that they are most comfortable speaking. If the older adult speaks a language foreign to the nurse, the client should be questioned as to whether or not an interpreter is desired or whether a family member would like to communicate the client's history. Attention should also be paid to the older adult's comfort with the amount of personal space, eye contact, and physical gestures of the health care provider. The relationship of the nurse to the client requires recognition of and sensitivity to cultural differences, because some cultural groups definitions of health and illness may differ from the examiners. These same cultural groups may also have their own health practices that are thought to promote health and cure illness within the

Cultural Focus

During the assessment, pay close attention to culturally appropriate behaviors. It is important to determine how the older adult would like to be addressed and the language that they are most comfortable speaking. If the older adult speaks a language foreign to the nurse, the client should be questioned as to whether or not an interpreter is desired or whether a family member would like to communicate the client's history.

group. All nurses should make efforts to modify health care according to the client's cultural beliefs in order to provide culturally competent care.

It is important to remember that although older clients may be part of a specific cultural group, they may have acculturated to a certain degree during their time in the United States. Therefore, a cultural history is an essential step in determining the basis of the client's health care beliefs and practices. Some health care facilities have begun to add cultural assessment questions to client's admission assessment. Sample questions to guide the assessment may be found in Exhibit 1.4. It is important to remember that all older adults should be treated with dignity and respect. Consequently, always use a client's formal title (Mr., Mrs., Dr.), or ask how they would like to be addressed. If the older client speaks a language with which the nurse is not familiar, determine if the older adult client would like an interpreter or whether a family member would like to communicate the individual's needs. It is important to note that the fast pace in which the American culture operates may be seen as a sign of disrespect to older adults from different cultural backgrounds. A quick approach to patient care, which is often essential in busy health care climates, often is perceived as uncaring and hasty. Recognizing this allows for nurses to approach the clients more slowly and with greater attention to caregiving and detail. The amount of personal space, the comfort with eye contact, and the use of physical gestures, such as hand-shaking, should also be assessed to determine the older adult's comfort with these common social norms.

When conducting assessments on older adults, it is also necessary to remember that some of the standardized assessment tools, such as the Geriatric Depression Scale and the Mini Mental State Examination, are available in different languages. Be cautious about interpreting a tool that has not been formally translated, as the meanings of many words change by cultural background. During the assessment, it is necessary to determine the decision maker in the family and respect the client and families wishes in sharing information. In some cultural backgrounds, older adults are prevented from hearing about their diagnoses, and family members are given this information. In addition, some diseases of

CULTURAL FOCUS

During the assessment, it is necessary to determine the decision maker in the family and respect the client and family's wishes in sharing information. In some cultural backgrounds, older adults are prevented from hearing about their diagnoses, and family members are given this information. Thus, it is essential for nurses to assess client's understanding of their role in the plan of care and whether or not the plan is consistent with cultural beliefs.

older adulthood, such as dementia and depression, are stigmatized in many cultures. While some older adults will participate actively in setting goals and objectives for care, as well as determining acceptable interventions and outcomes, others will be more comfortable relinquishing this task to family members and health care providers. Some cultures hold health care providers in high esteem and, in attempts to be respectful, may be unwilling to disagree with plans of care. Thus, it is essential for nurses to assess clients' understanding of their role in the plan of care and whether or not the plan is consistent with cultural beliefs.

HEALTH HISTORY

The health assessment always begins with a health history. This is usually the first time that the older adult and nurse have an opportunity to meet, and it marks the beginning of the therapeutic relationship. It is important at this time to focus on gaining the trust of the client. Consequently, a sufficient amount of time should be set aside for the health history so that the older adult does not feel rushed. Normal changes of aging result in an overall slowing down of response time to questions, not to mention that the older person being interviewed may have 80 or 90 years of health history to relate to the nurse. Because of the time period that the health history must cover, the older adult may have difficulty extracting dates and details from memory, so it is important for the nurse to be patient and understanding. Some older adults may find some information to be too distressing to discuss, such as the birth of a still-born child, or may fear the consequences of their health problems so they may withhold certain medical information. Memories of painful tests or the fear of a stressful diagnosis may also cause the older adult to minimize symptoms. They may also fear being a burden on the health care system or on their children and, thus, hide or minimize symptoms of disease for this reason.

A thorough health history, including past medical and surgical history, cultural background, sources of social and financial support, occupation, education, living arrangements, assessment of alcohol and tobacco, and prescription and over-the-counter medication usage (including herbal supplements) should be obtained. Nurses should request that patients bring medication bottles to the assessment in order to determine what medications the client is taking and whether or not the older client's prescriptions have been filled with a generic drug. As noted earlier in this text, herbal medications, while rising in popularity among all older cultural groups, may be the primary healing source among some Asian, Hispanic, and other cultures. Awareness of the use of CAM therapies allows nurses to assess for the interaction of these therapies with traditional medications among all cultural groups. An assessment of nutritional status, commonly obtained through the use of a 24-hour recall, and a history of present illness should be obtained.

Special attention should be focused on the common problems of aging. The assessment for subjective reports consistent with diseases such as dementia, depression, musculoskeletal disorders, and sensory changes should be part of every health history. For example, complaints of symptoms such as memory loss, forgetfulness, chronic fatigue, loss of appetite, pain, and difficulties with hearing or vision are common among older adults and should be included among all health histories. The health care provider may use a form to gather this information orally, but must also be observant of other symptoms of common aging problems, such as depression, reading disabilities, or a dry cough.

Following the health history, the nurse must perform a review of systems (ROS) to determine any signs or symptoms of disease in each body system. The ROS is a comprehensive collection of subjective symptoms, including cardiovascular, respiratory, peripheral vascular, abdominal, integumentary, genitourinary, neurological, and musculoskeletal systems. Questions regarding older adults' health within each of these systems should be posed. For example, within the abdominal system, the older adult may be asked if there are any problems with nausea, vomiting, or diarrhea. Within the neurological system, the client may be questioned regarding the incidence

---

CULTURAL FOCUS

As noted earlier in this text, herbal medications, while rising in popularity among all older cultural groups, may be the primary healing source among some Asian, Hispanic, and other cultures. Awareness of the use of CAM therapies allows nurses to assess for the interaction of these therapies with traditional medications among all cultural groups.

---

and prevalence of headaches. The health history and review of systems collectively form the basis of the subjective portion of the health assessment.

REMINISCENCE AND LIFE REVIEW

The term *reminiscence* has been in use for many years as a manner in which to help older adults experience memories of earlier times. It was originally defined as thinking about or relating past experiences, especially those personally significant (McMahon & Rhudick, 1961). The concepts of reminiscence and life review are often used interchangeably but are similar in their ability to help older adults recall memories from an earlier period of time in order to experience emotions associated with these memories, or reach resolution regarding past events. Haight (2005) suggests that one method of reminiscence or life review that may be helpful during the health assessment is the oral history or narrative therapy in which the client is asked to tell the story about a particular problem or reason for seeking health care. In the process of storytelling, new insights are gained by both the client and health care provider, and the storytelling becomes therapeutic. Reminiscence may also be accomplished by asking an older adult about their memories of certain events, smells, or photographs. In order to stimulate reminiscence, older adults may be asked to write about or tape record memories of past events, develop a family tree, or write to old friends. Tornstam's theory of gerotranscendence, discussed in Chapter 1, suggests that reminiscence contributes to the reconstruction of identity and the understanding of reality as a process of reorganization and reconstruction.

PHYSICAL ASSESSMENT

A head-to-toe physical examination should follow the health history and a complete review of systems. The physical assessment begins with the evaluation of vital signs, including temperature, pulse, respiration, height, and weight. Because of the potential for orthostatic hypertension, blood pressure should be evaluated in three different positions: sitting, immediate standing, and one-minute standing, especially if the older adult is currently taking antihypertensive medications. Decreases in blood pressure of more than 20 mm Hg, are indicative of orthostatic hypertension and require further evaluation. Blood pressure readings should follow the American Heart Association guidelines (see Chapter 6). Respirations should fall within the normal range of 12 to 18 breaths per minute with regular heart rates averaging between 60 and 100 beats per minutes. The temperature response to infection among older adults varies greatly; some older adults respond to infections with elevated temperatures and others with aggressive infections show no febrile response. Gathering information on clients' weight and height is also essential to develop a baseline for further comparison of nutritional and hydration levels, as well as bone loss. Body mass indexes (BMI) less than 25 are considered ideal and should be measured when possible.

Following the gathering of vital signs, a head-to-toe physical assessment is necessary. The client's skin should be evaluated for any unusual findings, including cherry hemangiomas, liver spots, skin tags, keratoses, and precancerous and cancerous lesions. The presence of herpes zoster and decubitus ulcers, which occur commonly in older adulthood, should be evaluated. Hair growth and nails should be assessed for uniformity, with diminished hair growth and fungal infections of the nails requiring further evaluation. Evaluation of the head and neck for the presence of lesions or trauma should occur next, including the evaluation of the sclera for whiteness and a notation of the arcus senilis, if present. Evaluation for cataracts and macular degeneration should also be conducted, as these conditions occur commonly in older adulthood. Visual acuity declines as people age, so evaluation of vision and proper referral to an ophthalmologist for follow-up of abnormal findings of the eye should occur. Tympanic membrane and the light reflex in the ear should be identified, and an evaluation of hearing should be conducted. The nose should be palpated for tenderness and signs and symptoms of infection. The mouth and teeth should also be evaluated for deviations from normal, and referrals should be made to a dentist for further management of mouth and tooth disorders. The thyroid gland should be palpated for enlargement and nodules.

The evaluation of the heart and lungs begins with the evaluation of the carotid arteries and jugular beings in the neck. The carotid arteries should be symmetrical, nonbounding, and absent of bruits and adventitious sounds. The jugular veins should not be distended. The heart should be inspected and auscultated beginning at the apex. The first two heart sounds should be auscultated and any adventitious sounds, murmurs, rhythms, and pulsations should be noted. The lungs should be inspected and palpated for tactile fremitus and equal expansion. The lung fields should be percussed for areas of hyper-resonance or dullness. Lung sounds should be evaluated in all fields and adventitious sounds noted.

Inspection and palpation of the musculoskeletal system should begin at the temporomandibular joint and proceed inferiorly to the feet. Each joint, bone, and muscle group should be evaluated for abnormalities, tenderness, bilateral equality, strength, and range of motion. The abdomen should be inspected for abnormal scars, pulsations, or distention, and bowel sounds should be auscultated in all four quadrants. Older women should also be examined for breast masses and gynecological abnormalities, and older men should undergo an annual examination for prostate enlargement or malignancies.

An important part of the physical exam is the evaluation of laboratory tests. The proper use of these laboratory tests in evaluating older adults requires both knowledge of the normal ranges for age and the nurses' awareness of the clients' health and medication history. These changes were discussed in relation to specific bodily systems among older adults in Chapter 3. Table 3.2 provides a list of laboratory values for the older adult with age-related changes described. Among older adults, altered lab values often put them at risk for the development of disease. For example, an increase in glucose as part of the normal aging process likely plays a role in the high incidence of Type 2 diabetes among older adults. Moreover, a decrease in serum calcium plays a role in the higher risk of older adults for osteoporosis. Consequently evaluation of appropriate laboratory tests should be conducted as part of the health assessment among older adults.

In addition to lab values, it is important for nurses to understand the normal physiological changes associated with aging and compare them with abnormal change detected in organ systems. Misidentifying an age-related change as disease-induced may lead to therapeutic attempts to reverse normal aging. This may result in iatrogenic harm to the older adult. For example, consider a 72-year-old man visiting a health care clinic. The admitting nurse takes a routine fasting glucose level and finds it slightly elevated. If the nurse did not understand that a slight increase in fasting glucose commonly occurs with aging, this client would be sent for more expensive testing and possibly costly and painful treatment for Type 2 diabetes. Conversely, incorrectly assuming it is an age-related change may lead to therapeutic neglect of potentially or possibly treatable conditions. For example, one of the common myths of aging is that all older adults are cognitively impaired. While becoming *cognitively impaired* as one ages is of large concern to the aging population and their families, many older adults live well into their 10th decade with high cognitive and intellectual functioning as they were in their twenties and thirties. Memory losses are common in older adulthood, but the development of dementia is not a normal change of aging. Instead, it is a pathological disease process used to describe over 60 pathological cognitive disorders. Refer to Chapter 3 for a detailed discussion of normal aging changes in the elderly.

Altered presentation of illness is another challenge in the physical assessment of older adults. Diseases may present with atypical clinical signs and symptoms that can be confusing. Severe, acute illnesses will often present with nonspecific or vague symptoms. Typical signs and symptoms may be absent, such as a cough in an older adult with pneumonia. At other times, disease may present merely as failure to thrive, changes in mental status, falls, anorexia, or self-neglect. All health care providers need to be aware of these differences. For enhanced discussion of the altered presentation of disease in the elderly, see Chapter 6.

CRITICAL COMPONENTS OF A COMPREHENSIVE GERIATRIC ASSESSMENT

A comprehensive geriatric assessment is an interdisciplinary approach to the evaluation of older adults' physical, psychological, social, and spiritual functioning. These types of assessments are generally conducted in teams that include nurses, physicians, social workers, and therapists that assess and plan care addressing the multiple needs of older adults. As discussed earlier, when multiple disciplines collaborate in care planning, this ensures the best communication and the most comprehensive and effective plan for older adults.

A comprehensive geriatric assessment should always involve family members and caregivers, as appropriate. Frequently, family members and direct caregivers can contribute information that might be overlooked if they are not included in the assessment process. Involving family members in the planning of care for older adults not only gives the nurse the opportunity to assess the status of their relationship with the older adult client, but it also allows the nurse the opportunity to involve the caregivers in planning, education, and decision making. It is important to mention the potential mistakes health care providers can make in regards to family/caregiver involvement. One common mistake is to ignore the client and focus primarily on the caregiver to answer all the questions, receive information, and make decisions. Nurses may make ageist assumptions, underestimate clients' abilities, and not allow them to be active participants in their own care. On the other hand, nurses may receive inaccurate information if they do not involve the family or caregivers when needed. Individuals with cognitive impairment may still be quite socially skilled and may make the health care provider think they are cognitively intact and able to give accurate information. Also, some older adults may overestimate their abilities out of fear that the health care provider might uncover certain information that could result in loss of independence or institutionalization.

There are two critical components of geriatric assessment that must be discussed here: function and cognition. When older adults experience the onset of disease, changes in function and cognition are often the first symptoms. A savvy clinician may detect these early symptoms, conduct

EVIDENCE-BASED PRACTICE

Title of Study: Congruence Between Disabled Elders and Their Primary Caregivers

Authors: Horowitz, A., Goodman, C., Reinhardt, J.

Purpose: To study the congruence between perceived relationships among the disabled elders and their caregivers from several perspectives.

Methods: 117 visually impaired elders and their caregivers were examined through correlation analyses, kappa statistics, and paired t tests. 4 target issues included: elders' functional disability, elders' adaptation to vision impairment, caregivers' overprotectiveness, and caregivers understanding of the vision problem.

Findings: Elders did not rate caregivers as overprotective as much as caregivers rated themselves. Caregivers assessed elders as more disabled than the elders rated themselves. The two factors that correlated with congruence across measures were the caregiver's assessment of the elder's status and the quality of the relationship between the elder and the caregiver.

Implications: The findings of this study emphasize the importance of addressing congruence by target issue, rather than as a characteristic of the caregiver relationship.

The Gerontologist, Vol. 44, No. 4, 532–542.

a thorough assessment, and diagnose disease at an early and often more treatable stage. The presence of cognitive dysfunction should be assessed, because acute decline in cognitive function often signals the onset of physiological disease. Detection of changes in cognitive function may help the older adult to receive earlier and, thus, more effective disease treatment. In addition, detection of chronic cognitive dysfunction allows for early planning to assure the safety, high functionality, and optimum quality of life for the older adult.

Function

An older adult's ability to independently complete activities of daily living (ADLs) is a benchmark for health. If an older adult becomes incontinent or unable to bathe themselves, this often requires a change in the level of care. Moreover, an acute decline in functional status frequently signals the onset of physiological disease among older adults. For example, consider an older female who generally eats and bathes independently. One morning she wakes up and requires assistance to get out of bed and eat. This should signal the presence of functional decline and begin the process of assessment to determine the cause of the functional deficit. In this case, the presence of infection, delirium, or depression may be the reason behind the sudden onset change in function. Consequently, special attention must be paid to the functional assessment of older adults.

Functional assessment is a systematic attempt to measure objective performance in ADLs, including bathing, dressing, toileting, eating, ambulating, and continence. Instrumental activities of daily living (IADLs) are the more complex tasks people need for independent living. The IADLs include being able to shop, cook, manage finances, climb stairs, manage transportation, do housework and laundry, and manage medications. Assessment of functional limitations in older adults is very important for detecting disease and dysfunction, selecting appropriate interventions, and evaluating the results of these interventions. With the older adult, the ultimate goal is to maintain optimal function and be as independent as possible. The geriatric interdisciplinary team works toward promotion and maintenance of functional independence with the goal of assisting the older adult to live independently as long as possible and preventing hospitalization and institutionalization.

A functional geriatric assessment begins with a major review of ADLs. The Katz Index is an excellent functional assessment tool that has been used widely in many health care settings that care for older adults (Wallace & Shelkey, 2007). IADL scales include the Lawton IADL.

Cognition

A decline in cognitive function frequently signals the onset of physiological disease among older adults. Nurses caring for older adults are often in a position to evaluate cognitive status and screen for the development of cognitive impairments, which will assist in differential diagnosis. For example, consider an older nursing home resident who is usually cognitively intact. This resident usually remembers nurses' names, knows the date, and is oriented to person, place, and time. One evening, during the med pass, the client calls the nurse his mother. Further brief cognitive assessment indicates that the client is disoriented. Among older adults, this rapid change in cognitive status should signal the presence of delirium and further assessment to determine the cause. In this case, the presence of infection, medications, or sensory deprivation may be the reason behind the sudden onset change in cognitive function. Changes in cognitive status occur both in cognitively intact and cognitively impaired older adults. For example, clients with Alzheimer's disease may experience a decline in cognitive function in response to the pathological disease processes listed previously.

Because altered cognitive status is one of the more commonly occurring symptoms of disease among older adults, cognitive assessment is an essential skill to be acquired by nurses caring for the older population.

There are many instruments that can be used to accomplish this purpose. One screening tool that has been used successfully to screen for the development of changes in cognitive function symptomatic of dementia is the Mini Mental Status Examination (MMSE; Folstein, Folstein, & McHugh, 1975). Based on a 30-point scale, the MMSE measures levels of awareness and orientation, appearance and behavior, speech and communication, mood and affect, disturbances in thinking, problems with perceptions, and abstract thinking and judgment. The higher the older adult scores, the more intact the cognitive status. When the scale is 23 or lower, the client has a problem with cognition and needs further evaluation. The tool is easy to use after a little practice and has been used for initial and subsequent evaluation of older adults in a variety of settings. However, the instrument has been criticized as being insensitive to culture, language, visual impairments, and low literacy. The most effective way to perform the assessment is to make the client comfortable and establish a rapport. Eliminating noise and promoting attention and concentration will allow clients to answer questions to the best of their ability. After the examination, the score can be computed and used as a basis for care planning.

SUMMARY

The assessment of older adults is the first necessary step in providing care to this population. Geriatric assessment begins with a health history, followed by a review of systems and a comprehensive physical examination. Knowledge of normal changes of aging and pathological diseases greatly enhances the nurses' ability to effectively assess older adults. Particular attention to changes in function and cognition are among the most important assessment parameters in the care of older adults.

Older adults present challenges to health assessment. They greatly benefit from having a health care provider who is able to evaluate their ability to function independently, both physically and cognitively. The comprehensive geriatric assessment provides an excellent means for fully assessing all areas of older adult function. Such comprehensive assessment can detect symptoms amenable to treatment resulting in the highest possible quality of life for older adults.

CRITICAL THINKING CASE STUDY

Mr. Baxter is an 86-year-old man who presents to a comprehensive geriatric assessment center with early signs of dementia. He lives alone, takes five daily medications, and until recently has been able to independently complete his ADLs. However, last winter his furnace broke and his home radiator was frozen for 5 days. His daughter came to visit and found him living in the cold.

1. What dimensions does a comprehensive geriatric assessment generally involve?
2. What challenges do you anticipate in assessing Mr. Baxter?
3. What normal changes of aging may further complicate your assessment of Mr. Baxter?
4. What are the most important components of assessment for Mr. Baxter?

REFERENCES

Amella, E. (2004). Presentation of illness in older adults. *American Journal of Nursing, 104,* 40–52.

Boult, C., Boult, L., Morishita, L., Dowd, B., Kane, R., & Urdangarin, C. (2001). A randomized clinical trial of outpatient geriatric evaluation and management. *Journal of the American Geriatrics Society, 49,* 351–363.

Burns, R., Nichols, L., & Martindale-Adams, J. (2000). Interdisciplinary geriatric primary care evaluation and management: Two-year outcomes. *Journal of the American Geriatrics Society, 48,* 8–13.

Folstein, M., Folstein, S., & McHugh, P. J. (1975). 'Mini-mental state,' a practical method for grading the cognitive state of patients for clinicians. *Journal of Psychiatric Research, 12,* 189–198.

Fulmer, T., Hyer, K., Flaherty, E., Mezey, M., Whitelaw, N., Orry Jacobs, M. et al. (2005). Geriatric interdisciplinary team training program: Evaluation results. *Journal of Aging and Health, 17*(4), 443–470.

Haight, B. (2005). Reminiscence and life review. In J. Fitzpatrick & M. Wallace (Eds.), *Encyclopedia of nursing research* (pp. 510–511). New York: Springer Publishing Company.

Hogstel, M. O. (2001). *Gerontology: Nursing care of the older adult.* Albany, NY: Delmar Thomson Learning.

Institute of Medicine. (2001). *Crossing the quality chasm: A new health system for the 21st century.* Washington, DC: National Academy Press.

Li, M., Porter, E., Lam, R., & Jassal, S. V. (2007). Quality improvement through the introduction of interdisciplinary geriatric hemodialysis rehabilitation care. *American Journal of Kidney Diseases, 50*(1), 5–7.

McMahon, M., & Rhudick, P. (1961). Reminiscence. *Archives of General Psychiatry, 10,* 292–298.

Wallace, M., & Shelkey, M. (2007) *Try this. Katz Index of Independence in activities of daily living (ADL). Try this: Best practices in nursing care to older adults, a series from the Hartford Institute for Geriatric Nursing.* Retrieved August 9, 2007, from www.hartfordign.org/publications/trythis/issue02.pdf

CHAPTER FIVE

Health Promotion

Learning Objectives

1. Differentiate between primary, secondary, and tertiary levels of prevention among older adults.
2. Identify risk factors, harmful effects, and treatment for excessive alcohol usage among older adults.
3. Identify the harmful risks and interventions to stop smoking for older adults.
4. Discuss risk factors, assessments, and interventions for poor nutrition among older adults.
5. List barriers and facilitators to exercise among older adults.
6. Identify the causes of sleep disturbance among older adults, and provide nursing interventions to restore sleep quality.
7. Identify risk factors and interventions for fall prevention and minimizing injury in older persons.
8. Plan the nursing care of older adults, utilizing nonrestraint strategies.
9. Discuss appropriate immunizations for older adults.
10. Identify interventions for the early detection of cardiovascular disease.
11. Identify interventions for early detection of diabetes.
12. State American Cancer Society guidelines for early detection of cancer.

Mrs. Martin is an 82-year-old woman who was admitted to the hospital after a recent fall. She claims that she tripped en route to the bathroom and woke up on the floor in the morning. She lives alone, has no prior history of falls, and states that her daughter calls her daily and visits on weekends. You are the RN performing a follow-up home visit for a home safety check.

Upon visiting the home you discover that although it is very neat and clean, she has a number of throw rugs covering the hardwood floor in her living room. In addition, the carpet in her bedroom is coming up along the edges. Likewise, there currently is no clear path from her bed to the bathroom. After your assessment you make a plan to discuss your suggestions with Mrs. Martin.

The story of Mrs. Martin typifies that of older adults today. Older adults have many health care needs. These needs have resulted from both normal and pathological changes of aging. Pathological changes of aging may result from poor health practices acquired early in life and continued into older adulthood. The Federal Interagency Forum on Aging-Related Statistics (2004) reported that in the year 2001, the most leading causes of death in the United States were heart disease, malignant neoplasms, cerebrovascular diseases, chronic lower respiratory diseases, influenza, pneumonia, and diabetes. These have an affect on all individuals at one time or another, therefore, older adults may still benefit from health promotion activities, even in their later years. In fact, health promotion is as important in older adulthood as it is in childhood. Older adults are never "too old" to improve their nutritional level, start exercising, get a better night's sleep, and improve their overall health and safety.

The U.S. Department of Health and Human Services developed National Health-Promotion and Disease-Prevention Objectives (http://www.health.gov/healthypeople) titled Healthy People 2010. These objectives are achieved through varying levels of prevention. Primary prevention involves measures to prevent an illness or disease from occurring, for example, immunizations, proper nutrition, and regular fluoride dental treatments. Secondary prevention refers to methods and procedures to detect the presence of disease in the early stages so that effective treatment and cure are more likely. Routine mammograms, hypertension screening, and prostate specific antigen (PSA) blood tests are a few examples. Tertiary prevention is needed after the disease or condition has been diagnosed and treated. This is an attempt to return the client to an optimum level of health and wellness despite the disease or condition, for example, physical, occupational, and speech pathology services following a cerebrovascular accident.

Despite the need to promote health among older adults and the clearly defined objectives, many barriers stand in the way of improved health among this population. One of the greatest barriers surrounds misconceptions about the benefits of health promotion for older adults. Another barrier lies in the challenge of separating the normal changes of aging from pathological illness. For example, joints normally stiffen as one ages, causing the older adult to use the joint less for fear that the stiffness may worsen. In actuality, this joint may benefit from increased activity, which would potentially reduce or reverse the normal change of aging as opposed to exacerbate it. A final barrier to improving the health promoting activities of older adults is their own motivation to change. In fact, this is the most important factor in improving health. The best health care in the world cannot make an individual do something they don't want to do.

Historically, older adults have not been targeted for educational programs regarding risk awareness or prevention, detection, and screening activities. Only recently have third-party payers begun to pay for some of the necessary screening activities. Older adults tend to have more difficulty attending cancer prevention, awareness, and screening activities because of lack of funds or transportation. Sensory and cognitive deficits may prevent them from understanding or utilizing the information that is given. Fatalistic attitudes that cancer treatment for older adults is hopeless also contribute to the problem.

EVIDENCE-BASED PRACTICE

Title of Study: Building a Model of Self-Care for Health Promotion in Aging

Authors: Leenerts, M., Teel, C., Pendelton, M.

Purpose: To identify the essential factors in self-care related to health promotion and well-being in aging. To organize these findings in a literature-based, integrated model with applicability in practice, research, and education.

Methods: From the databases of Medline, CINAHL, and PsycINFO, both theoretical and research articles from the past 10 years relating to self-care and health promotion in community-dwelling elders were accessed.

Findings: The topic of the elderly related to self-care and health promotion is multifaceted and includes: internal and external environment, self-care ability, education, and self-care activity. An education plan is presented focusing on the promotion of self-care and health improvement.

Implications: A model of self-care for health promotion for the elderly was composed. Suggestions for its use in clinical practice were made, as well as theory formation and hypothesis testing.

Journal of Nursing Scholarship, 34(4), 355–361.

PRIMARY PREVENTION

Ideal health promotion behaviors at the level of primary prevention, include: smoking cessation and limited alcohol consumption, good nutrition, exercise, adequate sleep, safe lifestyles, and updated immunizations. Special attention to health promotion practices of diverse cultural groups is necessary as some of these groups are at higher risk for diseases. A 2002 report released by the Institute of Medicine reports that health disparities are evident in morbidity and mortality statistics. For example, African American women are more likely to die from HIV and Hispanic American/Latinas are more likely to die from chronic Lyme disease. Moreover, hypertension is among the top 10 causes of death in Asian American/ Pacific Islander and Native Hawaiian women. Despite the increased risk, these populations tend to be less likely to receive regular blood pressure and cholesterol evaluations. This chapter will discuss areas of health promotion for older adults and provide recommendations for effective interventions to promote health among the older adult population in the primary secondary levels of prevention.

Alcohol Usage Among Older Adults

The Robert Wood Johnson Foundation (2001) estimates that the number of older adults abusing alcohol will increase from 1.7 million to 4.4 million by the year 2020. For women of all ages and men older than age 65, more than seven drinks per week or more than three drinks per occasion is considered a risk for problem drinking (The National institute on Alcohol and Alcoholism). Alcohol dependence and alcoholism have the potential for great consequences among older adults, including negative effects on function, cognition, health, and overall quality of life. Nurses' and health care professionals' failure to understand the prevalence of

---

CULTURAL FOCUS

Special attention to health promotion practices of diverse cultural groups is necessary, as some of these groups are at higher risk for diseases reports that health disparities are evident in morbidity and mortality statistics. For example, African American women are more likely to die from HIV and Hispanic American/Latinas are more likely to die from chronic Lyme disease. Moreover, hypertension is among the 10 top causes of death in Asian American/Pacific Islander and Native Hawaiian women. Despite the increased risk, these populations tend to be less likely to receive regular blood pressure and cholesterol evaluations.

---

alcohol abuse is one of the greatest barriers surrounding interventions to help older problem drinkers. This is partly due to the fact that symptoms of alcohol use, including alteration in mental status and function, resemble the symptoms of delirium, dementia, or depression, which occur frequently among older adults. Moreover, older adults often are no longer in the workforce where daily performance failures, common with alcohol usage, can be more readily detected.

Alcoholism is a greater problem for older adults because older adults are not able to physiologically detoxify and excrete alcohol as effectively as younger people. Older adults with alcohol problems who receive treatment are capable of achieving positive health outcomes (Blow, Walton, Chermack, Mudd, & Brower, 2000). In fact, when older adults receive effective treatment for their alcoholism, their prognosis is much better than it is for their younger counterparts. When alcohol abuse is suspected among older adults, it is necessary to refer them immediately to an appropriate program for effective treatment.

Smoking

It is impossible in one brief book to discuss all of the harmful effects of cigarette smoking. Currently, there is evidence to support that cigarette smoking causes heart disease, several kinds of cancer (lung, larynx, esophagus, pharynx, mouth, and bladder), and chronic obstructive pulmonary diseases, including bronchitis, asthma, emphysema, and bronchiectasis. Cigarette smoking also contributes to cancer of the pancreas, kidney, and cervix (U.S. Department of Health and Human Services, 2000). The current cohort of older adults is one of the first groups to have potentially smoked throughout their entire adult lives. The effects of smoking are silent and often occur slowly over time. Older adults do not always experience typical symptoms of disease until lung damage has occurred. Research has shown that because smoking begins and propagates disease development, it is one of the most critical negative predictors of longevity. Because of the large number of medications older adults often take, including over-the-counter (OTC) and herbal medications, the potential for these drugs to interact with the nicotine in cigarettes is high. Nicotine–drug interactions can cause many problems for the older adult.

Despite contrary belief, it is possible for older adults to experience the benefits of smoking cessation even in old age. Moreover, it is important to note that older adults may be more motivated to quit smoking than their younger counterparts, because they are likely to experience some of the damage that smoking has caused. Nurses are in an ideal position to assist older adults to quit smoking to promote health or while recovering from an acute illness or managing chronic illnesses.

Interventions to stop smoking usually surround behavioral management classes, and support groups are available to community-dwelling older adults. Nicotine-replacement therapy and anti-depression medications are also helpful in assisting the older adult to quit smoking.

Nutrition and Hydration

A large study was conducted among older adults aged 65 and older (n = 1113) to determine whether older adult diets met the Recommended Daily Allowance (RDA) and what factors contributed to dietary adequacy. The results showed that diets were inadequate in 16.7% of the older participants. Nutritional knowledge and the possession of positive attitudes and beliefs contributed to good diets in the older population (Howard, Gates, Ellersieck, & Dowdy, 1998). More recently, Odlund (2003) found diets to be inadequate in community-dwelling older adults and Ammerman, Lindquist, Lahr, and Hersey (2002) report that 4 of the 10 leading causes of death are related to poor diet.

EVIDENCE-BASED PRACTICE

Title of Study: Quality Assessment in Nursing Homes by Systematic Direct Observation: Feeding Assistance

Authors: Simmons, S. Babineau, S., Garcia, E., Schnelle, J.

Purpose: To develop and test a standardized observational protocol for routine use to evaluate feeding assistance quality.

Methods: Four feeding assistance quality indicators were defined and operationalized for 302 long-term residents in 10 skilled nursing homes. The quality indicators included: (1) staff ability to adequately record intake, (2) staff ability to adequately provide assistance to at-risk individuals during mealtime, (3) staff ability to provide feeding assistance to residents identified by the Minimum Data Set as requiring assistance during mealtime, and (4) staff ability to provide verbal prompt to residents who receive physical assistance at mealtimes.

Findings: A significant difference exists between facilities for 3 of the 4 quality indicators. Staff "failed" the quality indicators as follows: QI 1: 42–91%; QI 2: 25–73%; QI 3: 11–82%; QI 4: 0–100%.

Implications: A standardized, observational protocol can accurately measure the quality of feeding assistance in nursing homes. This can be replicated and shows significant differences exist between facilities.

Journal of Gerontology, Medical Sciences 2002, Vol. 57A, No. 10, M665–M671.

Risk Factors for Malnutrition

There are many factors that account for the high prevalence of nutritional deficiencies in older adults. The normal changes of aging place the older adult at a higher risk for nutritional deficiencies. In addition, a decrease in the smell, vision, and taste senses and the high frequency of dental problems makes it difficult for the older adult to maintain adequate daily nutrition. Lifelong eating habits, such as a diet high in fat and cholesterol, are other obstacles to maintaining optimal nutrition. Such a diet is a leading cause of coronary artery disease. The diminishing senses of taste and smell result in less desire to eat and may lead to malnutrition. Diminishing taste is also accompanied by a decline in salivary flow, which accompanies aging. The taste buds are sensitive to sweet, sour, salt, and bitter. Although some taste sensations probably decline with age, the sensitivity to sweet is apparently higher, which may account for the older adult's preference for sweeter foods.

Nutrition and hydration assessments are necessary to help older adults meet daily nutritional requirements. By middle age, eating patterns have become relatively fixed, and change may be difficult. Familiar food patterns serve as a security blanket. Distinctive ethnic, racial, and regional characteristics are still prevalent among older adults, and ethnic or racial identity can be reaffirmed by suggesting the use of traditional foods. To determine the cultural–religious influence on the client's diet, the caregiver should start with an in-depth history of the client's dietary habits. The client should be questioned closely on food likes and dislikes, ethnic preferences, and general nutritional knowledge. It is best to encourage the good food habits of the client's particular cultural group and to make improvements gradually rather than impose too many changes at once. When working with cultural and religious food patterns—whether they be Chinese, Japanese, Mexican, American, Italian, Indian, Jewish, or any other—the health care professional must have a thorough understanding of the client's cultural and religious preferences. These could significantly impact their food intake and nutritional status.

There are many risk factors for malnutrition that must be assessed to determine their impact on maintaining a healthy nutritional status. Limited income is a substantial concern among older adults and contributes to the poor nutritional status in the population. Income usually decreases sharply with age (see Chapter 1). Retirement, health problems that affect one's ability to work, and inflation are just a few reasons many older adults live below the poverty line. This lack of income results in the tendency to purchase lower cost foods, which may be less nutritious. Moreover, many adults live in environments of care that are absent of adequate food preparation and storage facilities, refrigeration space, and other elements necessary to maintain a good level of nutrition. Lack of transportation to purchase food and poor eating environments are other contributing factors of malnutrition. One option for adults without transportation is the Title III Meal Program. This program offers Meals-on-Wheels, which serves healthy, home-delivered, hot meals to older adults. The cost of this program varies depending on the older adult's ability to pay.

In addition, because eating is often regarded as a social experience, isolation from family members and friends often negatively impacts nutrition by making the eating experience lonely. This is especially true for long-term care environments where the older adult is often seated away from others, but is left to eat in a loud, undesirable environment. Malnutrition among older adults may be closely linked to loneliness, boredom, anxiety, fear, bereavement, general unhappiness, isolation, and depression.

Physiologically, older adults may experience malnutrition because of some of the normal and pathological changes of aging. For example, loss of teeth, which commonly occurs among older adults, greatly impacts the eating experience. Moreover, the loss of teeth and replacement with poorly fitting dentures may cause older adults to make poor food choices simply because they're easier to eat, such as ice cream, milk shakes, and other foods high in carbohydrates. The lack of insurance reimbursement for replacement dentures as the gum sizes change also contributes to this problem. Moreover, the presence of chronic disease among older adults, such as cardiovascular diseases and diabetes, further impact nutrition. In these cases, the addition of dietary supplements may be helpful.

Failure to Thrive (FTT)

Failure to Thrive (FTT) is a syndrome used to describe a client who experiences malnutrition in absence of an explanatory medical diagnosis. It was first recognized as a syndrome in the late 1980s and is derived from work with infants bonding with their mothers. In these studies, a lack of maternal bonding seemed to be the cause of FTT in infants (Hogstel, 2001). FTT in adults is thought to be similar in that it seems to result from a lack

---

CULTURAL FOCUS

Distinctive ethnic, racial, and regional characteristics are still prevalent among older adults. Ethnic or racial identity can be reaffirmed by suggesting the use of traditional foods. To determine the cultural–religious influence on the client's diet, the caregiver should start with an in-depth history of the client's dietary habits.

---

of physical touching or affection and meaningful care. Earlier work on touch indicates that when human beings lack touch, the experience is equivalent to malnutrition and may possibly cause psychotic breakdown (Colton, 1983). Because of the loss of partners and friends, as well as translocation and institutionalization of older adults, touch deprivation is highly likely to occur in this population. Gleason and Timmons (2004)) underscore the importance of touch as a continued need that may be fulfilled by health care professionals. However, the authors caution professionals to assess the resident's perception of touch in all cases.

FTT has often been found in conjunction with dehydration, impaired cognition, dementia, impaired ambulation, and difficulty with at least two activities of daily living. Neglect is a frequent cause of FTT and is usually accompanied by family dysfunction and stress. Nurses play an important role in the assessment of FTT and the timely implementation of interventions to prevent further malnutrition and promote client health and safety.

Interventions to Promote Nutrition

After identifying nutritional concerns and risk factors, it is necessary to plan care surrounding nutrition in the older adult. In light of the fact that there was limited nutritional information available to current older adults in their early and middle years, teaching is an essential intervention. In 2003, the U.S. Preventive Services Task Force (USPSTF) conducted a comprehensive review of dietary education programs. They found sufficient support to recommend dietary counseling to produce small to moderate changes in diet in primary care populations. They also found that the need to increase dietary counseling increased greatly in the presence of high cholesterol, obesity, diabetes, and hypertension. When counseling was provided to disease populations, medium to large changes in diet occurred. Consequently, once a dietary assessment has been conducted, it is essential to provide teaching on what food in the client's diet is healthy and should remain and which should be replaced with healthier alternatives.

One guideline that has been effective in this teaching is the Food Guide Pyramid. These Dietary Guidelines for Americans recommend 3 to 5 servings of vegetables or vegetable juices, 2 to 4 servings of fruits and fruit juices, and 6 to 11 servings of grain products daily. Moreover they recommend a diet with less than 10% of calories from saturated fat and less than 30% of calories from total fats with limited trans fats. Each food group provides some but not all of the nutrients one needs. Foods in one group cannot replace those in another, therefore, no one food group is more important than another; they are all necessary for good health. It is a convenient plan designed to help a person plan an adequate diet, because it allows you to evaluate the daily intake of milk and milk products, meat, fruits, vegetables, and bread, grains, and cereals. Many older adults can name the food groups but are unable to recall the amount of each food group that should be consumed per day.

It is essential to work with the older adults to help them identify which foods provide maximum nutrition without empty calories. It is also important to provide behavioral counseling to help patients set reasonable weight and body fat goals and increase self-esteem and social support to help to meet these goals.

Exercise

The role of regular exercise in promoting health and preventing disease cannot be underscored enough. There is overwhelming evidence that regular exercise results in improved sleep, reduced constipation, lower cholesterol levels, lower blood pressure, improved digestion, weight loss, and enhanced opportunities for socialization. A recent study by Melov, Tarnopolsky, Beckman, Felkey, and Hubbard (2007) found that six months of resistance exercise training resulted in reverses signs of aging in human skeletal tissue. Despite these seemingly wonderful results, a great deal of research shows that the amount of exercise performed by older adults in industrialized countries is reduced with age. This reduction occurs despite the absence of both physiological and psychological restrictions against exercise. However, normal changes of aging, diseases, and environmental changes often result in barriers to effective exercise among older adults.

Nurses are in an ideal role to teach the interventions necessary to help older adults to participate in exercise programs, beginning with the benefits of exercise. Helping older adults choose exercise programs that they will enjoy, as well as encouraging them to exercise with others, are key factors in motivating them to exercise. The ideal exercise program will combine strength training, flexibility, and balance. One of the most popular forms of exercise among older adults is walking. Walking transcends care settings, requires little equipment (except good shoes), and is accessible 24 hours a day. Other exercises popular among older adults include both weight-bearing and aquatic exercises. Weight-bearing and muscle-building exercises assist in maintaining functional mobility, promoting independence, and preventing falls. In addition, weight-bearing exercises have been shown to be very effective in reducing bone-wasting related to osteoporosis (Katz & Sherman, 1998). Aquatic exercises are a pain-free method of promoting health and increasing functional ability, especially for older adults with arthritis and osteoporosis. It is important that older adults who have not been regularly exercising have a complete health assessment prior to beginning a new exercise regime.

Sleep

Inability to fall asleep and sleep through the night are among the most frequent complaints of older adults. Kryger, Monjan, Bliwise, and Ancoli-Israel (2004) report that approximately 57% of older adults report one or more sleep problems. Sleep is affected by both normal and pathological changes of aging. Normal changes of aging include an increase in night-time awakenings and overall sleep deficiency, shorter periods of deep sleep, a decline in slow wave activity and longer time spent in stage 2 of the sleep cycle. Pain and medication side-effects are among the pathological contributors to poor sleep among older adults. Kryger et al. (2004) report that inability to get a good night's sleep results in: excessive daytime sleepiness, attention and memory problems, depressed mood, falls, use of sleeping medications, impaired health, and lower quality of life. A good night's sleep is essential to maintaining energy and function as well as motivation to continue a high quality of life. The first step toward achieving good sleep hygiene is to perform a comprehensive sleep assessment. Based on the results of the assessment, the nurse may provide teaching about the effects of normal changes of aging on sleep and reassure older adults that changes in sleep are not necessarily problematic. With this information, anxiety regarding "too little sleep" may be diminished. The following recommendations may help the older adult to enhance their quality of sleep:

- Increase physical activity during the day.
- Increase pain medication or alternative pain methods to help older adults suffering from painful conditions to get better rest at night.
- Examine the sleep environment. Adjustments in noise and lighting may help older adults to sleep better.
- Assess the stress in the lives of older adults. Identification and resolution of stressful life factors may help older adults to sleep more peacefully.
- Some believe daytime napping can interfere with a good night's sleep. Therefore, older adults who choose to nap during the day should acknowledge that it will likely reduce the total nighttime sleep needed.

Fall Prevention

Falls among older adults in every care setting are a large national problem. Vu, Weintraub, and Rubenstein (2004)) report that falls occur at a rate of 1.5 falls, per bed, per year. Many falls are benign and result in no injury to the older adult. However, when an older adult falls, the consequences may be devastating. They are likely to develop a fracture, which begins them on a spiral of iatrogenesis, which may end in death.

In fact, the CDC (2006c) reports that 13,700 older adults died from falls in 2003. While older men tend to die from falls, older women experience more hospitalizations for fall-related hip fracture (http://www.cdc.gov/epo/mmwr/preview/mmwrhtml/ss4808a3.htm).

Both normal and pathological aging changes, as well as unsafe environments, contribute to the high rate of falls among older adults and place them at higher risk for falls. Normal changes of aging surround sensory alterations, such as visual and hearing decline, as well as changes in urinary function. Pathological changes include neuromuscular and cognitive disorders, osteoporosis, strokes, and sensory impairments. Older adults who have fallen previously have a higher risk of experiencing another fall.

The first line of fall prevention among older adults is to conduct a comprehensive fall assessment. Once an older adult is determined to be at

---

EVIDENCE-BASED PRACTICE

Title of Study: Diabetes Mellitus as a Risk Factor for Hip Fracture in Mexican American Older Adults

Authors: Ottenbacher, K., Ostir, G., Peek, M., Goodwin, J., Markides, K.

Purpose: To examine diabetes and other potential risk factors for hip fracture in a sample of community-dwelling, older Mexican American adults (> 65 years old).

Methods: 3050 older Mexican American subjects participated in a longitudinal study. They were originally interviewed and tested to establish a baseline and then reassessed in 2-, 5-, and 7-year intervals. Incidence of hip fracture was noted for subjects over the 7-year follow up.

Findings: At baseline, 690 individuals were identified with diabetes. 134 subjects experienced a hip fracture during follow-up. Cox proportional hazard regression showed a greater hazard ratio for hip fracture for diabetic subjects compared to those without diabetes (when adjusted for age, body mass, smoking, and previous stroke). The hazard ratio for Mexican Americans taking insulin was 2.84 when adjusted for covariates.

Implications: In older Mexican Americans, it was found that an increased risk for hip fracture exists for persons with diabetes. Because the Mexican American population has a high incidence of Type 2 diabetes, further study is needed for the risk factors for this ethnic group.

Journal of Gerontology, Medical Sciences 2002, Vol. 57A, No. 10, M648–M653.

risk for falls, it is essential that a fall prevention program be implemented to prevent this from occurring. Fall prevention interventions include a thorough assessment of the environment in which the older adult lives. Area rugs and furniture that may be fall hazards should be removed and appropriate lighting and supports should be added to areas in which older adults ambulate. Many homes and facilities have placed a patient's mattress on the floor to prevent injuries from falling out of bed. The use of wall-to-wall carpeting also pads a patient's fall, resulting in less injury on impact. The use of an alarm for the bed or wheelchair to alert caregivers of an older adult's mobility may assist older adults who have had falls in the past. Shelkey (2000) reports that specially trained dogs may also prevent falls by alerting caregivers of the sudden mobility of an older adult.

Restraint Usage

In the need to prevent older adults from falling or harming themselves or others, physical restraints were developed and once commonly used by many nurses and health care providers in several environments of care. A

EVIDENCE-BASED PRACTICE

Title of Study: Changes in Postural Stability in Women Aged 20 to 80 Years

Authors: Low Choy, N., Brauer, S., Nitz, J.

Purpose: To identify the relationship between vision and postural stability in order to introduce fall prevention strategies.

Methods: Measurements of postural stability in 453 women aged 20 to 80 years using the Balance Master force-plate system, while performing the modified Clinical Test for the Sensory Interaction and Balance, and the Single-Limb Stance Test.

Findings: Women 60 to 70 years old were more unsteady than younger women in bilateral stance on a firm surface with eyes closed. Initial instability was noted in 40-year-olds when single-limb stance was tested with eyes closed. Further instability was evidenced in 50-year-olds when a foam surface was introduced. A further decline in stability was demonstrated for each subsequent decade when the eyes were closed in single-limb stance.

Implications: Age, visual acuity, and support surface were significant variables influencing postural stability in women. The cause(s) of this instability and subsequent decline in stability requires further investigation and research.

Journal of Gerontology, Medical Sciences 2003, Vol. 58A, No. 6, 525–530.

---

physical restraint is defined as a device or object attached to or adjacent to a person's body that cannot be removed easily and restricts freedom of movement. Several types of restraints are available and range from physical restraints, such as traditional side-rails on hospital beds, jackets, belts, and wrist restraints, to chemical restraints, such as sedatives and hypnotics. For a while in the 1980s, the fear of liability from falls was so high and the use of restraint alternative so low, that restraint usage sky-rocketed to the point where it was unusual to see an older adult without a restraint in hospitals or long-term care facilities. The Omnibus Budget Reconciliation Act (OBRA) of 1987 attempted to curtail restraint usage, but few alternatives were available to keep clients from falling, and the impact of the legislation was not as great as expected, but is improving.

Physical restraints greatly impact the physical, psychological, and cognitive function of older adults. In fact, evidence surrounding the negative effects of restraint is so disturbing that the mandate for restraint-free care can no longer be ignored. Older adults should only be restrained if they are in immediate, physical danger or hurting themselves or others and then for only a brief period of time. Restraint alternatives should be implemented to keep residents safe from falls. Some of the alternatives to restraints include placing an older adult's mattress on the floor so they are not injured while getting out of bed during the nighttime, as well as the use of wander-guards and chair and bed alarms to alert the caregivers when the client is attempting to get out of their bed or chair. As mentioned previously, dogs may also been trained to summon a caregiver when the client begins movement.

Adult Immunization

One of the greatest advances in primary prevention and public health has been the use of immunizations to prevent disease. People age 65 and older and persons of all ages with chronic diseases are at increased risk for complications from viral infections. During epidemic outbreaks, more than 90% of deaths attributed to pneumonia and influenza occurred among persons aged 65 and older. The few controlled studies of efficacy in persons age 65 and older suggest that when there was a good antigenic match between vaccine and virus, influenza vaccination prevented about 40% of hospitalizations and deaths caused by respiratory illness. See Figure 5.1.

Influenza

Influenza is a major cause of morbidity and mortality in older adults. The 80 and older population experiences an estimated 200,000 hospitalizations and 36,000 deaths per year due to flu (CDC, 2006a). Despite the increase in immunization rates and recent Medicare reimbursement for the vaccine, influenza immunization rates among older adults in senior housing is approximately only 30–60% while the number of older adults receiving the vaccine has improved greatly. The CDC (2006a) reports that influenza vaccination levels increased from 33% in 1989 to 66% in 1999 among older adults, surpassing the Healthy People 2000 objective of 60%. The influenza vaccine, which is composed of inactivated whole virus or virus subunits grown in chick embryo cells, can markedly reduce the incidence of complications, hospitalizations, and death from the disease (and should be given annually to all older adults, especially those with chronic conditions such as pulmonary or cardiac problems and those in long-term care facilities). Vaccination is contraindicated in people who have experienced a reaction to the vaccine in the past and caution should be exercised in administering the vaccine to older adults who have allergies to eggs. A Healthy People 2010 goal (#14–29 a-b) is to increase the number of older adults who are vaccinated annually against influenza and ever vaccinated against pneumococcal disease (U.S. Department of Health and Human Services, 2000).

Pneumonia

The effectiveness of pneumococcal vaccine in the general population has not been determined with certainty. However, there is some evidence, and the U.S. preventive task force has recommended that the pneumococcal vaccine be used in immunocompetent individuals age 65 and older at otherwise high risk for pneumococcal disease. Estimates indicate that pneumococcal infections resulted in death in approximately 7% of older adults hospitalized for the disease in 2004 (CDC, 2006b). Despite this high death rate, many older adults still remain unvaccinated. The CDC recommends that all older adults should get the pneumonia vaccination every 10 years. However, many barriers about pneumococcal vaccination, such as the prevailing lack of importance of the disease and vaccination and the myth that receiving the vaccination will result in the disease, prevent the older adults from receiving immunization.

Tetanus and Diphtheria

In contrast to pneumonia vaccination, the effectiveness of tetanus and diphtheria (TD) toxoids is established on the basis of clinical studies and decades of experience. Currently, adults aged 50 and older account for the majority of cases of tetanus, with persons age 70 and older having a 26% case fatality rate. The TD vaccine series should be completed for

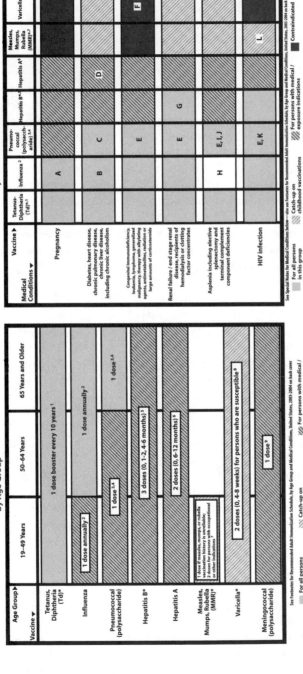

FIGURE 5.1 Immunization guidelines recommended by the CDC.

all clients who have not received the primary series, and all adults should receive periodic TD boosters. The optimal interval for booster doses is not established, but the standard regimen suggests a booster about every 10 years. Figure 5.1 presents immunization guidelines recommended by the CDC. Older adults often did not receive primary immunization against diphtheria and tetanus in their childhood years. Lack of immunization against these diseases leaves the older adult vulnerable to illness and possible death from these two toxoids.

SECONDARY PREVENTION

Adopting and maintaining healthy behaviors is the key to a high quality of life. However, the secondary level of prevention is also essential in detecting diseases at an early (often more treatable) stage. Strategies for detecting disease at an early stage involve annual physical examinations; laboratory blood tests for tumor markers, cholesterol, and other highly treatable illnesses; and diagnostic imaging for the presence of internal disease. Essential areas in which secondary prevention is especially important among the elderly include the early detection of cardiovascular disease.

Cardiovascular Disease

Cardiovascular disease (CVD) is a general term used for a wide variety of illnesses affecting this system. It affects approximately 50% of older women and 70% to 80% of elderly men (Williams, Fleg, Ades, Chaitman, et al. 2002). The CVDs most common among older adults include hypertension, coronary heart disease, and stroke. Early detection of CVDs will likely greatly impact treatment among older adults and has the potential to decrease morbidity and mortality.

In addition to screening for risk factors for cardiovascular disease, which include obesity, sedentary lifestyle, stress, alcohol, and smoking discussed in the previous section, the most significant nursing interventions necessary to detect cardiovascular disease are early and frequent blood pressure and cholesterol screening. The JNC–VII criteria for blood pressure are listed in Table 5.1. Frequent assessments should be conducted to determine a client's position within the provided ranges. When a client's blood pressure readings exceed the recommended limits, they should be referred to their primary health care provider for blood pressure management, including antihypertensive medications. The U.S. Preventive Services Task Force (USPSTF) recommends that older adults with normal blood pressure readings participate in blood pressure screening at least every 2 years.

TABLE 5.1   The JNC–VII Criteria for Blood Pressure

BP	Classification	SBP mmHG	DBP mmHG
Normal	<120	AND	<80
Prehypertensive	120–139	OR	80–89
Stage I Hypertension	140–159	OR	90–99
Stage II Hypertension	>160	OR	>100

The American Heart Association guidelines for cholesterol levels are listed in Table 5.2. Assessing cholesterol levels in clients within the normal range is important in order to reduce morbidity and mortality among this population. The USPSTF recommends that cholesterol levels be evaluated every 5 years after age 45. When clients' cholesterol levels exceed the recommended limits, they should be re-evaluated more often and referred to their primary health care provider for cholesterol management, including treatment with cholesterol-lowering agents. Lipid-lowering medications, known popularly as *statins,* are often effective in reducing further occlusion of the cardiac vessels. Statin medications, such as atorvastatin (Lipitor), fluvastatin (Lescol), lovastain (Mevacor), pravastain (Pravachol), and simvastatin (Zocor), are usually prescribed and must be taken daily. Nurses should instruct patients on proper administration of statins and also assist in the evaluation of their effectiveness through periodic laboratory evaluations. Primary prevention strategies are also recommended to reduce the effects of high cholesterol on cardiovascular disease. It is important to know that cultural backgrounds play an important role in cholesterol levels among older adults. For example, Mexican American men generally have higher cholesterol levels than any other ethnic group.

Diabetes

Type 2 Diabetes Mellitus (DM) is a chronic medical disease that occurs commonly among older adults. It is estimated that 20% of the U.S. popu-

TABLE 5.2   American Heart Association Guidelines for Cholesterol

	Mg/dl	Mg/DL	Mg/dl
Desirable	200	>40	<100
Borderline High Risk	200–239	>40	100–159
High Risk	>240	<40	>160

lation will develop Type 2 DM by the age of 75. The CDC reports that 17 million Americans have DM, and over 200,000 deaths occur each year from diabetes-related complications. DM is often a silent killer as the CDC estimates that 5.9 million Americans are currently unaware that they have the disease. As people age, there is a normal increase in insulin resistance and DM. As with cholesterol levels, cultural backgrounds effect the incidence of diabetes among older adults, with the highest rates of DM occurring in non-Hispanic Blacks. Identification of risk factors for Type 2 DM, such as cultural influence, obesity, low levels of activity, and poor nutrition, is the first step toward successful diagnosis and treatment of this disease.

Because Type 2 DM is manifested by an increase in blood glucose levels, screening for this disease is most efficiently accomplished by testing the blood for elevated glucose levels. Fasting glucose levels between 100 and 125 mg/dl are indicative of pre-diabetes and should be evaluated often. Higher levels are indicative of diabetes and must be referred to the primary health care provider for management. Management of DM often involves the administration of hypoglycemic medications, as well as insulin. Dietary management and weight loss are also recommended.

Cancer

Over half of cancer diagnoses in the United States occurs in those age 65 and older. The cancer incidence rate among people aged 65 to 69 is approximately double that for those age 55 to 59. Age is also an important predictor of cancer stage; those of advanced age often have their cancers diagnosed at later stages than do younger persons. Therefore, the positive outcomes of cancer treatment appear to diminish as age increases. For all age groups, lung cancer is still the number one cause of cancer mortality. For older men, the other major cancer killers, in order, are prostate, colon/rectum, and pancreas. For older women, colon/rectum cancer is the highest killer, followed by cancers of the lung, breast, pancreas, and ovary.

Screening for cancer among older adults is the most effective manner in which to detect the disease at the earliest possible stage. Consequently, early detection leads to the most effective treatment. Table 5.3 provides the American Cancer Society Recommendations on Screening for cancer. A detailed description of the tests is provided at http://www.cancer.org. It is important to note that many providers of care to older adults have debated the usefulness and ethical nature of screening older adults for cancer. Significant issues surround the cost effectiveness of these often expensive and painful diagnostic tests versus benefit in increasing life expectancy. Often cancer diagnosis among older adults results in treatment that greatly decreases quality of life and does not result in improved life expectancy.

TABLE 5.3 American Cancer Society Recommendations for the Early Detection of Cancer in Average-Risk Asymptomatic People

Cancer Site	Population	Test or Procedure	Frequency
Breast	Women, age 20*	Breast self-examination (BSE)	Beginning in their early 20s, women should be told about the benefits and limitations of breast self-examination (BSE). The importance of prompt reporting of any new breast symptoms to health professionals should be emphasized. Women who choose to do BSE should receive instruction and have their technique reviewed on the occasion of a periodic health examination. It is acceptable for women to choose not to do BSE or to do BSE irregularity.
		Clinical breast examination (CBE)	For women in their 20s and 30s, it is recommended that clinical breast examination (CBE) be part of a periodic health examination, preferably at least every 3 years. Asymptomatic women aged 40 and over should continue to receive a clinical breast examination as part of a periodic health examination, preferably annually.
		Mammography	Begin annual mammography at age 40.*
Colonocial	Men and women. age 50*	Fecal occult blood test (FOBT)†, or	Annual starting at age 50.
		Flexible sigmoidoscopy, or	Every 5 years, starting at age 50.
		Fecal occult blood test (FOBT)† and flexible sigmoidoscopy,‡ or	Annual FOBT and flexible sigmoidoscopy every 5 years, starting at age 50.
		Double contract barum (DCBE), or	DCBE every 5 years, starting at age 50.
		Colonoscopy	Colonoscopy every 10 years, starting at age 50.

140

Prostate	Men, age 50*	Digital rectal examination (DRE) and prostate-specific antigen test (PSA)	The PSA test and the DRE should be offered annually, starting at age 50, for men who have life expectancy of at least 10 years.
Cervix	Women, age 18*	Pap test	Cervical cancer screening should begin approximately 3 years after a woman begins having vaginal intercourse, but no later than 21 years of age. Screening should be done every year with conventional Pap tests or every 2 years using liquid-based Pap tests. At or after age 30, women who have had three normal test results in a row may get screened every 2 to 3 years. Women 70 years of age and older who have had three or more normal Pap tests and no abnormal Pap tests in the last 10 years and women who have had a total hysterectomy may choose to stop conical cancer screening.
Endometrial	Women, at menopause		At the time of menopause, women at average risk should be informed about risks and symptoms of endometrial cancer and strongly encouraged to report any unexpected bleeding or sporting to their physicians.
Cancer-related check-up	Men and women, age 20*		On the occasion of a periodic health examination, the cancer-related checkup should include examination for cancer of the thyroid, testicles, ovaries, lymph nodes, oral cavity, and skin, as well as health counseling about tobacco, and exposure, diet and nutrition, risk factors, sexual practices, and environmental and occupational exposures.

*Beginning at age 40, annual clinical breast examination should be performed prior to mammography.

†FOBT, as it is sometimes done in physicians' offices with the single sicot sample collected on a fingertip during a digital rectal examination, is not an adequate substitute for the recommended at-home procedure of collecting two samples from three consecutive specimens. Toilet bowl FOBT tests are not recommended. In companion with guaiac-based tests for the detection of occult blood, immunochemical tests are more patient-friendly and are likely to be equal or better in sensitivity and specificity. There is no justification for repecting FOBT in response to an initial positive finding.

‡Flexible sigmoidoscopy together with FOBT is preferred over FOBT or flexible sigmoidoscopy alone.

§Information should be provided to men about the benefits and limitations of testing so that an informed decision about testing can be made with the clinician's assistance.

Tertiary prevention and the treatment of acute and chronic diseases to prevent further disease progression and improve function will be discussed in Chapters 9 and 10, respectively.

SUMMARY

This chapter underscores the need for primary prevention among older adults to prevent and reduce the harmful effects of smoking and excessive alcohol usage and to prevent the effects of poor nutrition and sleep patterns, as well as sedentary lifestyles, on the health of older adults. Early detection of fall risk and implementation of strategies to prevent falls, as well as immunization against vaccine-preventable diseases, are additional primary prevention strategies to help maintain the health and quality of life of older adults. The early detection of disease is an essential secondary prevention strategy to decrease the morbidity and mortality of older adults. Nurses who care for older adults can do much to promote their health and well-being through education, research, and practice.

REFERENCES

Ammerman, A. A., Lindquist, C. H., Lahr, K. N., & Hersey, J. (2002). The efficacy of behavioral interventions to modify dietary fat and fruit and vegetable intake: A review of the evidence. *Preventative Medicine, 35*(1), 25–41.

Blow, F. C., Walton, M. A., Chermack, S. T., Mudd, S. A., & Brower, K. J. (2000). Older adult treatment outcome following elder-specific inpatient alcoholism treatment. *Journal of Substance Abuse Treatment, 19*(1), 67–75.

Centers for Disease Control. (2006a). *Key facts about influenza and influenza vaccine.* Retrieved July 19, 2007, from http://www.cdc.gov/flu

Centers for Disease Control. (2006b). *National hospital discharge survey: 2004 annual summary with detailed diagnosis and procedure data.* Retrieved August 8, 2007, from http://www.cdc.gov/nchs/data/series/sr_13/sr13_162.pdf

Centers for Disease Control. (2006c). *Preventing falls among older adults.* Retrieved July 19, 2007, from http://www.cdc.gov/ncipc/duip/preventadultfalls.htm

Colton, H. (1983). *The gift of touch.* New York: Seaview & Putnam.

Federal Interagency Forum on Aging-Related Statistics. (2004). *Older Americans 2004: Key indicators of well-being.* Washington, DC: U.S. Government Printing Office.

Gleeson, M., & Timmons, F. (2004). The use of touch to enhance nursing care of older person in longterm mental health care facilities. *Journal of Psychiatric & Mental Health Nursing, 11,* 541–545.

Hogstel, M. O. (2001). *Gerontology: Nursing care of the older adult.* Albany, NY: Delmar Thomson Learning.

Howard, J. H., Gates, G. E., Ellersieck, M. R., & Dowdy, R. P. (1998). Investigating relationships between nutritional knowledge, attitudes and beliefs, and dietary adequacy of the elderly. *Journal of Nutrition for the Elderly, 17*(4), 35–52.

Institute of Medicine. (2002). *Unequal treatment: Confronting racial and ethnic dispari-ties in health care*. Retrieved July 19, 2007, from http://www.iom.edu/Object.File/Master/4/175/Disparitieshcproviders8pgFINAL.pdf

Katz, W. A., & Sherman, C. (1998). Exercise is medicine. Osteoporosis: The role of exercise in optimal management. *Physician & Sportsmedicine, 26*, 39–42.

Kryger, M., Monjan, A., Bliwise, D., & Ancoli-Israel, S. (2004). Sleep, health, and aging: Bridging the gap between science and clinical practice. *Geriatrics, 59*(1), 24–30.

Mattiasson, A. C., & Heber, M. (1998). Intimacy—Meeting needs and respecting privacy in the care of elderly people: What is a good moral attitude on the part of the nurse/career? *Nursing Ethics, 5*, 527–534.

Melov, S., Tarnopolsku, M.A., Beckman, K., Felkey, K., & Hubbard, A. (2007). Resistance exercise reverses aging in human skeletal muscle. *Public Library of Science, 5*, 1–8.

Odlund, O. A. (2005). Nutritional status, well-being and functional ability in frail elderly service flat residents. *European Journal of Nutrition, 59*(2), 263–270.

Robert Wood Johnson Foundation. (2001). *Substance abuse: The nation's number one health problem*. Prepared by the Schneider Institute for Health Policy, Brandeis University. Available at http://www.rwjfliterature.org/chartbook/chartbook.htm. Princeton, NJ: Author.

Shelkey, M. (2000). Pet Therapy. In J. Fitzpatrick, T. Fulmer, M. Wallace, & E. Flaherty (Eds.), *Geriatric nursing research digest* (pp. 215–218). New York: Springer-Verlag, Inc.

U.S. Department of Health and Human Services. (2000). Healthy people 2010: National health promotion and disease prevention objectives. http://www.health.gov/healthy people.

U.S. Preventive Services Task Force. (2003). Behavioral counseling in primary care to promote a healthy diet: Recommendations and rationale. *American Journal of Nursing, 103*(8), 81–91.

Vu, M. Q., Weintraub, N., & Rubenstein, L. Z. (2004). Falls in the nursing home: Are they preventable? *Journal of the American Medical Directors Association, 5*(6), 401–406.

Williams, M. A., Fleg, J. L., Ades, P. A., Chaitman, B. R., Miller, N. H., Mohiuddin, S. M., et al. (2002). Secondary prevention of coronary heart disease in the elderly (with emphasis on patients ? > or = to 75 years of age). An American Heart Association scientific statement from the council on clinical cardiology subcommittee on exercise, cardiac rehabilitation, and prevention. *Circulation, 105*, 1735–1743.

CHAPTER SIX

Pathological Disease Processes in Older Adults

Leaning Objectives

1. Identify clinical presentation of, and interventions for, commonly occurring musculoskeletal disorders among adults.
2. Identify clinical presentation of, and interventions for, commonly occurring cardiovascular and respiratory disorders among adults.
3. Identify clinical presentation of diabetes among older adults.
4. Identify clinical presentation of, and interventions for, commonly occurring infectious diseases among older adults.
5. Identify clinical presentation of, and interventions for, cancer in older adults.
6. Identify clinical presentation of, and interventions for, Parkinson's disease in older adults.

Mr. Marse is a 75-year-old African American male who is extremely anxious when he comes into the emergency department with complaints of an intense crushing pain in his chest that has lasted for 30 minutes and has been unrelieved by nitroglycerin. As you take Mr. Marse and his wife to an examination area you notice that he is very short of breath, and he tells you that he is feeling dizzy. His wife tells you that he has been under a lot of stress recently and she is very worried about him. As a result of Mr. Marse's symptoms, you immediately call the doctor and take Mr. Marse's vital signs, which are as follows: BP 200/110, P 85, R 46, T 100.1°F. He tells you that he does not think that he can stand the pain much longer.

OA can be a primary disorder, or a secondary disorder, resulting from a previous anatomic abnormality, injury, or procedure, or from occupational factors. Nursing assessment for OA includes the evaluation of pain as the presenting symptom for most patients, and radiographic examination of the joints can help aid in the diagnosis and staging of OA. However, the progression of the disease as seen on X-rays does not always coincide with the symptoms. In fact, older adults with minor articular changes may experience profound pain. Treatment for OA is aimed at relieving pain and preserving or restoring function. Pharmacological treatments frequently include nonsteroidal anti-inflammatory drugs (NSAIDs) and acetaminophen, and narcotic pain relievers when necessary.

Various nutraceuticals aimed at reducing pain and improving function are used frequently among older adults with OA. Herbal supplements commonly used include vitamins C, D, and E, which have shown some evidence of reducing OA symptoms. Ginger and glucosamine have also been used extensively by older adults to reduce arthritis-related pain. Nurses must exercise caution in the administration of nutraceuticals and provide teaching regarding the possible danger of these herbal medications as little is known about their interaction with prescription medications. Acupuncture is becoming a more popular nonpharmacological OA management strategy, and anecdotal evidence supports its use. However, there is insufficient literature to fully support the use of these alternative strategies independently to reach treatment goals.

Joint replacement among older adults with osteoarthritis is gaining in popularity. These surgical procedures are used primarily to replace hip and knee joints that are dysfunctional because of the long-term effects of osteoarthritis. While the rehabilitation may be long and intense, more and more individuals in their eighties and nineties are having total joint replacements with the hope that the surgery will bring about new mobility and greatly improve their quality of life.

Osteoporosis

Osteoporosis is another of the most common chronic diseases of older adulthood. Physiologically, osteoporosis results from a demineralization of the bone and is evidenced by a decrease in the mass and density of the skeleton. A theory of the etiology of osteoporosis results from age-related changes in the synthesis of vitamin C resulting in decreased calcium absorption. The most common areas of bone loss are the vertebrae, distal radius, and proximal femur.

Osteoporosis affects approximately 44 million women and men aged 50 and older in the United States. It is estimated that this number will

EVIDENCE-BASED PRACTICE

Title of Study: Testing an Intervention for Preventing Osteoporosis in Post-menopausal Breast Cancer Survivors

Authors: Waltman, N., Twiss, J., Ott, C., Lindsey, Moore, T., Berg, K.

Purpose: To test a 12-month intervention for preventing or treating osteo-porosis in postmenopausal women who had completed treatment for breast cancer (except Tamoxifen) and for whom hormone replacement therapy was contraindicated.

Methods: The intervention was multifaceted and consisted of: (1) home-based strength and weight training exercises; (2) 5 or 10 mg alendronate per day, 1500 mg calcium per day, 400 IU vitamin D per day; (3) educa-tion on osteoporosis; and (4) strategies to promote adherence to interven-tions. Outcomes were rated categorically: (1) adherence to interventions, (2) dynamic balance, (3) muscle strength, and (4) bone mineral density (BMD) of the hip, spine, and forearm.

Findings: 95% adhered to calcium and vitamin D, aldendronate therapy was above 95%, and adherence to strength training exercises was above 85%. Over 1 year, the 21 participants showed significant improvements in balance; muscle strength for hip flexion, hip extension, and knee flexion; and BMD of the spine and hip. They also showed a signifi-cant decrease in BMD of the forearm. 3 out of the 21 women who had measurable bone loss at baseline had normal BMD after 12 months of intervention.

Implications: Significant increases in BMD of the hip and spine were found at 12 months, as well as a significant decrease in BMD of the forearm. The multicomponent intervention only lasted 1 year, and the time nec-essary for full bone modeling or remodeling is believed to be 4 to 6 months, respectively. BMD associated with exercise does not increase until several remodeling cycles have been completed, so it was recom-mended that this intervention be continued beyond 1 year. Data from this study was used in the planning of a study that was to last for 2 years.

Journal of Nursing Scholarship, Fourth Quarter 2003.

grow to over 52 million by the year 2010 (National Osteoporosis Foun-dation, 2003). In older adults with osteoporosis, the overall decline in bone mass weakens the bone making it vulnerable to even slight trauma. Normal changes of aging in the sensory system and in neuromuscular coordination combine with medications and environmental factors to place the older adult with osteoporosis at high risk for fall-related frac-tures. Fractures of the humerus and femoral neck are common, as are hip fractures in women over age 65. Fractures in older adults often position these individuals in a spiral of iatrogenesis, with an increased risk of impaired mobility, decubitus ulcers, pneumonia, and incontinence.

Older individuals who are at highest risk for osteoporosis include: (a) small, thin women who have fair skin and light hair and eyes; (b) older adults with a family history of osteoporosis; (c) postmenopausal women; (d) women over age 65; and (e) men over age 80. In addition, older individuals who consume a diet low in calcium, smoke, use excess alcohol or caffeine, or live a sedentary lifestyle are at higher risk for developing the disease.

Older adults with osteoporosis may develop Kyphosis late in the disease. Kyphosis is a convex curvature of the spine that causes loss of height and chronic back pain as well as abdominal protuberance, gastrointestinal discomfort, and pulmonary insufficiency. Bone density screenings can detect bone loss for those at risk for developing osteoporosis. However, as there are often no symptoms of this disease, osteoporosis is seldom diagnosed until a traumatic fracture is sustained. In the event a fracture occurs, one common treatment procedure is kyphoplasty, which involves the insertion of an inflatable bone around the fracture. This procedure has been effective at reducing the morbidity and mortality of this disease.

Nursing interventions for the prevention of osteoporosis include encouragement of diets high in calcium and a program of regular exercise. Diets high in calcium (1500 mg/day) and weight-bearing exercise are among key factors in preventing bone loss in normal individuals and those at risk. New medications, administered weekly or monthly, have been shown to prevent further bone loss in those diagnosed with osteoporosis. Alendronate Sodium (Fosamax®), risedronate (Actonel®), or Raloxifene (Evista®) have been shown to prevent further bone loss and develop new bone mass. While clients taking the daily form of bone resorption inhibitors do not have any special consideration, clients taking the weekly form of the medication should be instructed to take the medication with breakfast and stand or sit upright for 30 minutes after administration. The use of calcitonin (Calcimar®, Miaclcin®, Ostreocalcin®) to treat postmenopausal osteoporosis may be recommended. However, this medication must be administered intranasally or intramuscularly once daily. Consequently, once per week or month dosing is often preferred by clients.

In individuals with documented bone loss from osteoporosis, nursing interventions surround fall prevention strategies. Fall prevention interventions include a thorough assessment of the environment in which the older adult lives. Area rugs and furniture that may be fall hazards should be removed and appropriate lighting and supports should be added to areas in which older adults ambulate. Many homes and facilities have placed a patient's mattress on the floor to prevent injuries from falling out of bed. The use of wall-to-wall carpeting also pads a patient's fall, resulting in less injury on impact. The use of alarms on beds or wheelchairs to alert caregivers of an older adult's intent to ambulate may assist to prevent falls among older adults who have fallen in the past. Shelkey (2000) reports that specially trained dogs may be helpful in alerting caregivers of the sudden mobility of an older adult to prevent falls.

CARDIOVASCULAR AND RESPIRATORY DISORDERS

Hypertension

Hypertension (HTN), or abnormally high blood pressure, results from many nonmodifiable and modifiable risk factors and lifestyle behaviors, and is a serious risk factor for the development of many types of cardiovascular and renal diseases. Thus, the prevention and treatment of HTN in older adults is essential in order to maintain both health and function among the older population. Hypertension is considered a silent killer, because it has no signs and symptoms. While some older adults experience headaches from elevated blood pressure, older adults with this disorder may be unaware of it if they do not receive a blood pressure reading. In fact, approximately one-third of people with HTN are unaware they have it. The American Heart Association (2007) estimates that of those with HTN, at least 50% are not on medication while about 25% more are on inadequate hypertensive therapy.

The JNC-VII criteria for blood pressure are listed in Table 5.1. The guidelines define stage I hypertension as a blood pressure of 140/90 or above measured on three separate readings. It is important for older adults to undergo regular blood pressure screening and, if hypertensive, to follow the directions of their physicians. Hypertension treatment guidelines vary somewhat. Nevertheless, treatment of hypertension has been shown to reduce morbidity and mortality in both genders and in all ages and races (CDC, 2007b). Risk stratification is often used to make decisions about treatment for hypertension. In clients with low CV risk factors, even a blood pressure as high as 160/100 mm Hg may be treated with lifestyle modifications alone. The combination of diabetes and smoking together is more dangerous than either risk factor alone, related to the possibility of microvascular complications occuring (ACP, 2007). In contrast, in clients at high risk, such as those with diabetes, antihypertensive drug therapy may be recommended, even when the blood pressure is less than 140/90 mm Hg. The treatment target is a blood pressure of less than 130/80 mm Hg (JNC-VII).

The current guidelines for staging and treating hypertension are listed in Table 5.1. Nursing interventions for the treatment of hypertension generally begin with diet and lifestyle modification. Older adults with diagnosed hypertension are generally encouraged to follow a low sodium and low fat diet. Exercise is encouraged among older hypertensive clients and has been shown to reduce blood pressure. Despite these clearly obvious benefits of exercise, the majority of older adults do not exercise, and should be encouraged to choose culturally appropriate exercises that they enjoy, such as walking, tai chi, or yoga. The stress management effects of these therapies, as well as the cardiovascular benefits, are essential for disease management.

Once-daily dosing of medications and a gradual approach toward therapeutic leveling is essential. Drugs are increased very gradually until optimal control is attained. In general, first-line therapy consists of thiazide diuretics, such as hydrochlorothizide (HCTZ) or Diuril; and beta blockers, such as atenolol (Tenormin), labetolol (Normodyne), or propranolol (Inderal). Angiotensin-converting enzymes (ACE inhibitors), such as benazepril (Lotensin) or captopril (Capoten); and calcium channel blockers, such as amlodipine (Norvasc) and diltiazem (Cardizen), are used for first-line therapy only when the diuretics and beta blockers are contraindicated. It is important to note that one of the major side-effects of these medications is impotence. As a result of this side-effect, many men stop taking the medication. It is important for nurses to assess for this frequently occurring side-effect and determine its impact on medication compliance.

Congestive Heart Failure

Congestive heart failure (CHF) is a chronic medical condition that occurs more commonly as people age. In the United States, approximately 4.8 million people have CHF, and each year 400,000 new cases are diagnosed. Approximately 287,000 die each year from heart failure (CDC, 2006a). Both the presentation and outcome of CHF are often influenced by the presence of comorbidity, and about 80% of all clients with CHF are age 65 and older. CHF is a chronic illness that often presents as acute crisis. The amount of hospitalizations for heart failure rose from approximately 400,000 in 1979 to over 1.1 million in 2004 (CDC, 2006a).

CHF is a multifaceted disease exacerbated by normal changes in the heart that accompany aging. The individual structural (physical) and functional (performance) changes that typify this disease are broad and generally involve multiple body systems. CHF commonly occurs when the pumping ability of the heart is impaired and it can no longer deliver adequate blood circulation to supply the body's metabolic requirements.

CHF may be used to refer to either left ventricular failure (LVF) or right ventricular failure (RVF). Left ventricular failure is the cause of CHF in older adults (Hogstel, 2001). Left ventricular failure may lead to right ventricular failure causing fluid to accumulate in the lungs and heart, virtually drowning the cardiac muscle. Approximately 287,000 people died of CHF in 2006 (CDC, 2006a).

Many diseases result in CHF, but the CDC (2006a) reports that the most common causes are coronary artery disease, hypertension, and diabetes, with 7 of every 10 people presenting with CHF having a previous diagnosis of hypertension. CHF is an inclusive term for cardiac pathologies that obstruct circulation, causing excess fluid to build up in the lungs and body tissues. Blood backed up into the lungs creates pulmonary edema with accompanying dyspnea and fatigue. Fluid also becomes obstructed in the venous system where the excess pressure causes it to leak into body tissues. This fluid retention, in turn, creates edema, usually seen in the lower extremities.

The typical presentation of CHF is the sudden development of shortness of breath (dyspnea) with exertion (DOE). Fatigue and weakness are common. DOE often progresses to shortness of breath at rest, accompanied by both orthopnea and paroxysmal nocturnal dyspnea (PND), or dyspnea when lying down. In older adults, memory loss, confusion, diaphoresis, tachycardia, palpitations, anorexia, and insomnia may occur. Pedal edema and fluid in the lungs are common findings. Normal and pathological aging changes may often make the early assessment and treatment of CHF difficult. For example, pedal edema or weight gain of CHF may be confused with normal pedal edema that occurs with aging or the side effects of steroid treatment for COPD. Altered cough reflex may prevent early detection of pulmonary changes. Other symptoms such as chest pain or tightness, fatigue, general weakness, a nonproductive cough, insomnia, and other may be commonly attributable to other conditions of aging and orthopnea. For example, consider the case of an 89-year-old man with repeated incidents of anxiety attacks. Not until an EKG and chest X-ray were done during, or subsequent to, these attacks were cardiac and respiratory signs of CHF associated with these circumstances. The expected classic symptoms of CHF are not always exhibited in the older adult.

Nurses play an important and comprehensive role when caring for the older adults with CHF. The first role of nurses is to identify early symptoms of CHF. Nurses who treat elderly patients will likely encounter this disease and should be aware of its signs and symptoms and how they present in the older adult. Managing factors that will decrease hospital readmissions is the next role of nurses. In so doing, disease progression will be minimized resulting in a maximum quality of life. Nurses must educate clients about self-care and medication administration and involve the clients in their own care. Treatment for CHF usually involves a regimen of angiotensin-converting enzyme (ACE) inhibitors, digoxin, and diuretics. ACE inhibitors, such as benazepril (Lotensin) or captopril (Capoten), reduce mortality, relieve symptoms, and improve exercise tolerance, but they must be used cautiously in clients with an elevated serum creatinine clearance or renal impairment. Digoxin is commonly used, but it must be administered cautiously in clients on ACE inhibitors who are in sinus rhythm. Diuretics, such as furosemide (Lasix), are often used for CHF clients, and are most effective when sodium is restricted to less than 2g/day to reduce diuretic doses. Potassium supplements should be used, along with nonpotassium sparing diuretics. Anticoagulants, such as warfarin (Coumadin), are used if there is concern about thrombi or emboli. Vasodilators (nitrates) are often necessary (Hogstel, 2001). When an older client with chronic CHF develops mild to moderate symptoms of the disease, the administration of intravenous diuretics is usually started in order to decrease cardiac workload. Without further symptoms, and adequate urinary output, the older adults may be evaluated for several hours in the emergency department, home, or outpatient facility and then discharged. The persistence of symptoms or failure to reduce cardiac output requires further treatment and hospitalization.

Nurses can be instrumental in the treatment of CHF by assisting older adults with weight loss for obese clients, sodium restriction, alternating periods of activity and rest with avoidance of activity levels that exacerbate symptoms, and appropriate drug therapy. Although intense physical exercise should be avoided, moderate exercise to tolerance should be encouraged. Too much activity restriction can result in severe muscle and cardiac deconditioning, which can cause the older adult to become a cardiac cripple, that is, severely disabled and unable to tolerate normal levels of activity because of severe deconditioning. Clients should alternate aerobic activity and rest and avoid excessive walking or swimming, because these increase the cardiac workload.

Exacerbations and remissions are a common pattern with CHF. Failure to intervene in a timely manner can lead to further decline, disability, and premature death. It has been demonstrated that long-term care settings that implement a standardized interdisciplinary protocol for treating CHF can improve resident care and apply preventative responses that avoid hospitalizations (Martien & Freundl, 2004). It is important to maintain older clients with CHF at the highest possible level of wellness to avoid the development of absolute failure, pulmonary edema, or cardiogenic shock. The major causes of transition from chronic failure to acute failure and/or pulmonary edema in the older adult are often infection, exacerbation of other co-morbidities, surgery, trauma, and other severe stressors. Consequently, nurses must identify the role of these issues, coordinate services to maintain health, and assist the client to prevent precipitators of CHF to the extent possible.

Angina and Myocardial Infarction (MI)

Angina pectoris and myocardial infarctions (MI) are prevalent cardiac disorders among older adults. It is estimated that angina occurs in approximately 13.1% of older adults (CDG, 2007c). The Merck Manual reports that MI occurs in approximately 35% of older adults, and 60% of hospitalizations due to acute MI occur in persons 65 or older. A CDC study of 356,112 adults nationwide reported that 12.9 had a history of MI (CDC, 2007c).

A variety of factors can precipitate angina and MI among older adults; the most common of which is coronary artery disease (CAD). Other causes of MI include coronary thrombosis, coronary occlusion and coronary spasm (AHA, 2007). Angina results from a lack of oxygen supply to the heart muscle due to a reduced blood flow around the heart's blood vessels. It is the most common symptom of myocardial ischemia and is experienced commonly among older adults with coronary artery disease (CAD). The American Heart Association (2007) defines a myocardial infarction as "the damaging or death of an area of the heart muscle (myocardium) resulting from a blocked blood supply to that area" (AHA, 2007). It occurs when a part of the heart muscle dies because of sudden, total interruption of blood flow to that area.

The classic clinical presentation of MI, regardless of gender, is pain. The pain and dysrhythmias of MI are often more serious in older adults than in younger clients as a result of both normal and pathological aging changes. Moreover, older adults may not exhibit normal signs of MI, which include: (a) crushing, radiating chest pain; (b) gray, or cyanotic skin; (c) diaphoresis; (d) severe anxiety; (e) nausea and vomiting; and (f) hiccough. In some cases, there may be no symptoms of MI (silent heart attack). However, older adults may display several symptoms: (a) pain in the back, shoulder, jaw, and/or abdomen; (b) a diminished level of consciousness or acute confusion; (c) hypotension; (d) dizziness or syncope; (e) transient ischemic attack (TIA); (f) CVA; (g) weakness; (h) fatigue; (i) falls; (j) restlessness; or (k) incontinence. While research on clinical presentation of MI among younger populations has revealed gender differences in the clinical presentation of disease, a recent study by Rosengren et al. (2004) revealed that there are no gender differences in clinical presentation among older adults.

Nurses play an important and comprehensive role when caring for older adults with MI. The first role of nurses is to identify early symptoms of angina and MI. Both of these diseases may present as pain, so pain complaints must be considered seriously and proper assessment implemented. Nurse's beliefs that pain is a natural and expected part of angina or MI is among one of the most prevalent myths that prevent appropriate treatment. Other barriers include older adult's hesitancy to report pain, because they also expect it, think nothing can be done for it, or are afraid to bother their nurse. Objective pain is aided by the presence of many standardized tools for assessing pain in older adults. The most frequently used measure of pain evaluation is a numeric rating scale, in which the client is asked to choose a position on a scale of 1 to 10, with 1 being very little pain, and 10 being the worst pain imaginable. However, some research suggests that the abstract nature of these scales makes them difficult for some older adults, especially those with cognitive impairments, to complete. Visual Analogue Scales (VAS) are straight horizontal 100 mm lines with verbal pain descriptors on the left and right sides. Older adults are asked to indicate a position on the scale that represents their pain. These tests also are not perfect. The "Faces Scale" depicts facial expressions on a scale of 0–6 with 0 = smile and 6 = crying grimace, which is another alternative to objective pain assessment. Determining the right tool for each patient is a necessary step to utilizing these objective measures effectively. These scales may be used for baseline and subsequent pain assessments to evaluate effectiveness of treatment. For older adults with cognitive impairments, awareness of known painful conditions and evaluation of behavior is essential for effective assessment and management of pain. The five-item Pain Assessment in Dementia Scale has been demonstrated to be effective for assessing pain in this population (Warden, Hurley, & Volicer, 2003).

After pain complaints are validated, further symptoms of angina and MI should be evaluated in conjunction with the interdisciplinary team using EKGs and cardiac enzyme evaluation. MIs are a medical emergency and must be managed accordingly. Drug therapy for chronic angina usually involves the daily application of nitroglycerin patches (Nitrodisc®, Nitro-Dur®) to enhance perfusion to the cardiac vessels. Clients with chronic angina are usually encouraged to keep sublingual nitroglycerin pills (Nitrostat®, Nitrolingual®) with them. Proper teaching regarding the application of patches and the administration of sublingual nitroglycerin is necessary. Clients should be taught to remove the patch and clean the area before applying the next patch. Sublingual nitroglycerin must be placed under the tongue and allowed to dissolve.

Lipid-lowering medications, known popularly as *statins,* are often effective in reducing further occlusion of the cardiac vessels. Statin medications, such as atorvastatin (Lipitor), fluvastatin (Lescol), lovastain (Mevacor), pravastain (Pravachol), and simvastatin (Zocor), are usually prescribed and must be taken daily. Nurses should instruct patients on proper administration of statins and also assist in the evaluation of their effectiveness through period cholesterol level evaluation. The American Heart Association guidelines for cholesterol levels are listed in Table 5.2. Assessing cholesterol levels in clients is important in order to reduce morbidity and mortality among this population. Selective beta-blocker medications, such as acebutolol (Sectral) and atenonol (Tenormin), may also be prescribed to prevent MI in patients with angina. Like with CHF, nurses can be instrumental in the treatment of angina and MI by assisting older adults with weight loss for obese clients, developing a program of physical activity levels, and encouraging maintenance of a low cholesterol diet (see Chapter 5 for more details on these health promotion activities).

Obstructive Airway Diseases

The group of obstructive airway diseases collectively rank as the fourth leading cause of death in the United States, with an increasing mortality rate, especially among older adults who continue to smoke. The three major obstructive airway diseases found prevalently among older adults include chronic bronchitis, asthma, and emphysema, which collectively form the chronic obstructive pulmonary diseases (COPD). While the three diseases have distinct pathological processes, they all result in difficulty breathing and, when untreated, may escalate to medical emergencies. Chronic bronchitis is caused by the inflammation of respiratory passages and results in edema and the development of sputum, which tends to make breathing very difficult and, in some cases, impossible. Asthma is manifested by the onset of bronchospasm, mucosal edema, and large amounts of sputum production. Asthma is on the rise in the United States with the incidence and death rates of the disease increasing among all age groups, including older adults. Some older adults grow old with the disease, and some experience new onset asthma in their later years. Emphysema results from damage to the alveoli (the functional units in the lungs), which results in a reduction in the lung tissue available for aeration (alveolar-capillary diffusion interface).

While COPD may result from several factors, such as air pollution, smoking continues to be the number one cause. Even though there is no formula to calculate the number of cigarettes needed to produce COPD, small airway changes may begin as early as at about a 20-pack-year-history (packs per day times years smoked) (Hogstel, 2001). Persons who have COPD tend to ignore their symptoms for a long time, which means that clients may be admitted to the hospital, treated for other problems, or go to surgery without a clear diagnosis of COPD, even though it is present. As a result, they may develop unforeseen pulmonary problems along with whatever treatment is being given. Consequently, it is important for nurses to elicit a history of smoking or prolonged exposure to second-hand smoke and history of COPD symptoms from clients.

Nursing interventions for COPD vary by disease, but the goals of all disease therapies are to maintain clear airways. Suggested nursing therapy and management are similar across diseases. Teaching regarding the use of oxygen is an important nursing role; ordering and demonstrating the application of the nasal cannula, as well as instructions regarding operating the tanks, is often needed. Clients using oxygen must be cautioned not to increase the oxygen level beyond the prescribed dosage for fear of medical complications and the possibility of becoming dependent on higher levels of oxygen.

Treatment of both asthma and emphysema currently often entails the administration of steroid medications. These medications may be inhaled or administered orally. The side effects of these medications include skin disorders and hormonal interference. Inhaled bronchodilators, such as beta agonists or theophyllines, are also common treatments for obstructive pulmonary diseases. Teaching regarding the use of inhalers is often necessary as these are the preferred method of drug administration. Cough suppressants and antihistamines should be avoided among clients with obstructive respiratory disorders as these medications impair coughing ability and may cause fatal levels of sedation in respiratory compromised clients. In clients where palliative measures are warranted, these medications may be appropriate to facilitate peaceful death. In these cases, opioids have been supported as safe and effective in reducing terminal dyspnea and respiratory distress.

Cerebral Vascular Accident (Stroke)

Cerebral vascular accidents, commonly known as stroke, are among the leading cause of chronic disability in this nation. The risk of stroke occurring increases sharply as people age, with approximately 700,000 strokes occuring each year and 200,000 stroke deaths occurring among those aged 65 and older. The symptoms of stroke include sudden onset weakness or numbness in the face, leg, or arm on one side of the body; changes in vision, including the loss of vision in one eye; difficulty speaking or understanding language; or sudden onset, severe headache and dizziness. Unexplained falls may also be symptomatic for stroke.

Risk factors for development of stroke are similar to those of other cardiovascular diseases. Both modifiable and nonmodifable risk factors account for the high rate of stroke among older adults. Smoking, obesity, diabetes, and hypertension are among leading modifiable risk factors, while advanced age and African American racial background are major nonmodifiable risk factors for stroke development, the same as those for other CV diseases.

Strokes are caused by three distinct pathological processes that stem from risk factors for the disease. A hemorrhage results when a blood vessel in the brain ruptures and part of the brain tissue dies. Emboli or clots that form in one area of the body may also travel to the brain and cause brain death. Finally, the carotid arteries, which carry oxygenated blood to the brain, may become clogged preventing blood flow and resulting in tissue death.

Often older adults with and without risk factors for the disease experience "little strokes," or warning strokes, called transient ischemic attacks (TIAs). TIAs are manifested by lack of consciousness for a short period of time lasting from 20 minutes to 24 hours and have the potential to cause loss of blood flow to the brain. Consequently, reports of TIAs should be accompanied by a full assessment and the identification of risk factors and symptomatology for stroke. In addition, a plan of care to prevent strokes from occurring must be implemented immediately.

Prevention of strokes generally involves the facilitation of adequate blood flow to the brain. In clients with a history of emboli, anti-embolitic therapy should be implemented and evaluated regularly for therapeutic efficacy. In patients with occluded carotid arteries, carotid endarterectomy procedures may be implemented (cleaning plaque from the carotid artery) in order to enhance blood flow to the brain and reduce the chance of an embolus breaking off from the plaque and moving to the cerebral vasculature. Effective auscultation of the carotid arteries for bruits (the sound of turbulent blood flow) during routine health assessments greatly enhances the early detection of occlusions in the vasculature and facilitates stroke prevention.

Strokes may best be prevented by implementing nursing interventions to reduce risk factors, such as obesity and hypertension. Diet and nutritional management, exercise, and weight reduction are primary prevention strategies that have been effective in reducing the risk of stroke. Blood pressure management with these strategies, as well as prescription

---

CULTURAL FOCUS

Both the incidence and the mortality rates for strokes are higher for Blacks than for Whites. Consequently, nurses must consistently assess risk factors for strokes in these populations of older adults, including hypertension, smoking, diabetes, and obesity.

medications, also reduces the risk of stroke substantially. Nursing interventions to prevent strokes in high-risk clients, or those with family histories or TIAs, include the administration of one aspirin per day, ticlopidine (Ticlid), or warfarin (Coumadin) and management of hypertension.

When symptoms of a stroke are presented, a computed tomography (CT) scan, or carotid or cerebral angiography, is usually conducted, and the cause of the symptoms is identified. If the stroke is due to the development of a clot (or thrombus), tissue plasminogen activator (tPA), a clot-dissolving drug, may be administered immediately. The tPA may potentially dissolve the clot that caused the stroke and quickly restore blood flow to the brain (Hogstel, 2001). Nursing care for patients with stroke focuses on stabilization of the client and rehabilitation to the highest possible functional level.

DIABETES MELLITUS

Diabetes mellitus (DM) is a chronic medical disease manifested by an increase in blood glucose levels. The American College of Physicians (2007) reports that 1 in every 14 Americans has diabetes, resulting in over 200,000 deaths, 82,000 amputations, and 44,400 new cases of renal disease each year. Due to greater screening and educational efforts at the state and national levels, diagnosis rates for diabetes increased 49% from 1990 to 2000 and are expected to continue to rise (http://www.cdc.gov/diabetes/pubs/glance.htm#growing).

DM is a prevalent disease among older adults, manifested by an alteration in the production and use of insulin (Hogstel, 2001). In older adults, elevated blood glucose levels symptomatic of DM result from altered insulin availability. This is related to defects in the action and/or production of insulin. When the glucose levels are elevated (hyperglycemia) glucose spills into the urine, hence the name *diabetes mellitus*, which translates to *sweet urine*. There are two different types of diabetes mellitus: Type 1 and Type 2. Type 1 is also known as juvenile onset DM, or insulin dependent DM (IDDM). Type 2 DM generally appears during older adulthood and is known as adult onset DM (AODM), or more commonly, noninsulin dependent diabetes mellitus (NIDDM).

Diabetes and heart disease often go together with obesity and high cholesterol to form what is commonly known as the cardiovascular dysmetabolic syndrome. This syndrome involves a cluster of symptoms including dyslipidemia, hypertension, hyperglycemia, hyperinsulinemia, and endothelial dysfunction. Having diabetes raises the risk of cardiovascular complications because it can cause vascular changes. The insulin sensitivity thought to result in DM may precede disease development by several years and should be closely watched for by nurses caring for obese patients.

Smoking greatly affects the symptoms of cardiovascular dysmetabolic syndrome and is the greatest modifiable risk factor for preventing complications from diabetes. As reported in Chapter 5, smoking cessation even after many years of heavy smoking may result in health benefits in the older population and should be encouraged by nurses working with older clients.

Nursing interventions for diabetes must begin with a thorough assessment of functional ability, physical health, social support, financial support, and older adult's goals for treatment. The type of therapy should be tailored to the individual client's needs and issues. Overall goals aim at reduction of cardiovascular risk factors, smoking cessation, exercise, proper weight control, and control of hypertension. Diet and exercise are two important therapeutic options. Exercise is helpful in increasing insulin sensitivity (American College of Physicians, 2007), and many nursing homes and care facilities offer exercise programs.

Therapeutic goals for older adults with NIDDM focus on blood glucose control. This may be accomplished with low carbohydrate, diabetic diets and weight loss and exercise, as well as management of the disease with oral hypoglycemic medications and insulin when necessary. Complications of NIDDM resulting from poor blood sugar control include peripheral neuropathy, nephropathy, retinopathy, erectile dysfunction, foot ulcers, and kidney failure. The use of angiotensin-converting enzyme (ACE) is often recommended to minimize the damage to the kidneys from poor blood sugar control.

NIDDM among older adults is closely linked to obesity and physical inactivity in this population. Weight reduction is essential for managing NIDDM in obese older adults, and it is of great importance for older adults with NIDDM to develop healthy eating habits that will result in control of glucose levels. Self-management of NIDDM in the elderly includes a suitable diet, medication use, blood glucose monitoring, foot examination, and exercise. Certain age-related barriers may prevent older adults from following appropriate diets, adhering to medication and blood sugar regimens, and beginning and maintaining an exercise program. Examples of barriers to disease management include poor vision (can result from diabetic retinopathy or cataracts), co-morbidities, or decreased motor function. For more information on promoting exercise, dietary assessments, and nutritional counseling, see Chapter 5.

While educating older adults with NIDDM, it is important to note that medications may produce episodes of low blood sugar or hypoglycemia. Consequently, older adults should be encouraged to carry lifesavers or a sugary candy with them at all times to take in the event that they feel weak or dizzy from hypoglycemia. It is also important to teach patients how to monitor their daily blood sugar. The use of an alarm clock or wristband, blood sugar tests, and other medications or activities may help to increase adherence to blood sugar monitoring. Clinical management of NIDDM involves awareness of symptoms in elderly patients, establishment of healthy diet and exercise regimens, and maintenance of hypoglycemic or insulin medications necessary to control blood sugar and prevent complications.

INFECTIOUS DISEASES

Influenza

Influenza, commonly known as the flu, is a contagious viral disease that frequently infects the population in the winter months. The Centers for Disease Control (CDC, 2007d) report that between 10% and 20% of the U.S. population are infected with the influenza virus each year. The flu is often only a mild disease in healthy children and adults, manifesting symptoms such as fever, sore throat, dry cough, headache, and aching muscles. Older adults are more likely to develop life-threatening complications from the flu, such as changes in mental status, dehydration, pneumonia, extreme tiredness, and death. Each year, approximately 36,000 U.S. residents die from influenza, and 200,000 more are hospitalized from the disease (CDC, 2006b).

The influenza virus is spread via droplets through the air when someone infected with the virus coughs or sneezes. The viruses are spread quickly from one person to another, particularly in places where there is a large gathering of people. Carriers of the influenza virus may spread the disease even before they begin experiencing symptoms.

Similar to pneumonia and other acute and chronic illnesses, older adults may present with flu symptoms differently from their younger counterparts. The classic symptoms of cough, congestion, nausea, and vomiting may be absent or attributed to other disease processes. Older adults with the flu may present with acute confusion or delirium. Consequently, careful histories should be taken to differentiate symptoms of the flu from other illnesses, such as chronic dementia, depression, or psychosis. If the client has chronic confusion or dementia, the presence of influenza may cause deterioration of the baseline cognitive and functional status.

Evaluation of the symptoms of flu is essential when assessing older clients, especially during high-incidence seasons. Once an older adult develops the flu, nursing interventions include making sure that the client gets plenty of rest as well as maintaining nutrition and hydration. Symptomatic treatment of the disease with fever reducers, such as acetaminophen or ibuprofen, and cough suppressants is also often necessary. Because the flu can quickly develop into pneumonia in the older population, vigilant evaluation and treatment of the symptoms is imperative.

Vaccination remains the most commonly used method of preventing and reducing the impact of the flu. Vaccination is required each year, because the flu viruses change constantly and unpredictably. Due to the potential life-threatening complications of the flu, the U.S. Public Health Service strongly encourages all older adults to get an annual flu vaccination, which is currently reimbursed by Medicare. However, as noted earlier, all older adults do not have Medicare, especially those from various cultural backgrounds that may have recently immigrated to the United States. In these cases, some health departments, grocery stores, pharmacies, and senior centers offer free or low-cost vaccination clinics. Nurses should encourage all older adults to get annual influenza vaccinations. Contrary to popular opinion, receiving the flu vaccine *does not* cause the flu. The most frequent side effect of vaccination is soreness and redness around the vaccination site for 1–2 days. Reactions of low fever, malaise, and muscle aches occur infrequently and most often affect persons with no exposure to flu viruses, such as young children. Immediate reactions, which are usually allergic reactions such as hives, swelling of lips or tongue, and acute respiratory distress, only affect those who have a hypersensitivity to a component of the vaccine component, usually egg protein. Because the flu vaccine contains a small quantity of egg protein, individuals with severe allergies to egg should consult with their physician before receiving the flu vaccine. The vaccine takes approximately 2–3 weeks to begin working.

Pneumonia

Although pneumonia is a grave health concern for all populations, it is a substantial problem for older adults. Pneumonia results in the highest number of infectious disease deaths in the United States with an estimated 60,000 deaths each year (Institute for Clinical Systems Improve-

---

CULTURAL FOCUS

Medicare currently reimburses providers for annual influenza vaccinations. However, not all older adults have Medicare, especially those from various cultural backgrounds that may have recently immigrated to the United States. In these cases, some health departments offer free or low-cost vaccination clinics. Nurses should encourage all older adults to get annual influenza vaccinations.

---

ment [IGSI], 2003). The death rate from pneumonia is even higher among older adults who have had recent surgery or been weaned from mechanical ventilation, and it has a great impact on society because of the high costs involved in treating this disease (Hogstel, 2001). Moreover, the rates of pneumonia are projected to increase commensurate with the rise in the geriatric population.

Normal changes of aging, such as lowered immune status, and changes in respiratory function (Graf, 2006), including altered cough reflex and diminished airway clearance, play an important role in the increased risk of morbidity and mortality from pneumonia among older adults. The presence of chronic diseases such as COPD, CHF, GERD, impaired swallowing and tube feeding, and impaired mobility, as well as alterations in levels of nutrition, also are risk factors for pneumonia and resulting poor outcomes. Malnourished older adults, or those who have a low albumin (Hogstel, 2001), are also at high risk for pneumonia.

The symptoms of infection change with age, resulting in both delayed diagnosis and treatment of pneumonia among the elderly. These factors contribute greatly to the increased mortality rate of the disease among older adults. The delay occurs because pneumonia has a wide variety of presentations. The traditional symptoms include cough, fever, and dyspnea. Purulent sputum and pleuritic chest pain are often absent or difficult to assess among older adults, but most experience confusion or delirium, altered functional abilities, and/or decompensation of under-lying illnesses. These symptoms are often present, along with the atypical symptoms, but not in all cases. Amella (2004) reports that the fever and chills associated with infectious diseases, such as pneumonia, are often replaced with confusion and decreased functional status in older adults. Amella (2004) further reports that an increased respiratory rate, with decreased appetite and functioning, may be more sensitive for pneumonia in this population than traditional symptoms. The presence of changes in cognitive status among older adults as the presenting sign and symptom of disease cannot be stressed significantly enough. Consequently, when an older adult presents with acute confusion or delirium, or changes in baseline cognitive function, a careful history and physical exam should be undertaken in order to determine the causes of these cognitive changes. If pneumonia is suspected, diagnostic testing, including a chest X-ray and white blood count, should be initiated immediately.

Nursing assessment and management of pneumonia is based on assessment of the disease as well as identification of the cause of infection. Older adults with pneumonia may be treated at home or within an acute or long-term care setting, as long as symptom management is adequate in these environments. For older adults who require intravenous antibiotics and frequent respiratory therapy, or for older adults with a history of poor outcomes from pneumonia and other disease, hospitalization is necessary.

CRITICAL THINKING CASE STUDY

Mrs. Giovanetti was a 75-year-old woman who lived independently in her own home with her husband. She volunteered 2 days a week at a local food bank and remained an active member of the community. Three days into the new year of 2002, she began to feel weak and tired. She shook it off as the beginning of a cold and went to bed early. The next morning, she could not get out of bed to perform her activities of daily living; she was confused as to place and time and was short of breath. Her husband called an ambulance, and she was admitted to the hospital with acute viral pneumonia.

1. What critical changes in function and cognition were present in Mrs. Giovanetti as symptoms of her disease?
2. How common is the presence of pneumonia in the older adult population?
3. What is the role of the pneumonia vaccine in preventing the presence of this disease in the older populations?
4. What risk factors did Mrs. Giovanetti have for developing pneumonia?
5. What nursing interventions would you plan for Mrs. Giovanetti to ensure a full recovery from the disease and prevention of iatrogenesis during recovery?

Nursing interventions for the treatment of pneumonia include the administration of medications aimed at destroying the causative organism or virus. In addition, high protein diets and increased fluid intake are necessary to boost the immune system and provide adequate hydration to clear secretion. Hydration should be approached with caution in clients with CHF. Antihistamines and cough suppressants should be avoided among older adults unless they are needed to help induce sleep at night, as both can prevent the cough reflex necessary to clear pneumonia-related secretions (Hogstel, 2001).

Treatment of fever and discomfort with acetaminophen or NSAIDs is indicated for pneumonia. Respiratory therapy, such as postural drainage and percussion, may also be necessary. Clients should be evaluated frequently for symptom progression. Complications that require follow-up and/or further therapy include (a) dyspnea, (b) worsening cough, (c) the onset or worsening of chills, (d) fever occurring more than 48 hours after drug therapy is begun, or (e) intolerance of the medications (Hogstel, 2001). The recovery period for pneumonia may be extensive, lasting several months for some older adults (Hogstel, 2001).

Sexually Transmitted Disease and Human Immunodeficiency Virus/Acquired Immune Deficiency Syndrome

While health care providers are becoming increasingly knowledgeable regarding the unique needs of older adults, the sexuality of this population has continued to remain largely unrecognized. Consequently, nurses often ignore the sexuality of older adults during assessments, assuming that this aspect of human functioning is no longer applicable. The possibility of older adults contracting STDs, such as chlamydia, gonorrhea, HIV, or hepatitis, is not often considered. However, the original Janus Report on Sexual Behavior found that weekly sexual activity for both men and women continues past middle age (Janus & Janus, 1993). Moreover, a recent study of 179 residents of subsidized independent-living facilities, revealed that the majority had physical and sexual experiences in the past year (Ginsberg, Pomerantz, & Kramer-Feeley, 2005).

Despite the prevalent myths, sexual activity among older adults occurs frequently and is on the rise simply because there are so many more older, healthier adults than ever before (Hogstel, 2001). Sexual activity in men is heightened by the recent availability of erectile agents such as sildenafil citrate (Viagra), vardenafil HCL (Levitra), and tadalifil (Cialis). Howover, because older adults often are not educated regarding safe sex practices and no longer fear pregnancy, condom usage is low, resulting in a great rise in the number of STDs and new HIV cases diagnosed among older adults.

Nurses must include a sexual history in the health assessments of all older adults. Sexual assessments are challenging for both the nurse, who often has no education or experience concerning sexuality in older adults, and the older adult, who may not be comfortable discussing sexuality with health care providers. Lack of experience and general discomfort with sexuality among health care providers prevents geriatric professionals from assessing and managing the sexuality needs of older adults. In the case of most older adults, particularly those from certain cultures, sexuality was not openly discussed. Some older adults may be hesitant to verbalize their feelings for fear of being considered as lecherous or depraved.

A model to guide sexual assessment and intervention of older adults is available and has been well used among younger populations since the 1970s. The PLISSIT model (Annon, 1976) begins by first seeking permission (P) to discuss sexuality with the older adult. This permission may be gained by asking general questions such as "I would like to begin to discuss your sexual health; what concerns would you like to share with me about this area of function?" Questions to guide the sexual assessment of older adults are available on many health care assessment forms. The next step of the model affords an opportunity for the health care provider to share limited information (LI) with the older adult. In response to the increase in older adults with sexually transmitted diseases, it is essential to provide them with safe sex information at this time. In the next part of the model, specific suggestions (SS) are provided to older adults to help them fulfill their sexuality. These suggestions may focus on the use of CDC recommended safe sexual practices. The final part of the model allows for intensive therapy (IT) to be provided to the older adult regarding sexual issues that may arise during the assessment. This may include the discovery of sexually transmitted diseases, which require treatment.

The assessment of an older adult's sexuality should take place in a quiet area that affords the client necessary privacy. The establishment of a trusting relationship between health care provider and client is essential. The nurse must be respectful of the older adult's sexual beliefs and practices and prevent judgmental thoughts or comments. Appropriate history questions regarding sexuality include (a) the number and history of partners, (b) sexual practices, (c) physical signs and symptoms of sexual problems, (d) the level of satisfaction with current sexuality, and (e) the use of protection and precautions. The nurse must provide education on safe sex practices to all sexually active older adults, including the use of condoms.

In the older adult population, STDs, such as syphilis, genital herpes, and hepatitis, may remain from earlier years and be passed unknowingly to partners.

Ten percent of all AIDS cases are among people aged 50 and older; 25% are over age 60 (http://www.hivoverfifty.org). However, it is important to note that this number is most likely low due to misdiagnosis and will continue to increase as the population of older adults increases. The number of cases of other STDs and hepatitis are also likely to increase commensurate with the increasing elderly population. Due to the normal and pathological changes of aging, symptoms of HIV and AIDS may go undetected. For example, common problems of aging such as fatigue, alteration in function, or altered cognitive status (Hogstel, 2001), which could be symptomatic for HIV, also occur as a result of normal aging changes. The awareness of the possibility of STDs among older adults heightens the awareness of these potential disorders and focuses attention on the need for diagnosis. When sexual history questions lead the nurse to believe that the older adult is sexually active, especially with more than one partner,

CULTURAL FOCUS

Many cultural biases present barriers to discussion about sexual practices among older adults, which make assessment difficult. In some cultures, sexuality is not discussed. Nurses must identify these barriers to assessment and in a respectful manner assess older adult's sexual practices. This will provide nurses with the necessary information needed to implement interventions to prevent the transmission of sexually transmitted diseases.

diagnostic testing may include the presence of semen and vaginal cultures to rule out infection. These tests should also be conducted if positive symptomatology for STDs is present. However, STDs, such as chlamydia, gonorrhea, syphilis, and other diseases, often have few or no symptoms. Vaginal or penile pain, itchiness or tenderness, and discharge may be symptomatic of STD infections among older adults. Because HIV is often transmitted simultaneously with other STDs, the nurse should encourage clients diagnosed with an STD to be tested for HIV. The ELISA test may be used to diagnose the presence of the HIV virus. If this test is positive, the Western blot test may be conducted to confirm HIV infection.

If STD, HIV, or hepatitis are diagnosed among older adults, appropriate drug therapy is initiated. Nurses should provide teaching and medication administration as needed. In addition, the diagnosis of these diseases provides an opportunity to teach older adults safe sex practices, which is essential in order to prevent further, or repeat, infection.

CANCER

While the presence of cancer is seen in all populations, the incidence and prevalence of cancer is disproportionate to the population. In fact, approximately 75% of all malignancies in the United States occur among older adults, which, at present, constitute only about 13% of the population. Individuals aged 65 and older were found to account for 56% of all cases of breast cancer and 80% of all prostate cancer in 2002. Clearly, advanced age is a risk factor for the development of cancer. But, older adults are also more likely to be diagnosed with cancer at an advanced stage when the cancer is less amenable to treatment and increased morbidity and mortality are more likely. Cancer diagnosis and mortality are highly associated with factors such as race and socioeconomic status.

For both older men and women, lung cancer remains the highest cause of mortality, followed by prostate cancer and colorectal cancer for older men and breast cancer and colorectal cancer for older women. Prostate cancer accounts for 43% of all new malignancies diagnosed in the United States. Historically, older adults have not received such aggressive therapy as the younger populations. Ageism and myths of aging prevented older adults from being involved in clinical trials for new cancer treatments, and health care providers often perceived this population to be at high risk for adverse effects from cancer therapy. However, more recently, older adults have begun to receive more aggressive treatments for cancer and are tolerating these treatments well. While special consideration for the normal and pathological changes of aging must be made, older adults should be offered all treatments available to the younger populations.

Approximately 218,890 men will be diagnosed with prostate cancer in 2007 (ACS, 2007). Of all men diagnosed with cancer each year, approximately 27,000 will die. This rate is even higher for African Americans (American Cancer Society, 2007). As stated previously, prostate cancer deaths are second only to lung cancer deaths in the United States (ACS, 2007). While 1 man in 6 will get prostate cancer during his lifetime, only 1 man in 34 will die of this disease. Moreover, prostate cancer is nearly 100% survivable if detected early (US Too!, 2004). The availability of prostate specific antigen (PSA) testing for prostate cancer has greatly increased the detection and treatment of early-stage prostate tumors in older men. The American Cancer Society (2007) reports that over 230,000 men will discover this year that they have prostate cancer with a median age of diagnosis of 71 years; more than one-third of those newly diagnosed are older than 75. Treatment for prostate cancer includes the options of internal or external radiation therapy, radical prostatectomy, watchful waiting, and hormonal therapy for late stage disease. Nurses play an instrumental role in providing teaching during and after diagnosis with prostate cancer as well as referring clients to appropriate educational and support services. Nurses will also be involved in administering treatments aimed at reducing the symptomatology surrounding this disease as well as aiding treatment.

Among older women, over 200,000 new cases of breast cancer were diagnosed in the United States in 2004. Like prostate cancer in men, the risk of women developing breast cancer increases with age. Between 1986 and 2000, women aged 50 and older were the only group to experience an increased incidence of breast cancer. This is likely due to both the increased numbers of older women during this time period as well as the greater availability and attention toward breast cancer screening, such as self-breast examination (SBE) and mammography. The progression in lumpectomy and mastectomy procedures, as well as new developments in radiation and chemotherapy treatments, has sharply increased the survival rate for breast cancer for older women. The nursing role in screening and administering treatments for breast cancer is essential in promoting good outcomes for these older female clients.

Nurses play an instrumental role in both assessing for cancer and cancer management. In terms of primary prevention, nurses must educate, counsel, and encourage clients to engage in cancer prevention activities, such as the use of sunscreen, smoking cessation, good nutrition, and exercise. Secondary prevention strategies such, as self-breast examination, mammograms, and prostate cancer and skin cancer screenings, should be recommended and followed-up to determine compliance. Providing support and information during the diagnosis process is essential in treatment decision making.

Pain management is another important role of nurses in managing older adults with cancer. The most common pharmaceutical medications used to treat pain in older adults consists of acetaminophen, nonsteroidal and anti-inflammatory drugs (NSAIDs), and opioids. However, the frequency of adverse drug reactions among older adults and analgesic sensitivity in this population (Chapter 7) underscores the need for the old cliché to "start low and go slow" (AGS, 1998). For example, NSAIDs contribute to gastric ulceration and mask pain that leads to ulcer diagnosis. Older adults have also been found to respond to morphine as if they were given a larger dose, suggesting the need to decrease morphine dosages in this population. It is important to note that pain medication for older adults should be given on a regular basis, not PRN, or as needed (AGS, 1998). Collaborative pain medications, such as antidepressants, anticonvulsants, and anxiolytics, may also be helpful in pharmacologically reducing pain among older adults. Nurses must also administer radiation and chemotherapeutics and manage the difficult side effects of these medications, which include nausea, vomiting, fatigue, and changes to bodily image. Several medications are currently available to minimize these symptoms, but they must be administered with caution among older adults.

PARKINSON'S DISEASE

Parkinson's disease (PD) is one of the most common neurodegenerative disorders affecting the elderly population. It occurs in 1 of every 100 persons over the age of 60 (Lyons & Koller, 2001). Furthermore, it is estimated that 3% of those persons over the age of 65 have PD, suggest-

---

CULTURAL FOCUS

While self-breast examinations are among the most effective methods for detecting breast tumors, many older women avoid self-exams and mammograms because of attitudes that one does not touch oneself or expose one's breasts to others. This may be a cultural belief or a holdover from the teachings of prior generations. Nursing assessment of comfort levels with self-breast examination and demonstration of appropriate techniques are essential at enhancing compliance among older women of all cultural groups.

ing that the occurrence of the disease increases with age (Noble, 2007). It is estimated that, more than 1 million older adults in the United States live with PD every day, which is more than many less frequent neurodegenerative diseases combined (Hogstel, 2001).

Parkinson's disease affects men more than women and Whites more than Blacks or Asian Americans. Nurses who understand the disease, are aware of the signs and symptoms, know available treatment options, assess individual functionality, and advocate for the client are best able to implement plans of care for these clients (McMahon, 2004).

PD is a slow and degenerative nature that results from the death of dopamine-producing neurons in the brain. By the time symptoms are present, 70% to 80% of these neurons have already been destroyed (Hogstel, 2001). Dopamine is the critical chemical responsible for body movement and balance. It exists in balance with another chemical transmitter, acetylcholine, which is not destroyed by the disease. When acetylcholine levels exceed dopamine levels, symptoms appear.

The causes of PD have not been determined. Recently, a genetic component has been identified by research, and this is currently under investigation. The roles of environmental toxins, poisons, viruses, and medications have also been implicated in the development of PD, but these are also still under investigation. Some medications, including chlorpromazine and haloperidol, as well as reserpine, methyldopa, and metacolpramide, have been linked to the development of PD symptoms.

There are no objective clinical markers for PD. The signs and symptoms of the disease usually bring the client into the health care setting, where a thorough health assessment is conducted. The diagnosis of PD is most often determined by the presence of three motor signs: tremor, rigidity, and bradykinesia. Noble (2007) reports that patients present with either "tremor dominant" PD or "motor disorder" characterized by gait distruance, rigidity, and postural instability. Besides these common signs, clients with the disease may exhibit additional symptoms such as depression and autonomic dysfunction.

Identifying the signs and symptoms of Parkinson's disease may be accomplished during routine health assessment, but nurses must be aware of the signs that characterize this disease, because they can be very difficult to assess. For example, postural changes that are typical in PD may present as other musculoskeletal changes common with aging. Assessment of the signs and symptoms is crucial for symptom management.

Signs and symptoms of the disease may be detected through a functional assessment of older adults. For example, tremors make it difficult to get dressed in the morning, rigidity makes it hard to get out of bed in the morning, and bradykinesia may impair mobility. Overall, individual function may be dramatically altered, and that should serve as a major warning sign for nurses caring for older patients. The client's response to the medication levodopa may also aid in the diagnosis of PD.

There is no cure for PD. Therefore, symptom management is the primary focus of nursing care. It is imperative to make an early yet accurate diagnosis so that an appropriate course of treatment may be determined. Although the causes of PD are still unknown, a significant amount of information regarding the disease is available. The goal should be to isolate the signs and symptoms that typically characterize the disease and provide specific treatment options, both pharmacological and nonpharmacological. As advocates for patients, nurses must understand and present to clients all of the options available for treatment. It is important that nurses assess each individual for characteristic signs and symptoms of the disease. The overall goal of nursing care for PD clients is to provide support for individuals with this life-threatening disease and their families and to meet physical, psychological, social, and spiritual needs as the disease progresses.

Treatment of PD generally combines levodopa with carbidopa (Sinemet®). These medications assist in boosting the level of dopamine in the brain, thereby minimizing the symptoms of PD. As symptoms progress, the ability to perform activities of daily living decreases and the need for pharmacotherapy increases. Yet, the question remains as to when to begin medical treatment. Some physicians recommend starting medication as soon as the symptoms are diagnosed as PD; others may recommend waiting until symptoms interfere with functional ability and functional disability becomes apparent. Side effects of the medications can include confusion, hallucinations, hypotension, nausea, and vomiting, so patients may choose to utilize nonpharmacological treatment options or delay medical treatment, thus postponing potential discomfort from the unwanted side effects.

If motor abilities are relatively intact, nonpharmacological treatments may be extremely beneficial. Physical and occupational therapy may help those with a shuffling gait, focusing on the client's balance abilities and providing assistive devices where applicable. Nutritional therapy is also essential when caring for the Parkinson's patient. Immobility is a major contributor to constipation and, therefore, it is important to assess the dietary needs of PD clients to prevent severe constipation. Exercise is also extremely therapeutic for clients with PD by improving mobility, flexibility, posture, balance, and overall function, as well as decreasing the risk of falls related to the disease (Lyons & Koller, 2001).

SUMMARY

As the lifespan continues to increase, the incidence and prevalence of both acute and chronic disease rises. The interaction of normal changes of aging and co-morbidity often results in acute diseases developing into chronic conditions among older adults. The risk factors, presentation, and duration of both acute and chronic illnesses is often different among older adults than of their younger counterparts. Older adults are at a higher risk for developing serious chronic illnesses than any other age group. Moreover, as the older adult population continues to rise, the number of chronic illnesses among this population will also increase proportionally. The presence of chronic diseases among older adults presents the risk for functional decline in the older population, which may greatly impact quality of life.

This chapter presented some commonly occurring acute and chronic illnesses among older adults and the appropriate nursing care for these specific conditions. In order to appropriately manage chronic illnesses among older adults, attention must be paid to the special presentation of disease in this population and the most effective geriatric health care management of the disease. With quality nursing care, acute and chronic illnesses can often be prevented or detected at an early stage, when treatment is more successful. Ultimately, the risk for functional decline will be minimized and quality of life maximized. Older adults may continue to maintain a high functional ability despite many chronic illnesses. With the help of knowledgeable and skilled health care providers and appropriate disease management, functional independence becomes a very realistic goal for older adults with chronic illness.

REFERENCES

Amella, E. (2004). Presentation of illness in older adults. *American Journal of Nursing, 104*, 40–52.

American Cancer Society. (2007). *Overview: Prostate cancer. How many men get prostate cancer?* Retrieved July 18, 2007, from http://www.cancer.org/docroot/CRI/content/ CRI_2_2_1X_How_many_men_get_prostate_cancer_36.asp?sitearea=

American College of Physicians. (2007). *ACP diabetes care guide*. Philadelphia: American Colleges of Physicans.

American Geriatric Society (1998). Chronic pain management for the elderly, clinical practice guidelines. *Journal of the American Geriatrics Society, 46*, 635–651.

American Geriatrics Society Panel on Persistent Pain in Older Persons. (2002). Clinical practice guidelines: The management of persistent pain in older persons. *JAGS, 50*, S205–S224. Available at http://www.americangeriatrics.org/products/positionpapers/ persistent_pain_guide.shtml

American Heart Association. (2007). *What is a heart attack?* Retrieved July 18, 2007, from www. http://www.americanheart.org/presenter.jhtml?identifier=3038238

Annon, J. (1976). The PLISSIT model: A proposed conceptual scheme for the behavioral treatment for sexual problems. *Journal of Sex Education Therapy, 2*(2), 1–15.

Centers for Disease Control. (2006a). *Heart failure fact sheet*. Retrieved July 18, 2007, from http://www.cdc.gov/DHDSP/library/pdfs/fs_heart_failure.pdf

Centers for Disease Control. (2006b). *Key facts about influenza and the influenza vaccine*. Retrieved July 18, 2007 from http://www.cdc.gov/flu/keyfacts.htm

Centers for Disease Control. (2007a). *Arthritis Data & Statistics.* Retrieved July 18, 2007, from http://www.cdc.gov/arthritis/data_statistics/index.htm

Centers for Disease Control. (2007b). *High blood pressure facts and statistics.* Retrieved July 18, 2007, from http://www.cdc.gov/bloodpressure/facts.htm

Centers for Disease Control. (2007c). Prevalance of Heart Disease—United States 2005. *MMWR, 55*(6) 113–118.

Centers for Disease Control. (2007d). *Key facts about the flu.* Retrieved July 18, 2007, from http://www.cdc.gov/flu/keyfacts.htm

Federal Interagency Forum on Aging-Related Statistics. (2004). *Older Americans 2004: Key indicators of well-being.* Washington, DC: U.S. Government Printing Office.

Fulmer, T. (2001). Acute care. In J. J. Fitzpatrick, T. Fulmer, M. Wallace, & E. Flaherty (Eds.), *Geriatric nursing research digest* (pp. 103–104). New York: Springer Publishing Company.

Ginsberg, T. B., Pomerantz, S. C., & Kramer-Feeley, V. (2005). Sexuality in older adults: Behaviours and preferences. *Age and Ageing, 34*(5), 475–480.

Graf, C. (2006). Functional decline in hospitalized older adults. *American Journal of Nursing, 106*(1), 58–67.

Hogstel, M. O. (2001). *Gerontology: Nursing care of the older adult.* Albany, NY: Delmar Thomson Learning.

Institute for Clinical Systems Improvement. (2003). *Health care guideline. Community acquired pneumonia in adults.* Retrieved May 5, 2005 from http://www.icsi.org

Janus, S. S., & Janus, C. L. (1993). *The Janus Report on sexual behavior.* New York: Wiley Publishing.

Keller, H. H., Ostbye, T., & Goy, R. (2004). Nutritional risk predicts quality of life in elderly community-living Canadians. *Journals of Gerontology, Series A, Biological Sciences and Medical Sciences 2004, 59*(1), 68–74.

Lyons, J. M., & Koller, W. C. (2001). Parkinson's disease: Update in diagnosis and symptom management. *Geriatrics, 56,* 24–25, 29–30, 33–36.

Martinen, M., Freundl, M. (2004). Innovations in long-term care. Managing congestive heart failure in long-term care: development of an interdisciplinary protocol. *Journal of Gerontological Nursing, 30*(12), 5–12.

McMahon, T. (2004. Continuing professional development. Parkinson's disease, palliative care and older people: Part 2. *Nursing Older People, 16,* 22–26, 28.

National Osteoporosis Foundation. (2003). *America's bone health: The state of osteoporosis and low bone mass.* Retrieved July 18, 2007, from http://www.nof.org/advocacy/prevalence/index.htm

Noble, C. (2007). *Understanding Parkinson's Disease, Nursing Standard, 15*(12), 48–58.

Rosengren, A., Wallentinb, L., Anselm, K., Gittc, S., Behard, A., Battlere, F., et al. (2004). Sex, age, and clinical presentation of acute coronary syndromes. *European Heart Journal, 25,* 663–670.

Shelkey, M. (2000). Pet therapy. In J. J. Fitzpatrick, T. Fulmer, M. Wallace, & E. Flaherty (Eds.), *Geriatric nursing research digest* (pp. 215–218). New York: Springer Publishing Company.

Stanley, M. (1999, July–August). Congestive heart failure in the elderly. *Geriatric Nursing, 20*(4), 180–187.

Us Too! International. (2004). Informed brochure. Retrieved January 16, 2005, from http://www.ustoo.org

Warden, V., Hurley, A. C., & Volicer, L. (2003). Development and psychometric evaluation of the pain assessment in advanced dementia (PAINAD) Scale. *Journal of the American Medical Directors Association, 4*(1), 9–15.

CHAPTER SEVEN

Medication Usage

Learning Objectives

1. Describe the demographics of medication usage in older adults.
2. Identify physiologic changes of aging and their effects on medication absorption, distribution, and clearance.
3. Discuss the prevalence of medication–medication, medication–disease, and medication–nutrient interactions among older adults.
4. Identify special considerations for administration of medications to older adults.
5. Discuss demographics and strategies for enhancing medication adherence.
6. Describe the usage of herbal and illegal drugs among older adults.
7. List medications that should be administered with caution in the older adult population.

Mr. Turner is a 73-year-old man who has been admitted to the hospital after being found unresponsive at home by his wife. His VS upon admission were T 97.5, P 75, R 16, BP 160/96, and a blood glucose of 640. He has a history of Type 2 diabetes and HTN, but states that he is not on any meds at this time. His wife states that he had been taking "some pills" but that they were too expensive so he stopped taking them. When asked if he checks his blood sugar at home, he states, "No, I never know how to work that machine and I ran out of the stuff that goes with it." His physician plans to start him on oral hypoglycemics as well as an insulin regimen and antihypertensives. A social worker comes to speak with him and his wife about payment options, and you, as his nurse, plan to do some diabetic teaching.

The story or Mr. Turner typifies today's older adult. In the United States, treatment of multiple acute and chronic illnesses often takes the form of medication. For every symptom, ailment, or illness, there is usually a long list of available treatments from which to choose. These treatments include a number of prescriptions and over-the-counter medications. The use of prescription, nonprescription, over-the-counter (OTC), and herbal medications among older adults is substantial. The availability of multiple and effective medications to treat the numerous diseases among older adults undoubtedly plays an instrumental role in the increasing lifespan of this population.

The availability and substantial usage of medications among the elderly is both of benefit and concern among older adults and health care providers. In fact, the use of excessive, and often inappropriate, medications among older adults remains one of the most prevalent problems within the older population (Morley, 2003). In the United States, older adults spend approximately $3 billion annually on prescription medications. Moreover, as adults continue to age, the number of prescription medications rise. The Centers for Disease Control and the Merck Institute of Aging and Health (2004) report that the average older adult takes five medications each day. Although older adults make up only 13% of the population, they consume 34% of all prescription medications and 30% of all nonprescription medications.

In an effort to reduce the large amount of unnecessary medications used by older adults in long-term care facilities, the Federal government developed the Omnibus Budget Reconciliation Act (OBRA) in 1987 and implemented it in 1990 (Standard of Practice—OBRA-90). While there has been some success, use of both prescription and OTC medications by older adults is disproportionate to census findings. Older adults currently represent only 10% of the population, but they use 25% of all prescription medications. The Alliance for Aging Research (2002) reports that the average older adult uses five prescription drugs and many over-the-counter medications.

Medication usage among older adults is complicated by several issues. Normal changes of aging often influence the manner in which medications are utilized by older adults. These changes affect how medications are absorbed through the gastrointestinal tract, skin, or musculature; distributed via the circulatory system; metabolized by the liver; and cleared from the body through the kidneys. These four pharmacokinetic mechanisms are also influenced by acute and chronic illnesses common in older adulthood, which may further slow or impair the ability of organ systems to absorb, distribute, metabolize, and excrete medications. These changes are summarized in Table 7.1.

TABLE 7.1 Pharmacokinetic Changes With Aging

Pharmacokinetics	Changes Within Older Adults
Medication Absorption	• Increase in gastric pH and a change in the amount of fluid within the stomach. • Decrease in time required for emptying stomach contents. • Takes stomach longer to move nutrients across the membrane. • Increased time needed for medications to become effective. • Increased time may also increase amount of medication absorbed. • Vitamins A and C may be more readily absorbed.
Medication Distribution	• Reduced lean body mass. • Increase in percentage of body fat. • Total body intracellular and extracellular water decreases by 15%. • Alterations in plasma protein binding. • Cardiac output declines by 1% every year. • Blood flow to the liver declines from 0.3% to 1.5% a year.
Medication Metabolism	• Reduced blood flow to the liver. • Decrease in functional liver cells. • The enzymes used to break down medicines are reduced.
Medication Elimination	• Reduction in the mass and a reduction in the number and size of the nephrons. • Reduced glomerular filtration rate. • Decreased renal tubular secretion. • Increased medication half-life.

PHARMACOKINETICS AND PHARMACODYNAMICS

Pharmacokinetics focuses on the drug absorption, distribution, protein binding, hepatic metabolism (biotransformation), and renal excretion. Specifically, pharmacokinetics is the study of how normal and pathological aging changes affect how medications are received into the body, distributed throughout the body, changed to their active form, and excreted when they complete their role. Among older adults, pharmacokinetics is focused on how medications are absorbed through the gastrointestinal track, skin, or musculature. The normal changes of aging that result in a decrease in subcutaneous tissue and muscle mass are considered here. Pharmacokinetics also focuses on how medications are distributed via the circulatory system. Consequently, slow circulatory systems, common among older adults, result in changes in the drug distribution aspect of pharmacokinetics. How medications are metabolized by the liver and cleared from the body through the kidneys are also components of pharmacokinetic study. Pharmacokinetics has resulted in a number of clinical interventions for older adults. For example, knowing that older adults experience slower absorption of medications may result in the need for a greater time period to achieve desired drug effect. It is important for nurses caring for older adults to understand the impact of normal and pathological age-related changes of aging in order to provide the plan of care that will achieve optimal medication effectiveness.

Pharmacodynamics focuses on drug effects at the receptor level. This refers to how medications work once they get to where they are supposed to go. It has also been referred to as what a drug does to the body. Pharmacodynamic changes are often caused by normal aging, but these processes have been poorly studied and it is not well understood why some drugs reveal enhanced effectiveness, while others do not.

Pharmacodynamic changes among older adults are challenging for researchers, partly because specific organ responsiveness to medications changes as people age. However, some specific pharmacodynamic changes have been found among several drugs commonly prescribed for older adults. For example, the California Drug Registry (2005) reports that increased receptor responses have been documented for benzodiazepines (commonly used for sleep enhancement), opiates (used for pain relief), and warfarin (used for several conditions in which blot clots would commonly form). Because of the change in pharmacodynamics, older adults receiving these medications experience increased responses to these medications, including increased sedation with benzodiazepines, increased analgesia and respiratory suppression with the use of opiates, and increased anticoagulant effects with the use of Warfarin. Other organ systems have also been noted to result in changes in pharmacodynamics among older adults, including the central nervous system, bowel, bladder, and cardiac system. Changes in pharmacodynamics are of concern to nurses caring for older adults because they may result in both the increased effects of medication among older adults and a higher incidence of adverse drug reactions.

Medication Absorption

Several changes occur in the gastrointestinal system throughout life. These include an increase in gastric pH and a change in the amount of fluid within the stomach, as well as a decrease in the time required to empty stomach contents and move active products and nutrients across membranes. As part of the normal changes to the elderly circulatory system, there is a decrease in the intestinal blood flow and altered intestinal motility. Some studies have reported an approximately 20% decrease in the small intestine surface area. Currently, there is no research to support that drug absorption decreases as a result of normal aging. However, the slowing of many gastrointestinal symptoms leads health care professionals to believe that an increased amount of time is necessary for medications to become effective in older adults. It is important to note that increased time for absorption may also increase the amount of medication absorbed. For example, vitamins A and C may be more readily absorbed among older adults because they remain in the small intestine longer.

In addition to these normal changes of aging, it is important to consider the number of changes in nutritional levels and eating habits as well as various disease states that may affect drug absorption. There is a substantial prevalence of nutritional deficiencies among older adults, partly due to normal changes of aging. For example, decrease in smell, vision, and taste and the high frequency of dental problems makes it difficult for the older adult to maintain adequate daily nutrition. Furthermore, lifelong eating habits, such as a diet high in fat and cholesterol, are other obstacles to maintaining optimal nutrition. Such a diet is a leading cause of coronary artery disease. Nutrition and hydration assessment are necessary to help older adults minimize the effects of aging on drug absorption. Teachings regarding appropriate food choices, such as avoiding spicy foods, which may be irritating to the stomach lining, are essential to changing nutritional patterns and reducing the effects of nutrition on drug absorption. Taking small steps toward good nutrition, by slowly replacing unhealthy food choices with healthier alternatives, is the most appropriate nursing intervention to help achieve nutritional outcomes.

Several diseases occur more commonly in the older population and impact drug absorption. Achlorhydria, a disease that greatly reduces the acidity of the stomach, may make it difficult to dissolve medications for absorption. Other gastrointestinal disorders, such as gastroesophageal reflux disease (GERD), or surgery to the stomach or small intestine, may also alter drug absorption. Moreover, polypharmacy among the elderly plays an impact on drug absorption, as multiple medications compete for the same sites. For example, antacids, taken with some antibiotics or cardiac medications may decrease the absorption of the later.

To illustrate the effects of normal changes of aging on absorption, consider the case of a 75-year-old man in good health and residing in the community. He walks 2 miles each day, continues to work, and takes a daily multivitamin. He visits the primary care clinic for a routine physical examination and complains of fatigue, headaches, flushing, and difficulty sleeping. His history, health assessment, and physical exam do not reveal any acute or chronic medical problems. It is recommended that he discontinue the multivitamin, because his symptoms are consistent with vitamin A toxicity. When his blood values return from the lab, this diagnosis is confirmed. The patient discontinued the multivitamin, and the symptoms were relieved.

Medication Distribution

There are several factors that affect drug distribution among older adults. These include changes in fluid pH, plasma protein, and serum albumin concentrations; reduced lean body mass; a relative decrease in total body water; and an increase in the percentage of body fat, blood flow, and tissue–protein concentration. These normal aging changes have the potential to alter the distribution of the medication compared to the blood concentration. These anatomical and physiology aging changes have the potential to greatly impact medication distribution among older adults.

Total body intracellular and extracellular water decreases by as much as 15% among older adults. This reduces the distribution of water-soluble medications and increases the distribution of fat-soluble medications. For example, medications such as digoxin, lithium, aminoglycosides, and cimetidine, which are water soluble, have the tendency to become elevated among older adults. Consequently, administration of water-soluble medications must be done with caution. Increased caution should be used when administering any of these medications with diuretics, which further reduce fluid volume in the body. Additionally, lean body mass is reduced in older adults. The proportion of fat tissue increases with age from 18% to 36% in men and from 36% to 48% in women between the ages of 20 and 80 years. Consequently, fat-soluble medications, such as barbiturates, phenothiazines, benzodiazepines, and phenytoin, have the tendency to accumulate in the increased fat distribution of older adults resulting in a prolonged half-life of these medications.

Alterations in plasma protein binding, which may occur as part of the normal aging process, are of particular concern to nurses caring for older adults (Hogstel, 2001). This change could potentially alter the distribution of a medication significantly, as well as change the half-life of a medication and disrupt the steady flow of medication needed for disease management. As with drug absorption, this change is exacerbated by other medications, which compete for the same binding sites. Plasma protein binding can affect drug distribution, especially for drugs that are highly protein bound. This change is particularly important for older adults with multiple chronic illnesses that further reduce serum albumin

(Hogstel, 2001). When serum albumin is decreased, the number of available binding sites for medications is also decreased. This results in an increased amount of active medication in the circulation and the potential for drug toxicity as free medication is potentially absorbed.

The cardiac output, which decreases by about 1% each year after the age of 30, has further potential to alter medication distribution. Moreover, blood flow to the liver, which decreases from 0.3% to 1.5% per year, and blood flow to the kidneys must also be considered as metabolism and elimination of such medications is dependent on their distribution to these organs (Hogstel, 2001). With an altered blood flow, it is possible that medications will have an increased half-life.

To illustrate the effects of normal changes of aging on distribution, consider the case of a 95-year-old woman with a heel ulcer in need of debridement. The client has multiple medical illnesses, including a long history of heart failure (HF). The normal protocol is to administer pain medication 30 minutes prior to the procedure. However, as the procedure begins, the nurse realizes that the patient is experiencing pain. The nurse requests that the surgeon stop the procedure and try again in another 30 minutes. Sixty minutes after the administration of medication, the procedure begins again; this time the client remains pain free because the medication was given increased time for distribution to the site of pain.

Hepatic Metabolism

Normal changes of aging that affect the biotransformation of medications vary greatly among older adults. Unlike medication absorption and distribution, determining the function of the liver is difficult. Thus, while medication metabolism is dependent on adequate liver function, that function is difficult to determine. Consequently, in the absence of diagnosed liver disease, it is often challenging to project how medications will be metabolized among older adults.

Normal aging liver changes that affect medication metabolism include reduced blood flow to the liver and a decrease in functional liver cells, which have the potential to impact how effectively medications are transformed. There are two phases of metabolism within the liver that affect medication processes: phase I metabolism, which involves the use of enzymes to break down medications, is reduced among older adults; phase II metabolism, known as conjugation, is generally not affected by the aging process (Hogstel, 2001).

While normal aging changes impact liver function and consequently the metabolism of medication within this organ, pathological changes of aging and the presence of chronic illness and treatments further complicate the metabolism of medications in the liver. Specifically, the use of multiple medications, alcohol, caffeine, smoking, poor nutrition, and multiple disease processes have the potential to greatly affect liver function and reduce the metabolism of medications.

To illustrate the effects of normal changes of aging on medication metabolism, consider the case of an 83-year-old woman who recently lost her husband. A grief therapist who works in the client's community suggests that she take one or two over-the-counter Benadryl capsules to help her sleep during this difficult time. The client does as suggested. However, because this medication tends to be poorly metabolized by aging livers, the medication accumulates and causes a delirium to begin in the client over a period of several weeks. Consequently, the client must be admitted to a skilled nursing facility for safety reasons, until the delirium resolves.

Renal Elimination

Elimination of medications among older adults is one of the most well-studied and easily predictable age-related changes in medication pharmacokinetics. Older adults experience a normal reduction in the number and size of the nephrons, reduced glomerular filtration rate, and decreased renal tubular secretion. Thus, it is generally understood that older adults will eliminate medications more slowly than younger individuals, resulting in an increased medication half-life. However, it is important to note that these changes vary greatly among older adults.

While it is tempting to measure the glomerular filtration rate by testing creatinine clearance, there is often little change in serum creatinine concentration, despite normal aging changes. Consequently, creatinine clearance may not be the most reliable measure of renal function and elimination of medications among older adults. A more sensitive measure of medication elimination incorporates several variables, such as body build or weight, age, and gender. This formula, known as the Cockcroft-Gault formula, is used to calculate creatinine clearance (Cockcroft & Gault, 1976). It may also be used to calculate the correct dosage of medication for older adult clients. For example, opiate medications are often highly appropriate for older adults in pain, however, a reduction in the dosage of opiates is recommended. The Cockcroft-Gault formula may be useful in this case to calculate the necessary dosage to achieve pain management without unnecessary sedation and cognitive effects. Consequently, this formula may be helpful in calculating effect medication dosages across environments of care. However, it is important to remember that blood values for certain medications, such as digoxin, lithium, and procainamide, are also available and provide a more accurate measure of the medications levels within the body.

MEDICATION INTERACTIONS

Changes of aging and pharmacodynamics, as well as the presence of disease and the numerous prescription and OTC drugs taken by older adults (polypharmacy), makes this population at high risk for developing adverse reactions to drugs. In fact, older adults are estimated to be at 2–3 times higher risk for adverse reactions to medications than their younger counterparts. These adverse reactions result from drug-to-drug interactions, drug and disease interactions, and drug–nutrient interactions. The number of medications taken by older adults may independently predict the incidence of adverse reactions.

As the number of medications taken by older adults increases, there is a logical increase in the incidence of interactions between medications. Medication interactions occur when two or more medications are combined together, altering the strength and effectiveness of the medications. Many medication interactions may be predicted when administered to older adults based on previous knowledge of the drug. For example, the administration of vitamin K with warfarin is a well-known drug–drug interaction. In this case, the vitamin K increases the effect of warfarin, causing a potentially fatal reduction in clotting ability.

Despite the fact that the average older adult has three chronic diseases (Alliance for Aging Research, 2002), the number of older adults within clinical trials for new medications remains shockingly low. Townsley, Selby, and Siu (2005) report that older adults are significantly underrepresented in cancer clinical trials. While older adults are among the largest users of both prescription and OTC medications, the International Longevity Center-USA reports that 40% of clinical trials between 1991 and 2000 explicitly excluded people over 75 from participating. Consequently, information on the appropriate dosing, side effects, and medication interactions is not available to guide usage of these medications among the elderly.

Falman, Lynn, Finch, Doberman, and Gabel (2007) recently reported that the prescribing of inappropriate medications among older adults was common practice. In their study of 4,602 Medicare beneficiary patients over the age of 65, 44% were prescribed a medication that was known to be inappropriate among the elderly, and 15% were prescribed two such medications. The Beers criteria, developed from the HCFA Guidelines for potentially inappropriate medications in the elderly, presents medications known to place older adults at risk for developing adverse reactions (Table 7.2).

Medication–Disease Interactions

Because the average older adult has three chronic diseases, it is very common that the medications used to treat one disease potentially could affect management of another disease. This is especially true for patients with hypertension, congestive heart failure, diabetes, and renal failure. In patients with these diseases, the medication take for one can potentially impact the medication taken for another. For example, the use of several beta-blocker medications among older adults have reportedly contributed to increased episodes of already-existing impotence among older men. Another example may be the use of antihistamines, commonly prescribed or available over the counter for cold and allergy symptoms. In patients with benign prostatic hypertrophy (BPH), the medications may result in urinary retention (Hogstel, 2001). These drug–disease interactions may result in the need to discontinue a medication, or find an alternative that does not impact other disease processes.

Medication–Nutrient Interactions

Medications often interact with nutrients among older adults and have the potential to impact the nutritional status of the population in two specific ways. First, many medications have the tendency to impact appetite. For example, paroxetine, which is commonly prescribed for depression among older adults, may result in a decreased appetite and lead to weight loss and malnutrition. Conversely, several antipsychotic medications prescribed for bipolar disease or schizophrenia in the elderly may increase appetite resulting in the consumption of food poor in nutrients and obesity (Hogstel, 2001).

The second major interaction between medications and nutrients surrounds the impact of nutrients on the absorption, distribution, metabolism, and elimination of nutrients. In other words, nutrients have the potential to decrease absorption of medications, impair cardiac output, and alter liver and kidney function, which are critical for medication effectiveness. Moreover, older adults are at higher risk for medication–nutrient interactions because of normal and pathological aging changes, as well as higher rates of alcoholism and the use of restricted diets to treat disease. For example, the absorption medication may be affected by the intake of the medication with orange juice or milk.

Further difficulty in absorption may take place by the interaction of the medication with food. For example, some antibiotics may be rendered ineffective if combined with calcium or magnesium that was recently ingested during a meal. The use of nutritional supplements among the elderly, which contain many nutrients, may also potentially impact medication effectiveness. Administering medications via tube feedings results in a similar risk of nutrient–medication interactions (Hogstel, 2001). Moreover, certain nutrients may be excreted more quickly if they interact with medications, for example, diuretics, such as thiazide.

To reduce the risk of medication–nutrient interactions, it is important to pay close attention to the known interactions of medications. Medications should be administered with water, as opposed to orange juice, milk, or with nutritional supplements. Establishing an effective pattern of medication administration and evaluating medication effectiveness through assessments and care planning are the most appropriate nursing interventions to reduce medication–nutrient interactions.

GENERIC MEDICATIONS

With an increased emphasis on cost-effective health care for older adults over the past decade, the tendency to use generic medications is great. The decreased cost of these medications makes them very attractive to patients and third-party payers (such as Medicare). Generic medications must meet legal standards for effectiveness, safety, purity, and strength met by the original medication. Hogstel (2001) reports, "The total bioavailability of a generic medication may not vary from that of the brand drug by more or less than 20%" (p. 351); however, it is important to note that 20% can make a substantial impact on medication effectiveness, especially among medications with narrow therapeutic ranges. For example, generic forms of warfarin, which requires a narrow range for the effectiveness of clotting among older adults, may vary greatly from one generic formula to another. It is also important to remember that drugs within a given class may have differing side effects, which makes substituting one medication for another challenging. Moreover, physicians and nurse practitioners may not be aware that trade medications have been substituted for generics. For example, a generic medication may be chosen by a particular health plan that varies from the trade medication. There are clearly situations in which generic substitution should not be allowed. Consequently, it is the role of all health care providers to advocate for the most effective medication necessary to meet the needs of the client, and they should continually reassess the effectiveness of the medication. Nurses must request that patients bring medication bottles to the health care environment in order to determine if the older client's prescriptions have been filled with a generic drug or not.

INAPPROPRIATE MEDICATIONS

There are a number of medications that have been determined to be inappropriate for older adults and should be used with extreme caution. These are listed in Table 7.2.

TABLE 7.2   Beers Listing of Potentially Inappropriate Medications for the Elderly

amitriptyline (Elavil), chlordiazepoxide-amitriptyline (Limbitrol), and perphenazine-amitriptyline (Triavil)	disopyramide (Norpace, Norpace CR)	pentazocine (Talwin)	Antihistamines such as: single and combination preparations containing chlorpheniramine (Chlor-Trimeton), diphenhydramine (Benadryl), hydroxyzine (Vistaril, Atarax), PERIACTIN® (cyproheptadine HCl), promethazine (Phenergan), tripelennamine (PBZ), and dexchlorpheniramine (Polarmine)
	doxepin (Sinequan)	ticlopidine (Ticlid)	
barbiturates (all except phenobarbital)	meperidine (Demerol)	diphenhydramine (Benadryl)	INDOCIN® (indomethacin), INDOCIN SR® (indomethacin)
Long-acting benzodiazepines-chlordiazepoxide (Librium), chlordiazepoxide-amitriptyline (Limbitrol), clidinium-chlordiazepoxide (Librax), diazepam (Valium), and flurazepam (Dalmane)	meprobamate (Miltown, Equanil)	dipyridamole (Persantine)	methocarbamol (Robaxin), carisoprodol (Soma), chlorzoxazone (Paraflex), metaxalone (Skelaxin), FLEXERIL® (cyclobenzaprine), dantrolene (Dantrium), and orphenadrine (Norflex, Norgesic)
	ALDOMET® (methyldopa), ALDORIL® (methyldopa/hydrochlorothiazide)	ergot mesyloids (Hydergine), cyclandelate (Cyclospasmol), (other cerebral vasodilators)	
chlorpropamide (Diabinese)			phenylbutazone (Butazolidin)
digoxin (Lanoxin) >0.125 mg/day			reserpine (Serpasil), resperine combination products
			trimethobenzamide (Tigan)

Adapted from Beers, M. H. (1997). Explicit criteria for determining potentially inappropriate medication use by the elderly. *Archives of Internal Medicine, 157,* 1531–1536.

Consideration of normal aging changes in the amount of subcutaneous, fat, and muscle tissue should be considered when administering parenteral medications to older adults. With the decreasing muscle mass, it is possible that medications designed to reach the muscle may be injected deeper. This may result in damage to underlying tissues, as well as an alteration in expected response time to the medication. Assessment of a client's body composition and choice of needle size will help minimize harmful effects of parenteral medication administration to older adults. In addition, changes in vasculature may result in difficulty accessing peripheral intravenous sites for medication therapy. Providers skilled in challenging intravenous access should be consulted when alterations in vasculature prevent medication administration via this route.

MEDICATION ADHERENCE

It is generally reported that about one-half of all patients take the medications exactly as prescribed upon leaving the physician's office. The other half take the medications incorrectly, or not at all. Of those who take the medications incorrectly, one-third don't take it at all, one-third take some, and one-third do not even fill the prescription. Among the reasons for nonadherence to medication regimes is that health care providers fail to give clear instructions on use of the medication and when to take each dose. Moreover, the American Chronic Pain Association recently reported that 3 in 10 patients with chronic pain cannot fill their prescriptions because they cannot afford them; others simply forget to take it. Multiple prescriptions and complicated administration schedules, for example, medications that change dosages, contribute to lack of adherence (Hogstel, 2001). For example, many patients who wear daily nitroglycerin patches are not aware that one patch should be removed and the area cleaned, before applying the next patch.

CULTURAL FOCUS

The cultural backgrounds of older adults should be considered when choosing the route of medication administration. Some Vietnamese individuals may view medications administered via injection as more effective than those administered by mouth. Consequently, nurses caring for patients with this health belief may suggest an injectable form of a medication, if available.

Noncompliance rises along with the chronic illnesses commonly seen among older adults. As the older adult is asked to commit more time and resources to maintaining health, they are less likely to adhere closely to the recommended regimen. It is also important to note that older adults from various cultural backgrounds may not adhere to medication and treatment regimes because such plans conflict with their cultural healing beliefs. For example, a patient may be prescribed an oral medication to reduce blood pressure, but she may not take the medication, because her cultural background leads her to believe that oral medications are destroyed in the stomach and, thus, not effective. Enhanced understanding regarding older adults' health beliefs will result in improved medication adherence.

In order to promote maximum adherence, it is essential that nurses provide teaching regarding the recommended treatment regimen and assess patients' understanding, willingness, and capability to comply. In so doing, it is estimated that up to 23% of nursing home admissions, 10% of hospital admissions, and many physician visits, diagnostic tests, and unnecessary treatments could be avoided. Previous life experiences and cultural backgrounds can be very important in teaching older clients. Building on past experiences and integrating all aspects of life allows older adults to integrate new information on a familiar foundation. To aid in this teaching, many pharmacies provide information sheets with all new prescriptions that include:

CRITICAL THINKING CASE STUDY

Mrs. Johnson is a 90-year-old woman admitted to a skilled nursing unit for recovery from hip surgery. Medicare is paying for her 60-day anticipated stay. Her medications include: (a) Hydrochlorothiazide for hypertension; (b) vitamins E and C, and Aricept™ for early signs of dementia; (c) Zoloft for depression; (d) Darvocet™ PRN for arthritis-related pain; and (e) Restoril™ PRN for sleep. She generally takes her medications with orange juice each morning and PRN.

1. Which of Mrs. Johnson's medications are safe for her to take, and which should be administered with caution? Why?
2. What normal changes of aging may affect Mrs. Johnson's drug absorption, metabolism, distribution, and excretion?
3. What problems, if any, will Mrs. Johnson have in paying for her medications at the skilled nursing facility?
4. Do you anticipate any drug–drug or drug–nutrient interactions for Mrs. Johnson?

EVIDENCE-BASED PRACTICE

Title of Study: Congruence of Self-Reported Medications with Pharmacy Prescription Records in Low-Income Older Adults

Authors: Caskie, G., Willis, S.

Purpose: To examine the congruence of self-reported medications with computerized pharmacy records.

Methods: 294 members of a state pharmaceutical assistance program who also participated in ACTIVE, a clinical trial on cognitive training in nondemented elderly persons, participated by providing pharmacy records and self-reported medications. The average age of the sample participants was 74.5 years (range + 65–91); 87.8% were females.

Findings: It was found that 49% perfect agreement existed between self-reports and pharmacy records for major drug classes to 81% for specific cardiovascular and central nervous system drugs. Poorer health was consistently related to poorer self-reports.

Implications: Self-reported medications are more likely congruent with pharmacy records for medications prescribed for more serious conditions, for more specific classes of drugs, and for healthier persons.

The Gerontologist, Vol. 44, No. 2, 176–185.

- Name(s) of the medicine
- Ordered dose
- Directions for use
- Possible side effects
- Other drugs that should not be taken concurrently
- What to do if adverse effects occur

Low health literacy is currently considered a silent epidemic within the United States, affecting a substantial percentage of the population. Among the most at-risk populations for low health literacy are older adults who are also those most in need of health services. Healthy People 2010 defines health literacy as more than just an ability to read; it is action-oriented, leading to an improved capacity to be a full participant in one's health care. Health literacy requires that older adults not only be able to read information, but understand what they are reading, hear instructions, calculate medications, and communicate questions. Low health literacy often impacts the ability of older adults to fully understand medication instructions and health interventions. It disrupts clients' ability to effective prepare for diagnostic tests, make follow-up appointments, and maintain health. Moreover, low health literacy is a significant factor in noncompliance with health care treatments and medications. Kirsch, Jungeblut, Jenkins, and Kolstad (2002) estimate that more than 90 million Americans cannot understand basic health information. Nurses must be aware of the large prevalence of health literacy among today's cohort of older adults and assess their clients' ability to understand medication instructions fully in order to enhance adherence and health outcomes.

Easily opened containers are preferred by older adults and may be another intervention to increase adherence among older adults. Bold labeling of medications is helpful for visually impaired clients, and a review of medications should be conducted during each visit to a health care provider to encourage medication compliance. Clients should be encouraged to bring the actual medication container, as opposed to a listing. In this way, generic medications can be assessed, and the amount of medication remaining in the bottle can be measured against the prescription filled date. This process should include both prescription and over-the-counter medications.

Continual assessment of medication adherence and effectiveness is very important. Nurses should always know which medications their clients are taking, what these medications are prescribed for, and what the expected side effects and outcomes are. Changes in medication dosage and prescribing should be made when medications are found to result in adverse reactions, side effects, or are ineffective in meeting outcomes.

OVER-THE-COUNTER AND ILLEGALLY OBTAINED NARCOTICS AND HERBAL MEDICATIONS

The use of over-the-counter (OTC) and illegally obtained narcotic drugs and herbal medications among older adults is extremely prevalent and underdetected. Older adults use OTC medications and illegal drugs to treat pain, depression, gastric disturbances, anxiety, memory loss, and other disorders when they are unable to obtain or pay for effective treatment by health care providers. The use of these medications is often not assessed by health care providers, as older adults are assumed to be adherent to their prescription medication regime. However, the use of unprescribed medications among older adults is very widespread. Typical OTC medications used by older adults include analgesics (aspirin, Tylenol, Motrin), sleep aides (Tylenol PM, Benadryl), H2 agonists (Pepcid), laxatives, and antihistamines. Each of these medications has the potential to cause adverse reactions in the older adult population.

CULTURAL FOCUS

Older adults from various cultural backgrounds may be noncompliant with medication and treatment regimes because they conflict with their cultural healing beliefs. For example, a Hispanic client may be prescribed an oral medication, such as Vasotec™ to reduce blood pressure, but may not take the medication, because her cultural background leads her to believe that oral medications are destroyed in the stomach and, thus, not effective. Enhanced understanding regarding older adults' health beliefs will result in improved medication adherence.

A variety of medications is often used by older adults to reduce pain, enhance mood, or provide sedation. The use of illegal, narcotic medications is not a new problem to the older population, but this prevalent problem continues to be seldom recognized or evaluated by nurses and other health care professionals. Illegal and narcotic drug use among older adults results in great risk of harm to physical, psychological, and social functioning, and the effects may become long-term.

Nurses may fail to detect narcotic drug use because the symptoms of drug use, including alteration in mental status and function, mimic the symptoms of delirium, depression, and dementia, which occur frequently among older adults. Commonly used medications in these categories include morphine, codeine, Demerol, and marijuana, as well as other commonly used street drugs. While these medications may be prescribed by a physician or nurse practitioner and administered with appropriate evaluation of side effects and effectiveness, the use of these medications places older adults at very high risk for adverse reactions. Possible adverse reactions to OTC medications and illegally obtained narcotics include oversedation and respiratory arrest, falls, delirium, metabolic disturbances, and death.

The use of herbal medications to treat commonly occurring normal and pathological changes of aging has grown considerably over the past decade. The Gerontologocial Society of America (2004) reports that one-third of older adults used alternative medicine in 2002. Researchers in one California study also found that complementary and alternative medicine (CAM) was used by 38–50% of ethnic minority elders (Astin, Pelletier, Marie, & Haskell, 2000). Herbal medications may be preferred over traditional medications among many cultural groups including Chinese and other Asian cultures. Both the availability of these herbals, often referred to as nutraceuticals, and the anecdotal evidence of their effectiveness, have spawned the sudden growth in sales of these supplements. Nutraceuticals are also less expensive than prescription drugs.

EVIDENCE-BASED PRACTICE

Title of Study: Factors Associated With Illegal Drug Use Among Older Methadone Clients

Author: Rosen, D.

Purpose: To describe life stressors of exposure to illegal drug use and exposure of illegal drug use to older methadone clients.

Methods: The administrative data of a subsample of clients in a methadone clinic was reviewed. This study focused on African American and White clients who were over the age of 50. Respondents' age, gender, and race were socioeconomic control variables. Life stressors were defined as those variables that indicate economic well-being and living situations.

Findings: Exposure to methadone drug use within the client's social networks and neighborhoods significantly increased the likelihood of illegal drug use by the client.

Implications: Even though demographic trends show an increase in age of the methadone population the user numbers are also increasing. There is little research that shows their well-being and their needs.

The Gerontologist, Vol. 44, No. 4, 543–547.

The Gerontological Society of America (2004) reports that perceived effectiveness and lower cost resulted in 13% of older adults turning to herbal medications over prescription medication to treat medical problems.

Herbal supplements commonly used by older adults include vitamins C, D, and E, which have shown some evidence of reducing symptoms of osteoarthritis. Ginger and glucosamine have also been used extensively by older adults to reduce arthritis-related pain. Ginkgo biloba is widely used by older adults to enhance memory, and Saw Palmetto is used by many older men to reduce symptoms of enlarged prostate glands and to prevent prostate cancer. Ginseng is used by older adults to reduce stress, and St. John's wort is often used as an alternative or adjunct treatment for depression. A summary of the most frequently used herbal medications and their indications is provided in Table 7.3.

While these herbal medications promise older adults relief from their problems, they are not without danger. These medications may mask the diagnosis and progression of disease among older adults. For example, Saw Palmetto artificially reduces prostate specific antigen (PSA), the tumor marker for prostate cancer—leading to false negative results for diagnosis or progression of prostate cancer. Moreover, herbal medications have a high tendency to interact with other medications and conditions. For example, ginger interacts with warfarin, a commonly used blood thinner used by many older adults.

TABLE 7.3   Herbals and Herbal Components Under Study by the NTP*

Aloe vera gel	Widely used herb for centuries as a treatment for minor burns and is increasingly being used in products for internal consumption.
Bitter Orange	Bitter orange peel and its constituent synephrine are present in dietary supplements used for weight. Synephrine and other bitter orange biogenic amine constituents have adrenergic activity and may result in cardiovascular or other adverse effects similar to those induced by ephendra alkaloids.
Black cohosh	Used to treat symptoms of pre-menstrual syndrome, dysmenorrhea and menopause.
Bladder-wrack	A source of iodide used in treatment of thyroid diseases and also found as a component of weight-loss preparations.
Blue-Green algae	Claims to prevent cancer and heart disease and boost immunity. Use has been promoted for use in children to treat Attention Deficit Disorder
Comfrey	Used externally as an anti-inflammatory agent in the treatment of bruises, sprains, and other external wounds. Consumed in teas and as fresh leaves for salads. Based in part on NTP studies on the alkaloid components of comfrey, the FDA recommended that manufacturers of dietary supplements containing this herb remove them from the market.
Echinacea purpurea extract	Used as an immunostimulant to treat colds, sore throat, and flu.
Ephedra	Also known as Ma Huang. Traditionally used as a treatment for symptoms of asthma and upper respiratory infections. Often found in weight loss and "energy" preparations, which usually also contain caffeine. The Food and Drug Administration (FDA) has prohibited the sale of dietary supplements containing ephedra.
Ginkgo biloba extract	Ginkgo fruit and seeds have been used medicinally for thousands of years to promote improved blood flow, and short-term memory and to treat headache, and depression.
Ginseng and Ginsenosides	Ginsenosides are thought to be the active ingredients in ginseng. Ginseng has been used as a laxative, tonic and diuretic.
Goldenseal root	Traditionally used to treat wounds, digestive problems and infections. Current uses include as a laxative, tonic, and diuretic.
Green tea extract	Used for its antioxidative properties.
Kava kava extract	A widely used medicinal herb with psychoactive properties sold as a calmative and antidepressant. A recent report of severe liver toxicity has led to restrictions of its sale in Europe.

(continued)

TABLE 7.3   *(Continued)*

Milk thistle extract	Used to treat depression and several liver conditions including cirrhosis and hepatitis and to increase breast milk production.
Pulegone	A major terpenoid constituent of the herb pennyroyal. Has been used as a carminative, insect repellent, emmenagogue, and abortifacient. Has well-recognized acute toxicity to the liver, kidney and central nervous system.
Senna	Laxative with increased use due to the removal of a widely used chemical-stimulant type laxative from the market.
Thujone	Terpenoid is found in a variety of herbs including sage and tansy and in high concentrations in wormwood. Suspected as the causative toxic agent associated with drinking absinthe, a liqueur flavored with wormwood extract.

*Sales ranking from the *American Herb Association, 18*(3), 7.
From the National Toxicology Program Fact Sheet (2006). Retrieved August 2007 from http://ntp.niehs.nih.gov/files/HerbalFacts06.pdf

Safe usage of CAM by older adults requires health care providers to specifically assess their use during every health care encounter. Astin et al. report that 58% of those who use CAM did not mention their usage to their primary health care provider. Health care providers must understand the appeal of lower costs of these medications as opposed to the cost of prescription medications. An evaluation of the nutraceuticals and prescription medications used during the course of illness will provide the greatest safety for older adults. The most important nursing intervention to prevent adverse reactions from occurring with the use of OTC medications, alcohol, illegally obtained narcotics, and nutraceuticals is to assess their use then educate the client about the potentially dangerous effects of these medications.

SUMMARY

Older adults' utilization of medications is very high and will continue to rise throughout the twenty-first century. Medication usage in the older adult population is complicated by both normal and pathological changes in aging that affect drug absorption, metabolism, distribution, and excretion. Consideration must also be given to the interactions of various medications, including prescription, OTC, herbal, and illegal drugs, as well as alcohol and nutrients.

While much necessary attention has been focused on the excessive usage of prescription medication, the increased use of herbal medications

CULTURAL FOCUS

The use of herbal medications to treat commonly occurring normal and pathological changes of aging has grown considerably over the past decade. In addition, herbal medications may be preferred over traditional medication among many cultural groups, including Chinese and other Asian cultures. Both the availability of these herbals, often referred to as nutraceuticals, and the anecdotal evidence of their effectiveness have spawned the sudden growth in sales of these supplements. Safe usage of CAM by older adults requires health care providers to specifically assess their use during every health care encounter.

and illegal drugs by older adults will require additional attention and research in the future to determine the effectiveness and risks with these substances. Future study must also review ways to make necessary medications affordable for older adults.

REFERENCES

Alliance for Aging Research. (2002). *Ageism: How healthcare fails the elderly*. Retrieved October 16, 2003, from http:/www.agingresearch.org/content/article/detail/694

Astin, J. A., Pelletier, K. R., Marie, A., Haskell, W. L. (2000). Complementary and alternative medicine use among elderly persons: One-year analysis of a Blue Shield Medicare supplement. *Journals of Gerontology Series A: Biological Sciences & Medical Sciences, 55A*(1) M4–M9.

Centers for Disease Control and Merck Institute for Aging and Health (2004). *The state of aging and health in America*. Retrieved July 13, 2007, from http://www.cdc.gov/aging/pdf/State_of_Aging_and_Health_in_America_2004.pdf

Cockroft, D. W., & Gault, M. H. (1976). Prediction of creatinine clearance from serum creatinine. *Nephron, 16*(1) 31–41.

Fahlman, C., Lynn, J., Finch, M., Doberman, D., & Gabel, J. (2007). Potentially inappropriate medication use by Medicaid + choice beneficiaries in the last year of life. *Journal of Palliative Care Medicine, 10*(3), 686–695.

Gerontological Society of America. (2004, July 4). Alternative medicine gains popularity. *Gerontology News*, p. 3.

Hogstel, M. O. (2001). *Gerontology: Nursing care of the older adult*. Albany, NY: Delmar Thomson Learning.

Kirsch, I. S., Jungeblut, A., Jenkins, L., & Kolstad, A. (2002). *Adult literacy in America: A first look at the findings of the National Adult Literacy Survey* (3rd ed.). Vol. 201. Washington, DC: National Center for Education, U.S. Department of Education.

Morley, J. (2003). Editorial: Hot topics in geriatrics. *Journal of Gerontology Medical Sciences, 58A*, 30–36.

Townsley, C. A., Selby, R., & Siu, L. L. (2005). Systematic review of barriers to the recruitment of older patients with cancer onto clinical trials. *Journal of Clinical Oncology, 23*, 3112–3124.

CHAPTER EIGHT

Cognitive and Psychological Issues in Aging

Learning Objectives

1. Describe the prevalence of delirium, depression, and dementia in older adults.
2. Discuss the symptoms of delirium, depression, and dementia.
3. Identify the importance and components of mental status assessment.
4. Discuss treatment options for delirium, depression, and dementia.
5. Assess mood using a validated tool.
6. Contrast criteria for differentiating depression, delirium, and dementia in older adults.

Mr. Katz is a 75-year-old White male who enters his primary care provider's office very confused. He states that he needs to see the doctor "right now" and keeps repeating the request even though the nurse reassures him that the doctor will be right with him. As you take Mr. Katz to the exam room, he continues to be nervous and confused. His vital signs are stable. His wife says he was barely able to get dressed and out of the house this morning and has become increasingly able to do less for himself over the past several months.

One of the most prevalent myths of aging is all older adults will become senile, or demented as a result of the aging process. Becoming *demented* as one ages is of large concern to the aging population and their families and is the focus of a great deal of study in the older population.

Many assume that as people age they will ultimately become cognitively impaired. This image is perpetuated by the number of cognitively impaired older adults requiring care in nursing homes, in adult day care, or at home. However, this is not always the case. Many older adults live well into their 10th decade as sharp as they were in their twenties and thirties. While memory losses are common in older adulthood, the development of dementia is not a normal change of aging. Dementia is a term for a group of over 60 different pathological disease processes. These cognitive impairments develop as a result of disease, heredity, lifestyle, and perhaps environmental influences; they do not develop as normal changes of aging. Dementia is a chronic loss of cognitive function that progresses over a long period of time. Alzheimer's disease (AD) is the most common cause of dementia among older adults, making up about 50% of all dementia diagnoses, and there are approximately 4.5 million U.S. residents with AD. Dementia is a devastating occurrence for both older adults and loved ones, and much research is being conducted on the prevention, diagnosis, early detection, and treatment of AD and related dementias.

In older adults, three pathological cognitive and psychological conditions occur frequently that lead to cognitive impairment. These conditions are commonly known by those who care for older adults as the three Ds: delirium, depression, and dementia. It is important to understand the incidence, prevalence, causes, and treatment of these disorders in order to give appropriate treatment. Delirium, depression, and dementia occur from completely different disease processes, yet, they all tend to result in similar symptoms of cognitive decline. It is important to recognize the existence of these conditions in the older adult, screen for them appropriately, and refer the older adult for further evaluation and treatment at the earliest possible point of care. Key features of each of the three Ds are presented in Table 8.1. The following chapter reviews each of the three Ds in terms of the epidemiology, diagnosis, and treatment. They are presented in the order in which they may be assessed. In other words, if an older adult is experiencing signs and symptoms of impaired judgment, difficulty with language and calculation, disorientation or a change in behavior, then the nurse may consider delirium, followed by depression, then dementia.

Delirium

The typical scenario of delirium occurs as follows: an older adult is admitted to the hospital for necessary or elective surgery. When she arrives, the nurse asks her questions to complete the history, and she is able to quickly recall dates and procedures, such as the onset of arthritis or cataracts. She

TABLE 8.1 Comparison of the Clinical Features of Delirium, Dementia, and Depression

Clinical Feature	Delirium	Dementia	Depression
Onset	Sudden/abrupt: depends on cause; often at twilight of in darkness	Insidious/slow and often unrecognized: depends on cause	Coincides with major life changes: often abrupt but can be gradual
Course	Short, diurnal fluctuations in symptoms; worse at night, in darkness, and on awakening	Long, no diurnal effects; symptoms progressive yet relatively stable over time; may see deceits with increased stress	Diurnal effects typically worse in the morning; situational fluctuations, but less than with delirium
Progression	Abrupt	Slow but uneven	Variable: rapid or slow but even
Duration	Hours to less than 1 month: seldom longer	Months to years	At least 6 weeks can be several months to years
Consciousness	Reduced	Clear	Clear
Alertness	Fluctuates lethargic or hyper-vigilant	Generally normal	Normal
Attention	Impaired: fluctuates	Generally normal	Minimal impairment, but is distractible
Orientation	Generally unpaired severity varies	Generally normal	Selective disorientation

(continued)

199

TABLE 8.1 Comparison of the Clinical Features of Delirium, Dementia, and Depression (*Continued*)

Clinical Feature	Delirium	Dementia	Depression
Memory	Recent and immediate impaired	Recent and remote impaired	Selective or "patchy" impairment; "islands" of intact memory: evaluation often difficult due to low motivation
Thinking	Disorganized, distorted, fragmented, incoherent speech, either slow or accelerated	Difficulty with abstraction: thoughts impoverished; judgment impaired: words difficult to find	Intact but with themes of hopelessness, helplessness, or self-deprecation
Perception	Distorted: illusions, delusions, and hallucinations: difficulty distinguishing between reality and misperceptions	Misperceptions usually absent	Intact delusions and hallucinations absent except in seven cases
Psychomotor behavior	Variable hypokinetic, hyperkinetic, and mixed	Normal; may have apraxia	Variable; psychomotor retardation or agitations
Sleep/wake cycle	Disturbed: cycle reversed	Fragmented	Disturbed, usually early morning awakening
Associated features	Variable affective changes: symptoms of autonomic hyperarousal: exaggeration of personality type: associated with acute physical illness	Affect tends to be superficial, inappropriate and labile; attempts to conceal deficits in intellect; personality changes, aphasia, agnosia may be present; lacks insight	Affect depressed dysphonic mood exaggerated and details complaints; preoccupied with personal thoughts; insight present; verbal elaboration; somatic complaints, poor hygiene, and neglect of self

| Assessment | Distracted from task: numerous errors | Failings highlighted by family frequent "near miss" answers; struggles with test great effort to find an appropriate reply; frequent requests for feedback on performance | Failings highlighted by individual, frequent "don't knows": little effort; frequently gives up: indifferent toward test does not care or attempt to find answer |

Reprinted with permission from Springer Publishing Company. Forman, M., Fletcher, K., Mion, L., & Trygstad, L. (2003). Assessing cognitive function. In M. Mezey, T. Fulmer, & I. Abraham (Eds.), & D. Zwicker (managing ed.), *Geriatric nursing protocols for best practice* (2nd ed., pp. 102–103). New York: Springer Publishing Company.

is prepared for surgery, uneventfully undergoes the procedure, and is sent to the recovery room. Upon awakening from the anesthesia, she begins calling out for a person who is not present. She randomly pulls at her IV lines and pulls off her oxygen tube, alternating with periods of quiet rest. Because she is an older adult, the health care providers assume she is demented, give her sedative medications, and transfer her to a medical unit. In fact, although this scenario occurs frequently, the myths that surround the older adult's development of cognitive impairment could lead to inappropriate care for this woman. She is clearly experiencing the sudden onset, short-termed cognitive impairment known as delirium, but she may be diagnosed with dementia and sent to a nursing home for custodial type care. Due to the myths of aging and lack of knowledge about this cognitive disorder, delirium, like depression, is extremely under-diagnosed among older adults. Inouye et al. (2001) originally reported that nurses' sensitivity for detecting delirium in hospitalized elderly patients was low. McCarthy (2003) supported the need for strong environmental management of delirium in order to enhance patient outcomes.

Delirium is defined as a transient state of global cognitive impairment (American Psychiatric Association [APA], 1994) The diagnostic criteria for delirium includes (a) reduced ability to maintain attention to external stimuli and to shift appropriate attention to new external stimuli; (b) disorganized thinking; and (c) at least two of the following: (d) reduced level of consciousness; (e) perceptual disturbances; (f) disturbance of the sleep–wake cycle; (g) increased or decreased psychomotor behavior; (h) disorientation to person, place, or time; or (i) memory impairment. These symptoms of delirium, commonly thought of as acute confusion, usually develop over a short period of time (APA, 1994). Estimates of the incidence and prevalence of delirium in acute care settings show that approximately 16% of older adults experience this short-term cognitive disorder. Jacobson (1997) expected to see an increase in the amount of delirium reported as the population continues to age and the prevalence of dementia increases. Edwards (2003) reports that delirium is not a disease as much as a syndrome that may result from a variety of causes.

The symptoms of delirium are best classified using a delirium assessment tool, such as the Confusion Assessment Method (CAM). The specific symptoms of delirium that separate it from dementia are the acute onset and the fluctuating course of this disorder. In comparison, dementia develops over a long period of time, with fairly stable cognitive symptoms. For a diagnosis of delirium to be made, the older adult must also have difficulty concentrating on tasks, or conversations and either display disorganized thinking or altered level of consciousness. Delirium may develop in both cognitively intact and impaired older adults.

The cause of delirium is not fully known but is believed to be multifactorial (Balas et al., 2007). The presence of previous brain pathology, decreased ability to manage change, impaired sensory function, as well as the presence of acute and chronic diseases and changes in pharmacodynamic responses to medications, are all suggested causes. Cognitive impairment, a burden of comorbidity, depression, and alcohol use, have all been found to be independent predictors of delirium. Short and Winsted (2007) also found that medications, and surgical procedudres predicted delirium. Balas et al. (2007) report that older patients are at high risk for the development of delirium during acute care hospitalization.

Delirium has vast implications for older adults, their families, and the U.S. economy. Rizzo et al. (2001) report that delirium complicates hospital stays for more than 2.3 million older persons each year, involving more than 17.5 million hospital days and accounting for more than $4 billion of Medicare expenditures. The Harvard Health Letter ("Never Been the Same Since," 2007) reports that the presence of delirium has multiple negative outcomes and may and place older adults at risk for harm and permanent cognitive effects.

The most appropriate way to assess delirium is to understand its frequent occurrence in all settings, especially acute and long-term care. The use of a standardized delirium assessment tool, such as the Confusion Assessment Method (CAM), is essential for effectively detecting delirium.

Interventions to prevent delirium focus on best practices in care of older adults. While research on the causes and interventions for delirium is available, little has been done on work to prevent the onset of delirium in hospitalized older adults. Inouye et al. (2007) studied 491 patients age 70 years or older who were admitted to acute care units of large teaching hospitals. The researchers found that dementia, vision impairment, functional impairment, high comorbidity, and the use of physician restraints predicted delirium in the sample. Moreover, the authors stated that four of these five risk factors are amenable to clinical protocols that could be successfully implemented on the unit to prevent the onset of delirum in hospitalized patients, were implemented on the intervention units, and delirium was measured daily on all subjects. The researchers suggest that prevention of delirium is the most effective treatment strategy.

If delirium is assessed and determined to be the cause of cognitive impairment, the first line of treatment is to identify and remove the cause of the delirium. Delirium is a temporary and reversible condition, and full recovery is possible. A change in one medication is often the reason for the development of delirium, and a comprehensive analysis of medication should be conducted. While medications themselves may not

CULTURAL FOCUS

Language barriers common to various cultural groups within the United States may precipitate delirium, as well as sensory deficits and sensory overload or underload. All of these factors should be considered in assessing the older adult for delirium. Immediate detection and removal of the cause of delirium will enhance the patient's recovery. While the delirium is resolving, it is important to keep the older adult safe.

be the cause of the delirium, the interaction of a medication with another medication or with nutrients may trigger a delirium in an older adult. Translocation syndrome, resulting from a change in surroundings from a home to a nursing home or assisted-living facility, may also trigger the onset of delirium. Language barriers common to various cultural groups within the United States may precipitate delirium, as well as sensory deficits and deprivation. The onset of acute or chronic medical conditions, such as a urinary tract infection, or fracture, often precipitates a delirium among older adults, as well. Waszynski (2007) also reports that alcoholism and sensory impairment may cause delirium to begin among older adults. These frequent causes should be examined in the older adult with new onset cognitive impairment. If a new medication is added and an interaction is suspected, remove the medication, if possible, to allow the delirium to resolve. If a change in environment was the trigger, adding familiar items to the new environment and having family around may resolve the delirium. The older adult should also be assessed for the presence of infection or fractures and treated appropriately. If alcoholism is determined to be the cause, the removal of alcohol and the detoxification of the older adult will likely see the resolution of the delirium. Immediate detection and removal of the cause of delirium will enhance the patient's recovery to the quickest extent.

While the delirium is resolving, it is important to keep the older adult safe. This may include installing detection systems, such as chair and bed alarms, to alert caregivers of wandering behavior. Shelkey (2000) reports that specially trained dogs may be helpful in alerting caregivers of the sudden mobility of an older adult with delirium or dementia. Implementing fall prevention strategies, such as putting the mattress on the floor and ensuring that the older adult is in the most familiar environment possible, with appropriate translators, is essential. A calm, soft-spoken approach to care is necessary, and the delirious older adult should not be forced to participate in bathing or other behavior that frightens them. A sponge bath with warm water and a lotion massage may be more soothing and comforting than a shower for a delirious older adult. This calm

CRITICAL THINKING CASE STUDY

Mrs. Ortega was admitted to the hospital for repair of her left hip after a fall down her front porch steps. When admitted, she was alert and oriented and had a pleasant affect. The surgery went as planned, and Mrs. Ortega was transferred to the recovery room. Upon awakening from her anesthesia, she was highly disoriented. She began yelling, attempting to remove her IV, and trying to get out of bed. The nurses tried to calm her down, but without success. She was finally administered a sedative medication and transferred to a surgical unit.

1. Which of the three Ds does Mrs. Ortega most likely have? Why do you think this?
2. If Mrs. Ortega's pre-op status was not communicated to the surgical unit nursing staff, which of the three Ds would Mrs. Ortega most likely be assumed to have?
3. What risk factors did Mrs. Ortega have for developing this cognitive impairment?
4. What interventions could be put into place for Mrs. Ortega in the hospital and to make sure that this situation does not reoccur?

and understanding approach to care will speed the resolution of the delirium and prevent injury. Frequently reassuring families of the temporary nature of this illness is also necessary and essential for the emotional stability of the family and the continued support for the older adult.

DEPRESSION

Older adults experience many losses, including health, home, job, friends, family, spouse, and financial resources. These frequent losses are blamed for the high incidence of depression among older adults. It is not uncommon for a nurse or health care professional to state: "Of course they're depressed! I would be depressed too, if I went through what they did." In fact, one of the most prevalent myths of aging is that depression is a normal response to the many losses older adults experience. Older adults have the highest rates of depression within the U.S. population, and this is often attributed to the frequent occurrence of loss within the older population. While it is true that the situational life events mentioned previously play a role in the development or severity of depression, recent research on depression indicates that there is more to the development of depression than the experience of loss. In fact, the nature versus nurture controversy has uncovered the role of neurotransmitters

EVIDENCE-BASED PRACTICE

Title of Study: Delirium Among Newly Admitted Postacute Facility Patients: Prevalence, Symptoms, and Severity

Authors: Kiely, D., Bergmann, M., Murphy K., Jones, R., Orav, E., Marcantonio, E.

Purpose: To describe the prevalence of delirium, delirium symptoms, and severity assessed at admission to postacute facilities.

Methods: Subjects from seven Boston area skilled nursing facilities specializing in post acute care were assessed using the Mini Mental Status Exam, Delirium Symptom Interview, Memorial Delirium Assessment Scale, and Confusion Assessment Method (CAM) Diagnostic Algorithm. Delirium status was categorized: (1) full, (2) two or more symptoms, (3) one symptom, and (4) no delirium. Descriptive statistics were calculated, and chi-square analysis and analysis of variance were used to examine delirium characteristics by delirium group.

Findings: Among 2,158 subjects, approximately 16% had full CAM-defined delirium at admission, 13% had two or more symptoms, approximately 40% had one delirium symptom, and 32% had no symptoms of delirium.

Implications: Results indicate that 16% of persons admitted to post acute facilities have CAM-defined delirium, and more than two-thirds had at least one delirium symptom. The detection and management of delirium in post acute settings warrants the development and testing of strategies to detect delirium.

Journal of Gerontology, Medical Sciences 2003, Vol. 58A, No. 5, 441–445.

---

in the development of depression among older adults. Because of the many physiological changes in aging, this older adult population is more susceptible to the effects of altered neurotransmission than in any other age group. In fact, *Healthy People 2010* (U.S. Department of Health and Human Services, 2000) reports that older adults have the highest rate of depression, and the rate is even higher among older adults with coexisting medical conditions. Moreover, 12% of older persons hospitalized for problems such as hip fracture or heart disease are diagnosed with depression. Rates of depression for older people in nursing homes range from 15% to 25%.

It is now generally agreed that chemical imbalances caused by the decrease of certain neurotransmitters are the primary cause of depression among older adults. Both depression and suicide occur more frequently in older adults with a family history of the disease (Hogstel, 2001). Moreover, the National Institute of Mental Health (2007) reports that while more women have depression than men, non-Hispanic older white men are the most likely to die by suicide with a rate of 49.8 suicides per 100,000 older men. Hogstel (2001) reports a strong relationship between depression/suicide and drug and alcohol abuse. While a chemical component is the most likely cause of depression, role changes in aging, such as retirement, translocation, illness, and loss, may precipitate depression in at-risk individuals. The National Institute of Mental Health (2007) reports that 75% of older clients who successfully committed suicide had visited their health care provider within one month of the suicide. This indicates the great need for nurses to effectively assess for depression and suicidal ideation among older adults.

Changes in mood and thinking are the primary characteristics of depression. The DSM-IV criteria for a diagnosis of major depression disorder may be helpful in detecting depression. Just as there are differences among individuals, clients with depression differ in their emotional states. These differences may be based on cultural, ethnic, religious, or gender factors. For example, Aroian, Khatutsky, Tran, and Balsam (2001) reported that providing support services for depression and loneliness was essential among elderly immigrants to the United States. Physical symptoms of sleep impairment and appetite changes could easily be indicative of serious medical conditions, therefore, it is necessary to first rule out any primary medical concerns.

A complete history, including family history, is essential to begin the assessment of depression and should include questions about usual activities of daily living and any recent lifestyle changes. Use of the diagnostic criteria for depression is one way to ask about symptoms. There are also several depression scales, such as the Geriatric Depression Scale, which are easy to administer and assist with assessment of the client's condition. As stated earlier, depression often manifests itself as an alteration in cognition among older adults. The National Institute of Mental Health

---

CULTURAL FOCUS

Just as there are differences among individuals, clients with depression differ in their emotional states. These differences may be based on cultural, ethnic, religious, or gender factors. For example, Aroian, Khatutsky, Tran, and Balsam (2001) reported that providing support services for depression and loneliness was essential among elderly immigrants to the United States.

(2007) reports that in older adults with depression-related memory loss, drug treatment for the disease resulted in improvement. This syndrome, known as pseudodementia (Brown, 2005), may occur in both cognitively intact and cognitively impaired older adults.

There are many treatment options for depression, including medication and psychotherapy as well as electric shock therapy. The most frequently used form of treatment is medication. Not all older adults are afforded the opportunity for therapy that may greatly improve their levels of depression. Medication intervention in depression is extremely helpful and may be used independently or in conjunction with psychotherapy. There are several classes of antidepressants, including selective serotonin reuptake inhibitors, tricyclic antidepressants, monoamine oxidase inhibitors, and other atypical antidepressants. It is important to note that antidepressant medications taken in large amounts may result in death. In older individuals with depression, the risk of suicide is real; Hogstel (2001) reports the need to dispense medications cautiously in older adults who exhibit suicidal ideation to avoid overdosing.

Selective serotonin reuptake inhibitors (SSRIs) are a relatively new class of medications, and they work by inhibiting the reuptake of serotonin, thus increasing its concentration in the space between nerve cells. Fluoxetine (Prozac), paroxetine (Paxil), and sertraline (Zoloft) are examples of SSRIs. These antidepressant medications have an overall lower side effect profile than their predecessor antidepressants, but they are not perfect. The most common side effects of SSRIs are nausea, diarrhea, dry mouth, tremors, and insomnia. Because of these effects, SSRIs are usually taken in the morning right after breakfast, when clients are encouraged to be up and about, and the SSRIs help give them an early morning boost. Caution should be excercised when administering SSRIs to patients with Parkinson's disease, and possibly other tremulous disorders, because SSRIs may exacerbate their condition to the point of inducing Parkinsonian crisis (Hogstel, 2001). Because tremors are one of the more common side effects of SSRIs, it might be wise to consider another class of antidepressant for these clients.

Tricyclic antidepressants (TCAs) are still used commonly to treat depression among older adults, but they are increasingly replaced by newer classifications of antidepressant medications. These medications, including amitriptyline (Elavil), imipramine (Tofranil), and nortriptyline (Pamelor), typically are poorly tolerated among the older population because of the high side effect profile. They function by blocking the reuptake of selected neurotransmitters, such as norepinephrine and serotonin, which allows them to remain in the synaptic junction (the space between the neurons) for a longer period of time. The most frequently reported side effects of these medications include dry mouth, constipation, tremors, blurred vision, postural hypotension, and sedation (Hogstel, 2001). Administering the medications before bedtime often decreases the client's risk for falls.

Monoamine oxidase inhibitors (MAOIs) are rarely used because of their high risk of medication interactions and side effects. Examples of these include phenelzine (Nardil) and tranylcypromine (Parnate). They function by preventing selected forms of monoamine oxidase, which breaks down the chemicals norepinephrine, serotonin, and dopamine, and like the TCAs, MAOIs remain in the neuroleptic synapse for a longer period of time. Hogstel (2001) reports that common side effects include orthostatic hypotension, tachycardia, edema, dizziness, and agitation. It is essential that clients taking MAOIs adhere to a strict diet low in tyramines (found in aged cheeses, for example) and avoid specific medications (such as those containing ergotamine). Atypical antidepressants include trazadone (Desyrel) and bupropion (Buspar). Similar to SSRIs and TCAs, trazadone inhibits serotonin reuptake, and bupropion blocks the reuptake of dopamine, norepinephrine, and serotonin. Hogstel (2001) reports that side effects of these medications also may include dry mouth, dizziness, and drowsiness, as well as some gastrointestinal problems, such as nausea and vomiting, and an increase in the incidence of seizures. Stimulants such as dextroamphetamine (Desedrine or Destrostat) and methylphenidate (Concerta, Methylin, Methylin SR) may also be helpful in treating depression that is not responsive to newer generations of antidepressants.

Electroconvulsive therapy (ECT) is often poorly regarded among the lay public because of negative media attention surrounding it. However, despite its poor reputation, ECT is often an effective form of therapy among older adults. ECT may replace the use of multiple antidepressant medications and may benefit clients who have treatment-resistant depression. Prior to receiving ECT, older adults are administered an anesthetic and a muscle relaxant. Side effects include some initial confusion and disorientation, which typically resolves within a few days of treatment. The ECT treatments are usually given every other day for 6–12 treatments, with rapid resolution of depression exhibited.

Suicide

Untreated depression has the unfortunate capacity to end in suicide among older adults. It is estimated that 15% of severely depressed people commit suicide. The rate of suicide among older adults is disproportionate to the population; while older adults currently account for only 12% of the population, they commit almost 20% of all suicides. Early reports on suicide among older adults have revealed that while women make more suicide attempts, men are three times more successful at completing suicide. Moreover, if there is a family history of suicide, risk increases (Yesavage, 1992).

Diagnosis of depression is the highest risk factor for suicide. In addition, the relocation of older adults from home to long-term care institutions, living alone, and widowhood are also high risk factors for suicide among older adults. Nurses must be aware of these risk factors and take action when suicidal ideation is vocalized. Phrases such as, "I'm ready to die; I wish the good Lord would just take me," demonstrate feelings of helplessness, hopelessness, and worthlessness consistent with depression. Evidence has consistently revealed that approximately 80% of all people who have committed suicide told someone about it first, often a primary care provider. These types of statements require further evaluation with a standardized geriatric depression scale.

DEMENTIA

Decline in the cognitive function of older adults is one of the most prevalent concerns and a major focus of study in the older population. While normal changes of aging result in a decrease in brain weight and a shift in the proportion of gray matter to white matter, the development of dementia is not a normal change of aging. In fact, dementia, a general term used to describe over 60 pathological cognitive disorders, occurs as a result of disease, heredity, lifestyle, and, perhaps, environmental influences. It is commonly believed that all older adults will develop dementia as they age, but this is not the case. Memory losses are common to older adulthood, but they are often falsely labeled as dementia. Dementia is a chronic loss of cognitive function that progresses over a long period of time. The characteristics of dementia differentiate it from delirium (see Table 8.1), which has a sudden onset and acute duration. Dementia, as defined by the Alzheimer's Association (1999), is a "loss of mental function in two or more areas such as language, memory, visual and spatial abilities, or judgment severe enough to interfere with daily life" (p. 1). A commonly used scenario to discriminate between common memory loss and dementia is: If you lose your car keys, you simply experienced memory loss. If you find them and don't know what they are for—this may mean cognitive trouble.

Alzheimer's Disease (AD)

While Alzheimer's disease (AD) is not the only dementia affecting older adults, it is certainly the most common, making up about 50% of all dementia diagnoses. There are approximately 4.5 million U.S. residents

EVIDENCE-BASED PRACTICE

Title of Study: Memory Club: A Group Intervention for People With Early-Stage Dementia and Their Care Partners
Authors: Zarit, S., Femia, E., Watson, J., Rice-Oeschger, L., Kakos, B.
Purpose: To investigate the immediate and long-term consequences of dementia by examining afflicted individuals in the early stages of dementia while they can still participate in decision making.
Methods: A 10-session group program, Memory Club, is comprised of people with dementia and their care partners. Structured sessions of dyads, as well as separate meetings with other people with dementia and other care partners.
Findings: Participants evaluated this program very positively.
Implications: This study indicates that the person facing the long-term effects of dementia, as well as those who care for the afflicted individuals, found it helpful to converse with other persons in their same situation.

The Gerontologist, Vol. 44, No. 2, 262–269.

---

with AD. Some other types of dementia are multi-infarct dementia, Parkinson's-related dementia, Huntington's disease, Creutzfeldt-Jakob disease, Pick's disease, and Lewy Body dementia. Each dementia substantiates the classic definition given previously, including loss of mental function, but there may be different cognitive symptoms depending on the area/s of the brain affected by the disease.

Currently, the cause of AD is unknown. Research has supported only two risk factors for the development of AD—advanced age and a family history of the disease. Obviously, both of these risk factors are nonmodifiable. Consequently, the most effective treatment for AD is not risk factor modification, but early disease detection.

The Alzheimer's Association (http://www.alzheimers.org) reports that there are 10 early warning signs of AD, including (a) misplacing items, (b) loss of initiative, (c) changes in personality, (d) poor judgment, (e) changes in mood or behavior, (f) disorientation to time and place, (g) memory loss that affects job skills, (h) difficulty performing familiar tasks, (i) difficulty with finding the right words, and (j) problems with abstract thinking. In the early or mild stage of AD, clients still have many functional abilities, including the ability to perform certain tasks until they are completed (Baum & Edwards, 2003), therefore, AD may be difficult to detect by family and friends at this early stage, as older adults with the disease are often able to interact appropriately in a social environment.

Most often, the first sign of AD occurs when more difficult tasks need to be completed, such as writing checks to pay bills, scheduling appointments, or using the bus to get from one location to another. As the moderate stage of AD develops, the older adult will experience difficulty (a) finding the proper words to articulate thoughts or needs (aphasia); (b) performing fine motor tasks, such as household tasks or ADLs (apraxia); and (c) remembering (agnosia). Baum and Edwards (2003) report that older adults may have a limited capacity to learn and problem solve at this stage of the disease. All of these changes may create frustration for the older adult. While the older adult may have difficulty recognizing some familiar faces at this stage of the disease, they may still function well socially. As the disease progresses, the aphasia, apraxia, and agnosia are enhanced; older adults in the final stage of AD often do not speak at all, or it is garbled and incoherent. AD patients may become very functionally limited, incontinent, and unable to ambulate. Finally, there is often no memory left, and the patient's level of consciousness declines into a stuporous or comatose state (Baum & Edwards, 2003).

Effective evaluation of the cognitive function of older adults is the benchmark of excellence in geriatric nursing care. Frequent evaluation of cognitive status will allow the presence of delirium and dementia to be detected at an early stage, which facilitates the most effective possible treatment. If cognitive decline is detected, consistent reassessment of the progression of the disease and development of a plan of care is necessary for appropriate disease management. The use of a standardized cognitive assessment instrument, such as the Mini Mental State Examination (MMSE), is essential. If the older adult's score on the MMSE is consistent with low cognitive function, further diagnostic testing should occur to rule out other causes of cognitive impairment, such as delirium or depression. Moreover, further cognitive evaluation will provide data to make a more effective differential diagnosis.

Definitive diagnosis of all but multi-infarct dementia formerly was limited to post-mortem brain autopsy. However, recent advances in computed tomography (CT) scans, magnetic resonance imaging (MRI), and, most importantly, positron emission tomography (PET) scans have improved the ability to diagnose AD with more than 90% accuracy. In a consensus report prepared by the Neuroimaging Group of the Alzheimer's Association (Alzheimer's Association, 2005), researchers found that neuroimaging, such as MRI and CT, provided an accurate diagnosis of AD. However, PET is another type of imaging technology that uses a tracer called F-fluorodeoxyglucose (FDG), and in patients with AD, the PET scan showed that their brain activity had a marked reduction in

FDG uptake. Thus, PET scanning may also be quite significant in evaluating the progress of AD.

If older adults score low on screening instruments for cognitive impairments, such as the MMSE, they should be referred for a comprehensive geriatric assessment to aid in the diagnosis of AD and to rule out delirium and depression as possible causes of altered cognitive function. Many major hospitals have such assessment centers, and these can be a valuable resource for individuals and families coping with decline in cognitive status. The Alzheimer's Association is also a valuable source of information about further diagnosis and treatment for the disease.

Symptoms of dementia include difficulty communicating, forgetfulness, inattentiveness, disorganized thinking, altered level of consciousness, perceptual disturbances, sleep–wake disorders, wandering psychomotor disturbances, and disorientation. Working with older adults with cognitive disorders is very challenging and often frustrating. The focus is on maintaining function and independence as much as possible, while keeping the older adult safe. Nurses who work with older adults are developing interventions to increase the quality of life for those who suffer from dementia, including environmental manipulations, such as camouflaging doors and installing door alarms, applying wander guards, and providing safe wandering areas. Restraints are not an appropriate alternative for cognitively impaired older adults. Instead, placing mattresses directly on the floor, using carpeting to decrease injury from falls, and using commonly recalled signs and symbols to orient the older adult to the environment are a few of the appropriate interventions. The Alzheimer's Association (2000) recommends the techniques in Table 8.2 for caring for older adults with dementia.

One of the most important considerations in working with the AD population is the need to plan for structure and consistency. Maintaining a specific daily schedule may aid in reducing frustration or uncertainty, because environmental changes or alteration in daily routines may exacerbate dysfunction and worsen behavioral symptoms (Souder & Beck, 2004). Once a patient progresses beyond the mild to moderate stages of AD, increasing amounts of direct care and supervision are often needed. Translocation from one environment to another may potentially upset the patient, so attempting to transition the patient smoothly to this environment is important. One intervention is to maintain calm and comfort and to reassure his or her safety (Souder & Beck, 2004). Remember to speak directly to the older client with AD and listen respectfully, observing cues in facial expression, tone, and repetitive phrases or behaviors to obtain insight into what the patient is feeling (Souder& Beck, 2004).

TABLE 8.2   Tips for Assessing and Managing Troubling Behaviors of Cognitively Impaired Older Adults

Assess	Intervene	Evaluate
Identify the troublesome behaviors: • What was the behavior? • What happened just before or after the behavior? Did something trigger it? • What was your reaction?	Explore potential solutions: • Are there unmet needs of the person with dementia? Are they sick, in pain, or sexually unfulfilled? • Can you adapt the environment instead of the person? • Can you change your reaction or approach to the behavior?	Did your intervention help? • Do you need to explore other potential causes and solutions to the behavior?

Adapted from the Alzheimer's Association *Steps for Understanding Challenging Behaviors* (2000).

Maintaining function as long as possible is an important goal in the care of AD clients. This may require cuing or modeling when the client attempts to complete tasks such as ADLs (Souder & Beck, 2004). Environmental factors may also contribute to the patient's well being. For example, placing a patient who needs a quiet environment in a room close to a busy nursing station can overwhelm that patient and cause problematic behaviors (Souder & Beck, 2004).

Several medications known as cholinesterase inhibitors have recently been developed over the last decade to increase the levels of acetylcholine in the brain. These medications include donepezil (Aricept), galantamine (Reminyl), rivastigmine (Exelon), and tacrine (Cognex). These medications work to prevent further loss of cognitive function and to improve cognitive status in older adults with dementia. They are most effective when started in the early stages of the disease. Another medication that has shown some promise in treating AD is Namenda®, or memantine. The action of memintine differs from that of the cholinesterase inhibitors, but it works well in combination with this classification of drugs and appears to be well-tolerated. In addition, research to develop an AD vaccine is ongoing. Preliminary studies suggest that the vaccine is effective at reducing cognitive decline. Unfortunately, early studies of the vaccine showed the presence of brain inflammation among study participants, so further research is necessary. However, a recent report by the Alzheimer's Association (2005) indicates that an attenuate version of the vaccine currently undergoing clinical trial shows signs of effectiveness in 20% of patients enrolled in the study, and no adverse effects have been reported. Lithium has also been suggested as a possible medication to suppress the development of the beta-amyloid responsible for plaque formation among AD patients. However, the cardiovascular and central nervous system side effects of this medication make its use difficult.

Besides administering and evaluating the effect of medications, nursing interventions include physical and emotional support to the client and the family. There are many cultural variations in the care decisions made for older adults. Some cultural backgrounds lead to the belief that older adults with cognitive disorders, such as AD, must be cared for at home, by family. The traditional Western medicine model is more accepting of institutionalization of older adults. The Profile of Older Americans (Administration on Aging & U.S Department of Health and Human Services, 2005) reports that 54.7% (10.7 million) of older noninstitutionalized persons lived with their elderly spouses, and it is estimated that family members provide approximately 80% of the care for older adults.

The majority of care for patients with AD is often delegated to a specific caregiver. In many cases, the caregiver is also an older adult, most often a woman, with health problems of her own. The experience of caregiving is very stressful and has been shown to result in the onset of depression, grief, fatigue, decreased socialization, and health problems (Sullivan, 2007). Meeting the basic needs for nutrition, hygiene and grooming, and continued functioning and mobility are essential. The nurse, in conjunction with the caregiver, must also assess, document, and report any changes in physical and mental status of the client immediately so that interventions can be initiated to minimize short- and long-term

---

CULTURAL FOCUS

Some cultural backgrounds lead to the belief that older adults with cognitive disorders, such as AD, must be cared for at home, by family. The traditional Western medicine model is more accepting of institutionalization of older adults. The Profile of Older Americans (AARP, 2002) reports 54.7% (13.7 million) of older noninstitutionalized persons lived with their elderly spouses, and it is estimated that family members provide approximately 80% of the care for older adults. The nurse, in conjunction with family caregivers, must also assess, document, and report any changes in physical and mental status of the client immediately in order to implement interventions to minimize short- and long-term disease effects. In addition, care for the caregiver is often part of the nurse's role.

disease effects. In addition, care for the caregiver is often part of the nurse's role. More information on caregiving can be found in Chapter 9.

SUMMARY

As the population of older adults continues to rise, an increase will be seen in the number of cognitive and psychological disorders among this population. Although the presence of delirium, depression, and dementia are not normal changes of aging, they occur commonly in this population and threaten a large number of older adults. The presence of cognitive and psychological disorders among older adults markedly affects the ability of this population to independently complete activities of daily living. In addition, the presence of these illnesses is extremely costly, both emotionally and financially, for clients and their families.

This chapter discusses three frequently occurring conditions among older adults, commonly known as the three Ds: delirium, depression, and dementia. The incidence, prevalence, causes, and treatment of these disorders was reviewed. While delirium, depression, and dementia are the result of completely different disease processes, they all produce symptoms of cognitive decline. It is challenging to determine which condition is causing the problem, and it is of utmost importance to assess changes in cognitive function and to refer the older adult for further evaluation and treatment at the earliest possible point of care. This will ensure that older adults receive the most effective management of cognitive and psychological disease.

REFERENCES

Administration on Aging & U.S. Department of Health and Human Services. (2005). *A profile of older americans*. Retrieved July 12, 2007, from http://assets.aarp.org/rgcenter/general/profile_2005.pdf

Alzheimer's Association. (1999). *Alzheimer's disease and related dementias fact sheet*. Retrieved on July 13, 2007, from http://www.alz.org/documents/national/FS-Related Diseases.pdf

Alzheimer's Association. (2000). *Steps to understanding challenging behaviors*. Retrieved on July 13, 2007, from http://www.alz.org/national/documents/C-EDU-Stepsto UnderstandingChallengingBehaviours.pdf

Alzheimer's Association. (2005). *Basics of Alzheimer's disease*. Retrieved on July 13, 2007, from http://www.alz.org/documents/national/basics_of_alz_low.pdf

American Association of Retired Persons. (2005). Profile of Older Americans. Retrieved July 14th, 2007 from http://assets.aarp.org/rgcenter/general/profile_2005.pdf

American Psychiatric Association. (1994). *The diagnostic and statistical manual of mental disorders* (4th Edition). Washington, DC: Author.

Aroian, K. J., Khatutsky, G., Tran, T. V., & Balsam, A. L. (2001). Health and social service utilization among elderly immigrants from the former Soviet Union. *Journal of Nursing Scholarship, 33,* 265–271.

Balas, M. C., Deutschman, C. S., Sullivan-Marx, E. M., Stumpf, N. E., Alston, R. P., & Richmond, T. S. (2007). Delirium in older surgical intensive care unit. *Journal of Nursing Scholarship, 39*(2) 147–154.

Baum, C., & Edwards., D. F. (2003). What persons with Alzheimer's disease can do: A tool for communication about everyday activities. *Alzheimer's Care Quarterly, 4*(2), 108–118.

Brown, W. A. (2005) Pseudodementia. *The Pyschiatric Times, 22*(13), 83.

Edwards, N. (2003). Differentiating the three D's: Delirium, dementia, and depression. *MedSurg Nursing, 12*(6), 347–357.

Hogstel, M. O. (2001). *Gerontology: Nursing care of the older adult.* Albany, NY: Delmar Thomson Learning.

Inouye, S. K., Zhang, Y., Jones, R. N., Kiely, D. K., Yang, F., Marcantonia, E. R. et al. (2007). Risk factors for delirium at discharge: Development and validation of a predictive model. *Archives of Internal Medicine, 167*(13), 1406–1413.

Jacobson, S. A. (1997). Delirium in the elderly. *The Psychiatric Clinics of North America, 20,* 91–110.

McCarthy, M. C. (2003). Detecting acute confusion in older adults: Comparing clinical reasoning of nurses working in acute, long-term and community health care environments. *Research in Nursing and Health, 26,* 203–212.

National Institute of Mental Health. (2007). *Older adults: Depression and suicide facts.* Retrieved August 9, 2007, from http://www.nimh.nih.gov/publicat/elderlydepsuicide.cfm

"Never been the same since": Delirium in older people might have permanent effects on the brain. (2007). *The Harvard Health Letter, 32*(6), 4.

Rizzo, J. A., Bogardus, S. T., Leo-Summers, L., Williams, C. S., Acampora, D., & Inouye, S. K. (2001). Multicomponent targeted intervention to prevent delirium in hospitalized older patients: What is the economic value? *Medical Care, 39,* 740–52.

Shelkey, M. (2000). Pet therapy. In J. Fitzpatrick, T. Fulmer, M. Wallace, & E. Flaherty (Eds.), *Geriatric nursing research digest* (pp. 215–218). New York: Springer-Verlag.

Short, M., & Winstead P. (2007). Delirium dilemma. *Orthopedics, 30*(4), 273-276.

Souder, E., & Beck, C. (2004). Overview of Alzheimer's disease (includes abstract). *Nursing Clinics of North America, 39*(3), 545–559.

Sullivan, T. (2007). *Try this: The Caregiver Strain Index revised.* Hartford Institute for Geriatric Nursing. Retrieved July 12, 2007, from http://www.hartfordign.org/publications/trythis/issue14.pdf

U.S. Department of Health and Human Services. (2000). *Healthy people 2010: National health promotion and disease prevention objectives.* Retrieved from http://www.health.gov/healthypeople.

Wallace, M., & Shelkey, M. (2007) Try this. Katz Index of Independence in activities of daily living (ADL). *Try this: Best practices in nursing care to older adults, a series from the Hartford Institute for Geriatric Nursing.* Retrieved August 8, 2007, from www.hartfordign.org/publications/trythis/issue02.pdf

Waszynski, C. (2007) Try this. The Confusion Assessment Method. *Try this: Best practices in nursing care to older adults, a series from the Hartford Institute for Geriatric Nursing.* Issue 13. Retrieved August 8, 2007, from www.hartfordign.org/publications/trythis/issue13.pdf

Yesavage, J. A. (1992). Depression in the elderly. How to recognize masked symptoms and choose appropriate therapy. *Post Graduate Medicine, 91*(1), 255–258, 261.

CHAPTER NINE

Ethical Issues of Aging and Independence

Learning Objectives

1. Discuss ethical issues inherent in the aging process.
2. Define ethical principles used to guide ethical decision making.
3. Discuss problems and solutions associated with older adult drivers.
4. Use an ethical framework to explore issues related to older drivers.
5. Identify barriers and interventions to sexuality among older adults.
6. Use an ethical framework to explore issues related to sexuality among older adults.
7. Describe the incidence of problem and pathological gambling and its impact on the health of older adults.
8. Use an ethical framework to explore issues related to gambling among the elderly.

Mr. Larry is a 92-year-old healthy man. He lived in his own apartment and is completely independent in ADLs and IADLs. On June 14, 2000, he left his apartment complex at 8:09 a.m. to go to the store. While backing out of his driveway, he failed to see a school bus passing on the intersecting street and his car struck it on the passenger side. One child was killed and six others were injured. Residents and city officials are outraged, with many questioning why Mr. Larry was still driving.

Chronic illnesses that occur during the aging process frequently cause nurses to encounter ethical issues in the care of this population. Chronically ill older adults may experience cognitive disorders, suffer from pain and discomfort, endure poor quality of life, or need to cope with end-of-life issues. As nurses care for older adults, ethical dilemmas surrounding these issues of older adulthood arise daily and are often in need of immediate resolution. Moreover, these issues present great challenges to nurses and other members of the health care team.

Ethics are defined in *The American Heritage Dictionary of English Language* (2007) as "The study of the general nature of morals and of specific moral choices." *The American Heritage Dictionary of the English Language* (2007) defines bioethics as "The study of the ethical and moral implications of new biological discoveries and biomedical advances, as in the fields of genetic engineering and drug research." Issues surrounding the ethical care of older adults are complex and often require the integration of personal values and morals, as well as other factors specific to the nurse, the client, and the situation. Each person in the situation (client/resident, nurse, case manager, discharge planner, social worker, physician, family, and lawyer) has a personal perspective on effectively managing the situation based on their individual values, life experiences, education, and other factors. Each person also brings a set of morals and values used to identify right from wrong.

This chapter will explore the ethical issues inherent in the aging process. It begins with a discussion of ethical principles used to guide ethical decision making. These ethical principles will be applied to three

---

EVIDENCE-BASED PRACTICE

Title of Study: Our "Increasing Mobile Society"? The Curious Persistence of a False Belief

Authors: Wolf, D., Longino, C.

Purpose: Overall mobility has actually declined since 1950, so the topic of "increased mobile society" in the United States is examined.

Methods: Simple regression method analysis is used to estimate the size and significance of mobility trends in the United States.

Findings: In all age groups, overall mobility has declined. The largest decline is noted in the age group of 20–29 year olds, and the rate of those 65 years and older is also large. Interstate mobility has also declined or remained constant between adults aged 45 and 65 years.

Implications: Increased geographic mobility does not appear to be a contributing factor in predicting declining care for the elderly relatives.

The Gerontologist, Vol. 45, No. 1, 5–11.

---

specific issues of independence among older adults, including driving, sexuality, and gambling. At the conclusion of the chapter, students will have an increased understanding of the ethical and legal issues that older adults encounter and the resources used to assist with decision making when these issues occur.

ETHICAL PRINCIPLES

While there are many complex and challenging decisions ahead for nursing students and nurses in the care of older adults, it is important to know that nurses are not alone in making these decisions. Nurses are members of health care teams composed of physicians, social workers, therapists, clergy, and others who all bring unique perspectives to the care of older adults. In many ethical situations, the team is called together to discuss the situation and make decisions jointly. The nursing profession is consistently guided by the American Nurses Association (ANA) code for nurses. This document is a guideline for the goals, values, and ethical decisions of nurses. It is considered nonnegotiable and supersedes the policies of individual institutions in regard to nursing practice and ethical decision making. The code for nurses provides a number of interpretive statements specific to health care situations frequently encountered in the care of older adults. For example, the ANA has a position statement on polypharmacy among older adults and nurses' participation in end-of-life care. These statements can provide great support and resources during difficult ethical encounters throughout nurses' careers. The ANA code for nurses and interpretive statements may be found at http://www.nursingworld.org.

The ethical practice of nurses and other health care professionals involves the application of ethical principles to each situation. Ethical principles provide a framework for understanding the ethical issues that frequently arise among the care of older adults. For example, consider Mrs. Jones, a highly functioning 79-year-old widow recently admitted to a nursing home with mild cognitive impairment (MCI). Mrs. Jones began a friendship with Mr. Carl, who is cognitively intact and wheelchair bound. Mr. Carl is married to a woman who resides outside the facility. The nursing staff has noticed more and more intimate touches among the two residents and is concerned about whether Mrs. Jones is competent to make the decision to participate in this increasingly intimate relationship. The staff is also concerned about the moral and ethical issues surrounding Mr. Carl's relationship with a woman other than his wife. The availability of ethical principles can be extremely useful to guide nurses' actions within the situation. Understanding and effective use of ethical principles is essential to ethical decision making and the resolution of ethical dilemmas. In bioethics, four principles guide ethical deliberations: autonomy, beneficence, nonmaleficence, and justice.

Autonomy

Autonomy conveys a respect for the person's ability to govern self or to freely choose one's actions as long as these choices do not interfere with the autonomy or rights of other persons. This principle has also been called self-governance or self-determinism (Hogstel, 2001). World Reference.com defines self-determinism as the determination of "one's own fate or course of action without compulsion." Decisions involving autonomy or self-determination must consider the patient's right to choose for themselves, regardless of the consequences. Issues surrounding autonomy or self-determination are seen frequently in clinical areas, when patients refuse medications, treatments, and surgical procedures that are likely to improve their health. For example, clients of particular cultural and religious backgrounds do not believe in blood transfusion and, thus, will not consent to this procedure, even though it may be necessary to save lives. Enhanced understanding regarding older adults' health beliefs will result in improved capacity to make ethical health care decisions.

In the case of Mrs. Jones, the right to autonomy is complicated by the presence of mild cognitive impairment (MCI) and must be explored further. The question remains: Is she competent to make the decision to participate in an intimate relationship, or must another person be asked to do this? In Mr. Carl's case, the nursing staff must highly consider the resident's right to autonomy, even when the moral values and life experiences of the nurses lead them to believe his relationship with Mrs. Jones is wrong.

Ethical issues and dilemmas that surround this principle also include informed consent. Informed consent is defined by worlddictionary. com as the "consent by a patient to a medical or surgical treatment or to participate in an experiment after the patient understands the risks

---

CULTURAL FOCUS

Clients from diverse cultural and religious backgrounds may have health care beliefs that play a significant role in ethical decision making. Enhanced understanding regarding older adults' health beliefs will result in improved capacity to make ethical health care decisions.

involved." Informed consent must be obtained in order for a patient to undergo a medical treatment and/or participate in research studies. Informed consent is a required component of all health care procedures and research studies and shows respect for persons by supporting autonomous choice. From an ethical and caring perspective, informed consent decreases anxiety about health care interventions and encourages health care professionals, including nurses and researchers, to act responsibly during clinical practice and research. Numerous violations in informed consent have resulted in a great deal of mistrust of health care professionals and researchers from the perspective of older adults. The Tuskegee Syphilis studies conducted among African American men in the 1930s and '40s were one such example of the violation of multiple rights of one particular ethnic group. In this case, men were enrolled in a study, without their consent, and prevented from receiving penicillin for the treatment of syphilis. Many men died from the disease, because even though treatment was available, participants in this study were denied access. As a result of these atrocious violations of autonomy and self-determination, informed consent has become a standard component of health care and research. Informed consent has the potential to increase the willingness of patients and research participants to collaborate with nurses based on a trusting relationship between the nurse and the recipient of care.

In order to implement this principle safely in health care institutions where research is conducted, institutional review boards (IRBs) are established. The role of IRBs is to protect clients from unethical behavior on the part of researchers and clinicians. In so doing, IRBS ensure that research participants provide informed consent prior to participation in research, that the participants' results are confidential, and that no manipulation or coercion occurs.

CULTURAL FOCUS

The Tuskegee Syphilis studies conducted among African American men in the 1930s and '40s were one such example of the violation of multiple rights of one particular ethnic group. In this case, men were enrolled in a study, without their consent, and prevented from receiving penicillin for the treatment of syphilis. Many men died from the disease, because even though treatment was available, participants in this study were denied access. As a result of these atrocious violations of autonomy and self-determination, informed consent has become a standard component of health care and research.

Beneficence

Beneficence is defined as "doing good or participating in behavior that benefits a recipient of care." This ethical principle forms the basis of professional codes of practice for many health care disciplines. For example, Mr. James, a 79-year-old man is admitted to a medical–surgical unit for unexplained rectal bleeding. He has a history of two previous suicide attempts over the past year, since his wife died. The physician diagnoses a nontreatable malignancy. Out of concern that this diagnostic information will result in another suicide attempt, the health care team chooses to withhold this medical information from Mr. James until they are certain that his depression is stabilized and safety can be assured. In this case, the principle of beneficence assumed prominence over the person's right to self-govern. In the case of Mrs. Jones and Mr. Carl earlier in the chapter, the actual and projected outcomes of the intimate relationship would require assessment to determine what nursing actions are required regarding this relationship. If an assessment of Mrs. Jones finds that she is incapable of understanding the consequences of her relationship with Mr. Carl, then she must be prevented from being taken advantage of. However, if the assessment leads nurses to believe that Mrs. Jones and Mr. Carl understand the risks and consequences of their relationship, then the right to autonomy prevails. The difference between the two cases is revealed in each patient's ability to act autonomously. Both Mrs. Jones and Mr. James have questionable abilities to do this based on the presence of MCI and the history of two suicide attempts, respectively. In these ethical dilemmas and all others, nurses and other health care professionals must weigh the ability and right to act autonomously with the good and the bad of each considered action and then render a decision based on which action would be the most beneficial to the client and, thus, meet the health care goals.

Nonmaleficence

Nonmaleficence focuses on the health care provider's mandate to "above all, do no harm." This principle prevents nurses from aiding in physician-assisted suicide and/or causing pain or suffering to another person. Nonmaleficence provides the legal and correctional framework. It places value on all human life and freedom, the importance of each person's life and the need to honor the human dignity and choices of each person (Hogstel, 2001). Discussions of active and passive euthanasia involve the principle of nonmaleficence. Active euthanasia, committing a fatal act on an ill person, is not morally acceptable in most societies. However, passive euthanasia, letting a person die by omitting treatment (such as food, medication, or surgery to maintain life) and allowing the disease or injury to cause death, is practiced in this country and in other societies.

As stated earlier, the ANA code for nurses provides specific guidelines regarding nursing actions in a variety of ethical situations. These actions supersede facility policy and are nonnegotiable. Among other interpretive statements within the code, nurses are guided by the ANA (1994) position statement on assisted suicide. This position statement explicitly prohibits nursing involvement in active euthanasia or the intentional ending of another's life. However, there are examples of nurses practicing passive euthanasia in certain situations. The recent case of a younger woman in Florida who was brain damaged years earlier provides an interesting perspective on nurses' involvement in ethical end-of-life care issues. In this case, the client's husband had petitioned courts to remove his wife's feeding tube. After multiple court battles, his petition was successful, and the tube was removed. While nurses may have had differing ethical views on the decision, the ANA does not prohibit involvement in removal of life-sustaining treatment in some cases. Nurses in this case played an important role in providing compassion and care, as well as keeping the client comfortable during her last few days.

As with all ethical dilemmas, the decision to omit treatment needed to sustain life involves the analysis of ethical principles and the use of excellent communication with all involved individuals, including the client, health care providers, and family. In other situations, such as the case of intimacy between older nursing home residents discussed earlier, failure to assess Mrs. Jones's ability to consent to participate in an intimate relationship with Mr. Jones could be termed nonmaleficence. While nurses are often uncomfortable and lack knowledge in assessing and managing sexual issues among older adults, failure to do so in this case has the potential to cause harm to both residents. Use of the nursing process, as well as consultation with family and members of the health care team, generally result in effective decisions.

Justice

"The principle of justice supports the fair allocation of resources to individuals or the provision of an equal share of available resources to each person" (Hogstel, 2001, p. 540). This principle has specific application to older adults who must consistently fight against ageism. As discussed earlier in this text, ageism is defined as a negative attitude or bias toward older adults, resulting in the belief that older people cannot, or should not, participate in societal activities or be given equal opportunities afforded to others (Holohan-Bell & Brummel-Smith, 1999). In the case of Mrs.

Jones and Mr. Carl, failure to recognize the sexual needs of older adults, and manage these needs with similar priority to other physical needs, is a violation of the ethical principle of justice. Ethical issues that arise from the principle of justice and are influenced by ageism involve the distribution of health care resources at local and national levels, including micro allocation and macro allocation, respectively. For example, approximately 60% of patients cared for today are older adults, yet only 34% of nursing schools require a course in geriatric nursing. Nurses caring for older adults understand that ageism has great potential to impact the health care of older adults and their access to services. Moreover, ageism has the power to destroy the dignity and respect of older adults and impacts policies and care decisions for this population. Nurses must work consistently to identify ageism and mitigate its ability to influence policies and care decisions that will affect the quality of life of older adults. In so doing, nurses play an instrumental role in preventing the consequences of aging on older adults. This includes making sure that older adults are not discriminated against in selection for medical procedures or resources.

Consistent with the principle of justice is the issue of whether or not health care is a right for all persons, or a privilege for those who can afford it. While the United States has discussed a national insurance program, many other countries have implemented it in the spirit of justice.

DRIVING

As the percentage of older adults living in the United States continues to increase, the number of older drivers will rise. In fact, if the current trend in the number of older drivers continues, by 2026 this number could possibly exceed 2.5 times the 1996 levels. Moreover, conservative estimates indicate that between 1990 and 2020, the total annual mileage driven by older male drivers will increase by 465% and by older female drivers by 500% (Burkhardt, Berger, Creedon, & McGavock, 1998).

The risk for injuries, hospitalizations, and death from automobile accidents is increased in the older adult population because of the many normal and pathological changes in the neuromuscular and sensory systems. Consequently, the ability to respond to emergency driving situations may be slowed. Table 9.1 summarizes normal changes of aging that affect driving ability. It is estimated that the number of elderly traffic fatalities will more than triple by the year 2030, exceeding the number of alcohol-related fatalities in 1995 by 35% (Burkhardt et al., 1998). In addition, the increase in older drivers presents additional problems, because cars, roads, and highways were not developed to accommodate

TABLE 9.1   Normal Changes of Aging That Affect Driving Ability

System	Normal Aging Changes
Senses	Eyes • Visual acuity declines. • Ability of pupil to constrict in response to stimuli decreases. • Peripheral vision declines. • Lens of the eye often becomes yellow. Ears • Increased prevalence of hearing disorders.
Neurological	• Slower response time to stimuli. • Shift in the proportion of gray matter to white matter. • Loss of neurons. • Increase in the number of senile plaques. • Blood flow to the cerebrum decreases.

normal changes of aging among older drivers. This results in a large number of older adults unable to safely drive.

There are many ethical issues surrounding the decision about whether older adults should continue to drive. These issues are summarized in

CRITICAL THINKING CASE STUDY

Mr. Larry is a 75-year-old healthy man. He lives in his own apartment and is completely independent in ADLs and IADLs. On June 14, 2000, he left his apartment complex at 8:09 a.m. to go to the store. While backing out of his driveway, he failed to see a school bus passing on the intersecting street, and the passenger side of his car struck it broadside. One child was killed and six others were injured. Mr. Larry is now charged with manslaughter.

1. What normal or pathological changes of aging were involved in Mr. Larry's inability to see the school bus before colliding with it?
2. What do you think should be the resolution for this accident? Should Mr. Larry face criminal charges, lose his license, or both?
3. What effect would the revocation of a license have on Mr. Larry's ability to function independently?
4. Do you feel that accidents like Mr. Larry's underscore the need for older adults to be retested in order to drive? Should older adults have a mandatory license suspension?
5. What changes to vehicles and personal adaptations should be made so that driving is safer for older adults and other drivers?

TABLE 9.2 To Drive or Not to Drive?

Ethical Principle	Application to Issue of Independence
Autonomy (Self-Determination) The right to govern self or to freely choose one's actions as long as these choices do not interfere with the autonomy or rights of other persons.	The right to drive is complicated by normal changes in aging that effect senses and response time. What impact these changes have on Mr. Larry's ability to drive must be assessed. It is important to determine if these changes impacted the accident or whether the failure of Mr. Larry to see the school bus was independent of these normal aging changes. In clients with acute and chronic illness, the impact of these diseases on driving ability must also be assessed and weighed against the client's right to autonomy.
Beneficence Doing good or participating in behavior that benefits a recipient of care.	Putting Mr. Larry's safety first requires a full assessment of his physical, psychological, and emotional health to determine if it is in his best interest to continue driving or whether he would be safer without a driver's license. In this case, a driver's refresher course may be in the client's best interest.
Nonmaleficence Above all, do no harm.	Failure to assess the impact of normal and pathological changes on Mr. Larry's ability to drive puts both Mr. Larry and society at risk. With knowledge regarding the potential impact of normal and pathological aging on driving among older adults, it is a nurse's duty to be sure to assess these changes and implement interventions to promote the maximum safety for clients and society. Failure to do so in this case has the potential to cause harm to both.
Justice The fair allocation of resources to individuals or the provision of an equal share of available resources to each person.	The role of ageism in society often makes it easy to assume that older adults should not drive. However, while normal changes of aging impact driving ability, there are many ways in which to compensate for these changes. Consequently, full regard for the rights of autonomy must be adhered to in order for justice to prevail in the case of Mr. Larry and other older adult drivers.

Table 9.2. One ageist solution that has been suggested is to revoke their license to drive at a certain age. In fact, this has been considered as a viable solution to the problem. However, this will result in a great loss of independence among this population, and considering the ethical principles stated earlier, it is important to discuss ways in which older adults may be assisted to maintain their safety and independence as long as possible, while still protecting the safety of other drivers, passengers, and pedestrians. Consider the case study in this chapter using the ethical principles outlined earlier.

Nurses can play an essential role in helping older adults to maintain safe driving practices and ensure the safety of the community by assessing normal and pathological changes of aging in the older adult. The implementation of strategies to reduce the effects of normal aging and manage disease are also important components of safe driving. In addition, nurses should recommend that patients learn to drive again, adapting to their neuromuscular and sensory changes. Nurses working with older adult drivers should encourage them to take driver refresher classes that are run by the American Association of Retired Persons (AARP). Completion of the AARP driver refresher course often allows older adults to save money on car insurance.

SEXUALITY IN OLDER ADULTS

One of the most prevalent myths of aging is that older adults are no longer interested in sex. Because sexuality is mainly considered a young person's activity, often associated with reproduction, society doesn't usually associate older adults with sex. In the youth-oriented society of today, many consider sexuality among older adults to be distasteful and prefer to assume sexuality among the older population doesn't exist. However, despite popular belief, sexuality continues to be important in the lives of older adults. A survey of 1,126 older adults by Matthias, Lubben, Atchison, and Schweitzer (1997) found that 30% had participated in sexual activity over the past month. The need to continue sexuality and sexual function should be as highly valued as other physiological needs. Because much of society believes sexuality is not part of the aging process, nurses and other health care providers rarely assess sexuality, and few intervene to promote sexuality of the older population. Nurses may avoid the discussion because they lack knowledge about sexuality in older adults, or simply because they're inexperienced and uncomfortable with the issue.

The fulfillment of sexual needs may be just as satisfying for older adults as it is for younger people. However, several normal and pathological changes of aging complicate sexuality among older adults. Older adults may experience performance anxiety and may not be familiar with the risks of sexually transmitted diseases and appropriate prevention. Negative self-concepts and role changes that frequently occur in response to chronic illness may impact the experience of sexuality for older adults and could result in fear of rejection or failure, as well as boredom or hostility about sexual performance. The past sexual history of older adults may also play a role in sexual health. Delays in sexual development or a history of sexual abuse may continue to impact sexuality in the later years. Despite difficult issues and the great need to assess older client's sexuality, many older adults are reluctant to discuss sexual issues with health care providers.

Normal physiological changes of aging among women result in a decrease in circulating estrogen, which results in a thinning of the vaginal epithelium, the labia majora, and the subcutaneous tissue in the mons pubis. The vaginal canal shortens and loses elasticity. Follicular depletion of the ovaries as a result of a decrease in circulating estrogen leads to a further decline in the secretion of estrogen and progesterone (Masters, 1986). In response to these physiological changes, dyspareunia (painful intercourse), orgasmic dysfunction, and vaginismus may result (Meston, 1997).

Viropause, andropause, or male menopause are new and controversial terms to describe the physiological changes that affect the aging male sex response. The syndrome, usually beginning between the ages of 46 and 52 is characterized by a gradual decrease in the amount of testosterone (Kessenich & Cichon, 2001). The loss of testosterone is not pathological and does not result in sexual dysfunction. However, men may experience fatigue, loss of muscle mass, depression, and a decline in libido (Kessenich & Cichon, 2001).

In his work on the aging sexual response, Masters (1986) indicated that the reduced availability of sexual hormones in both male and female older adults result in declines in the speed and overall responses to sexual arousal. The physiological changes in hormone secretion affect four areas of sexual response: (1) arousal, (2) orgasm, (3) postorgasm, and (4) extragenital changes (Masters, 1986). In men, these changes are seen in the increased time needed to develop an erection and ejaculate. Erections also may require direct penile stimulation (Araujo, Mohr, & McKinlay, 2004). The volume of semen declines, and a longer period of time is needed between ejaculations. For women, in addition to the decline in vaginal lubrication and painful intercourse, the aging female may also experience fewer orgasmic contractions or painful uterine contractions during sexual activity (Harvard Medical School, 2003). Infrequent rectal sphincter contractions and a postcoital need to urinate may also be present (Harvard Medical School, 2003).

EVIDENCE-BASED PRACTICE

Title of Study: Andropause: Knowledge and Perceptions Among the General Public and Health Care Professionals

Authors: Anderson, J., Faulkner, S., Cranor, C., Briley, J., Gevirtz, F., Roberts, S.

Purpose: This study assesses the knowledge and perceptions of andropause, the natural age-related decline in testosterone in men, among health care providers and the general public.

Methods: Health care providers and members of the general public participated in brief surveys via a medical information telephone line. Trained clinical interviewers administered the questionnaire and documented the findings.

Findings: Of 443 general public participants, 377 (85%) agreed to participate in the survey. Of these, 77% had heard of andropause—male menopause—and 63% had taken TRT (testosterone replacement therapy). Out of 88 health care provider callers, 57 (65%) participated in the survey. Of these participants, 65% were pharmacists, 80% had patients with low testosterone symptoms, and 50% reported that patients rarely or never spoke of low testosterone. Among HCPs and the general public, respectively, 98% and 91% knew that low testosterone is treatable with medication, and 60% and 57% knew that it results in osteoporosis. Only 25% of HCPs and 14% of the general public knew that low testosterone does not cause loss of urinary control.

Implications: Some health care providers, as well as members of the general public, are knowledgeable about some aspects of low testosterone and have misconceptions about others. Therefore, it is clear that education is needed in this area.

Journals of Gerontology Section A, Biological and Medical Sciences, 2002 Dec, 57(12), M793–M796.

The normal changes of aging may alter or delay the sexual response of older adults, but sexual dysfunction is not a normal process of aging. The frequent occurrence of chronic illnesses and the use of multiple medications among older adults, however, frequently interfere with the normal sexual function of older men and women. Morley and Tariq (2003) report that medication usage, diseases such as diabetes and depression, and surgery to structures involved in the sexual response (e.g., prostate, breast) are all factors that result in sexual dysfunction among older adults. In these cases, removal of the medication causing the dysfunction, treatment of the chronic medical illness, and psychological therapy are interventions that may contribute to the resolution of sexual problems

(Morley & Tariq, 2003). Medications, vacuum erection devices, and surgery are options for resolving erectile impotence when other interventions fail.

The assessment and management of sexual problems of older adults is often complicated by ethical issues. As seen in the case of Mrs. Jones and Mr. Carl earlier in this chapter, normal and pathological aging changes, as well as the role of families, are important factors to consider when addressing sexual issues in this population. Moreover, a nurse's lack of knowledge and experience and general reluctance to assess and plan care related to sexuality issues has a substantial impact on the older adult's health and functioning. A summary of the ethical issues involved in this case are presented in Table 9.3.

As discussed earlier, older adults experience many physiological changes in their reproductive systems that impact their ability to function sexually, including changes in vaginal lubrication, response time, and body image. Moreover, the presence of depression and diabetes, as well as medications, such as beta blockers for hypertension, impact sexual response. The loss of partners in older adulthood also significantly impacts sexuality. However, because the topic of sexuality was not widely discussed in previous decades, older adults do not always fully understand these changes and their impact on sexuality. Despite older adults' lack of knowledge about sexuality, education that addresses normal and pathological aging changes, as well as the impact of role changes on sexuality, and interventions to compensate for these changes, is rarely provided. Consequently, older adults may stop functioning sexually, because they think they are *abnormal* or ill, and no one is available to counsel them otherwise.

A sexual assessment is the first step to discussing sexuality of older adults. The PLISSIT model (Annon, 1976) begins by first seeking permission (P) to discuss sexuality with the older adult. This permission may be gained by asking general questions such as, "I would like to begin to discuss your sexual health; what concerns would you like to share with me about this area of function?" Questions to guide the sexual assessment of older adults are available on many health care assessment forms. The next step of the model affords an opportunity for the health care provider to share limited information (LI) with the older adult. In response to the increase in older adults with sexually transmitted diseases, it is essential to provide them with safe sex information at this time. In the next part of the model, specific suggestions (SS) are provided to older adults to help them fulfill their sexuality. These suggestions may focus on the use of CDC recommended safe sexual practices. The final part of the model allows for intensive therapy (IT) to be provided to the older adult regarding sexual issues that may arise during the assessment. This may

TABLE 9.3 Is This Sexual Relationship Safe?

Ethical Principle	Application to Issue of Independence
Autonomy (Self-Determination) The right to govern self or to freely choose one's actions as long as these choices do not interfere with the autonomy or rights of other persons.	The right to autonomy is complicated by the presence of mild cognitive impairment (MCI) and must be explored further. The question remains: Is Mrs. Jones competent to make the decision to participate in an intimate relationship, or must another person be asked to make the decision for her? In Mr. Carl's case, the nursing staff must highly consider the resident's right to autonomy, even when the moral values and life experiences of the nurses lead them to believe his relationship with Mrs. Jones is wrong.
Beneficence Doing good or participating in behavior that benefits a recipient of care.	The actual and projected outcomes of the intimate relationship would require assessment to determine what nursing actions are required regarding this relationship. If an assessment of Mrs. Jones finds that she is incapable of understanding the consequences of her relationship with Mr. Carl, then she must be prevented from being taken advantage of. However, if the assessment leads nurses to believe that Mrs. Jones and Mr. Carl understand the risks and consequences of their relationship, then the right to autonomy prevails in this case.
Nonmaleficence Above all, do no harm.	Failure to assess Mrs. Jones's ability to consent to participate in an intimate relationship with Mr. Carl could be termed nonmaleficence. While nurses are often uncomfortable and lack knowledge in assessing and managing sexual issues among older adults, failure to do so in this case has the potential to cause harm to both residents. Use of the nursing process, as well as consultation with family and members of the health care team, generally result in effective decisions.
Justice The fair allocation of resources to individuals or the provision of an equal share of available resources to each person.	In the case of Mrs. Jones and Mr. Carl, failure to recognize the sexual needs of older adults and manage these needs with similar priority as other physical needs is a violation of the ethical principle of justice.

include the discovery of sexually transmitted diseases, which requires treatment.

It is important to educate older adults about normal and pathological aging changes in reference to sexuality. Interventions to promote sexuality among older adults may focus on the use of touch to create intimacy, as opposed to sexual intercourse. As older adults relocate to more supportive environments, privacy may also be an issue to address in order to help clients pursue sexuality in a dignified and respectful manner. In promoting privacy, it is essential to consider client safety. It may be the nurse's role to order the necessary equipment, such as grab bars and condoms, and demonstrate proper use to the older couple in order to promote safety.

For older adults with dementia, it is essential to conduct highly accurate assessments and document their ability to be involved in the decision-making process. As seen in the earlier case study, if a client is not capable of making competent decisions, then the nursing staff must prevent them from being taken advantage of by a spouse, partner, or other residents. Problematic sexual behaviors may occur in response to unmet sexual needs in older adults with dementia. These may include public masturbation or exposure, or making sexually inappropriate comments or gestures to nurses or other clients. While these behaviors are disturbing, they rarely go away when ignored. Further assessment and planning of care can help the older adults to meet their sexual needs in a dignified and respectful manner and will likely eliminate the behavior.

GAMBLING

Pathological, problem, and at-risk gambling has increased significantly over the past several decades. This is partially due to the widespread growth of state-sanctioned gambling in the form of lottery tickets and the growth of casinos. The incidence of gambling among older adults has risen from 61% of the population in the 1960s to 80% in 1991. Levens, Dyer, Zubritsky, Knott, and Oslin (2005) report that of 843 older adults studied, 69.6% of the sample had gambled at least once in the last year, and 10.9% were identified as at-risk gamblers. Wiebe and Cox (2005) showed that in their study of 1,000 older adults, 74.7% gambled, with 1.6% gambling at problem levels. Older adults are at greater risk for problem gambling because (a) they often have financial problems that they hope gambling will resolve, and (b) the multiple losses experienced by older adults is often soothed by the excitement of casinos.

Gambling is often very problematic for the health of older adults and may result in increased stress, alcohol use, and depression. In addition, gambling often results in a great loss of income, which could further trigger medication noncompliance, malnutrition, and safety risks. In order to prevent the possibly harmful effects of gambling among older adults, nurses should assess for problem gambling during routine health encounters. The *Diagnostic and Statistical Manual of Mental Disorders (DSM–IV)* classifies pathological gambling as a psychological disorder and has established 10 criteria in classifying pathological gambling behaviors (Table 9.4, NGISC, 1999).

Consider the case of Mr. Diamond, a 76-year-old man with a history of poorly controlled Type 2 diabetes and alcoholism. During his most recent visit to the veteran's administration primary care clinical, the nurse noted that Mr. Diamond was tearful during his physical examination. Mr. Diamond's fasting blood sugar was 641, and his HgA1C was

TABLE 9.4   *DSM–IV* "Diagnostic Criteria for 312.31 Pathological Gambling"

Persistent and recurrent maladaptive gambling behavior as indicated by five (or more) of the following:

(1) is preoccupied with gambling (e.g., preoccupied with reliving past gambling experiences, handicapping or planning the next venture, or thinking of ways to get money with which to gamble)

(2) needs to gamble with increasing amounts of money in order to achieve the desired excitement

(3) has repeated unsuccessful efforts to control, cut back, or stop gambling

(4) is restless or irritable when attempting to cut down or stop gambling

(5) gambles as a way of escaping from problems or of relieving a dysphoric mood (e.g., feelings of helplessness, guilt, anxiety, depression)

(6) after losing money gambling, often returns another day to get even ("chasing" one's losses)

(7) lies to family members, therapist, or others to conceal the extent of involvement with gambling

(8) has committed illegal acts such as forgery, fraud, theft, or embezzlement to finance gambling

(9) has jeopardized or lost a significant relationship, job, or educational or career opportunity because of gambling

(10) relies on others to provide money to relieve a desperate financial situation caused by gambling

TABLE 9.5 Ethical Decision-Making Framework

Ethical Principle	Application to Issue of Independence
Autonomy (Self-Determination) The right to govern self or to freely choose one's actions as long as these choices do not interfere with the autonomy or rights of other persons.	Mr. Diamond clearly has the right to gamble. However, what variables in his life interfere in this decision? Is he lonely, or financially compromised? Further assessment of these issues will help Mr. Diamond make a more informed decision regarding his gambling behavior and its impact on disease management.
Beneficence Doing good or participating in behavior that benefits a recipient of care.	It is important for the nurse to assess Mr. Diamond's gambling behavior and its impact on his health. This is an appropriate nursing action that is in the best interest of the client. While assessment may be embarrassing for Mr. Diamond, it is essential to prevent further risk to his health.
Nonmaleficence Above all, do no harm.	Failure to assess Mr. Diamond's gambling behavior and its impact on his health would be termed nonmaleficence. While nurses often do not feel that gambling is a health care issue, it has several health care consequences, such as stress and loss of financial resources, which could greatly impact health. Use of the nursing process, as well as consultation with family and members of the health care team, generally result in effective assessment and interventions.
Justice The fair allocation of resources to individuals or the provision of an equal share of available resources to each person.	In light of the rising incidence of problem and pathological gambling in older adults, assessment and management of gambling must take place at every health care encounter.

elevated. The nurse made several recommendations to Mr. Diamond on how to evaluate his blood sugar and take the medications. During the teaching session, Mr. Diamond glanced at his watch and began to hurry the appointment along. The nurse asked him what the rush was, and Mr. Diamond responded that he had to catch the bus for the casino. The nurse gained quick insight into an additional barrier to meeting Mr. Diamond's health care goals. Table 9.5 uses the ethical decision-making framework to examine Mr. Diamond's gambling.

Nursing interventions aimed at reducing pathological and problem gambling are focused on support for this addictive behavior and reduction of the health-related consequences of gambling. In the case of Mr. Diamond, referral to gamblers anonymous (http://www.Gamblers anonymous.org), and assistance with purchasing diabetes supplies and medications were obtained. Unwin, Davis, and DeLeeuw (2000) suggest a six-step approach to helping problem and pathological gamblers beginning with (1) screening for gambling using a standardized instrument or the DSM–IV criteria, (2) immediate intervention if the client is suicidal, (3) referral to Gamblers Anonymous, (4) enlisting the help of family members to support treatment adherence and effectiveness, (5) counseling, and (6) actively participating in the treatment plan with subsequent assessment for relapses.

SUMMARY

In the care of older adults, many ethical, legal, and financial issues will continue to arise. These issues range from who should receive services to who should make the decisions and how health care bills will be paid. These issues are complex and in great flux. Changes to laws governing health care decisions influence how these decisions will be made in the future. Moreover, the increasing older adult population is retiring later thereby impacting the health care and financial status of older adults.

There are several ethical principles that may be used to guide ethical decision making. When health care team members use these principles as the basis for discussion of ethical issues, they are better able to help clients make efficient and beneficial decisions. Furthermore, the use of legal and medical resources to plan for the financial and health care future of older adults is essential to ensuring maximum quality of life throughout older adulthood.

REFERENCES

The American Heritage Dictionary of the English Language (4th ed). (2007). Ethics. Retrieved July 14, 2007, from http://dictionary.reference.com/browse/ethics

American Nurses' Association. (1994). *Position statement on assisted suicide*. Washington, DC: Author.

Annon, J. (1976). The PLISSIT model: A proposed conceptual scheme for the behavioral treatment for sexual problems. *Journal of Sex Education Therapy, 2*(2), 1–15.

Araujo, A. B., Mohr, B. A., & McKinlay, J. B. (2004). Changes in sexual function in middle-aged and older men: Longitudinal data from the Massachusetts male aging study. *Journal of the American Geriatrics Society, 52*(9), 1502–1509.

Burkhardt, J. E., Berger, A. M., Creedon, M., & McGavock, A. T. (1998). *Mobility and independence: Changes and challenges for older drivers.* Washington, DC: Department of Health and Human Services (DHHS), under the auspices of the Joint DHHS/DOT Coordinating Council on Access and Mobility.

Harvard Medical School. (2003). *Sexuality in midlife and beyond: A special report from Harvard Medical School.* Boston: Harvard Health Publications.

Hogstel, M. O. (2001). *Gerontology: Nursing care of the older adult.* Albany, NY: Delmar Thomson Learning.

Holohan-Bell, J., & Brummel-Smith, K. (1999). Impaired mobility and deconditioning. In J. Stone, J. Wyman, & S. Salisbury (Eds.), *Clinical gerontological nursing: A guide to advanced practice* (pp. 267–287). Philadelphia: W. B. Saunders.

Kessel, B. (2001). Sexuality in the older person. *Age and Ageing, 30,* 121–124.

Kessenich, C. R., & Cichon, M. J. (2001). Hormonal decline in elderly men and male menopause. *Geriatric Nursing, 22,* 24–27.

Koeneman, K., Mulhall, J. P., & Goldstein, I. (1997). Sexual health for the man at midlife: In-office workup. *Geriatrics, 52,* 76–86.

Levens, S., Dyer, A. M., Zubritsky, C., Knott, K., & Oslin, D. W. (2005). Gambling among older, primary-care patients. An important public health concern. *American Journal of Geriatric Psychiatry, 13,* 69–76.

Masters, W. H. (1986, August 15). Sex and aging—expectations and reality. *Hospital Practice,* 175–177.

Meston, C. M. (1997). Aging and sexuality. *Western Journal of Medicine, 167,* 285–290.

Morley, J. E., & Tariq, S. H. (2003). Sexuality and disease. *Clinics in Geriatric Medicine, 19*(3), 563–573.

Unwin, B., Davis, M., & DeLeeuw, J. (2000). Pathological gambling. *American Family Physician, 61,* 741–749.

Wiebe, J. M. D., & Cox, B. J. (2005). Problem and probable pathological gambling among older adults assessed by the SOGS-R. *Journal of Gambling Studies, 21*(2), 205–221.

CHAPTER TEN

Quality of Life Issues Among Older Adults

Learning Objectives

1. Identify quality of life dimensions of older adulthood.
2. Describe the epidemic of elder mistreatment.
3. Describe the types, indicators of, and contributing factors to elder mistreatment.
4. Discuss strategies for the assessing reporting, treatment, and prevention of elder mistreatment.
5. Identify the incidence of pain and barriers to pain assessment in older adults.
6. Assess pain using client self-report and/or a validated pain instrument.
7. Identify strategies and considerations in treating pain in older adults.
8. Identify benefits and challenges of grandparenting.
9. Describe spirituality as an important component of quality of life.

Ms. Long, an 89-year-old White female, is admitted to your unit for a fracture of the right wrist and a dislocated right shoulder, which she claims to be the results of falling off a chair. She has a history of hypertension and coronary artery disease. Her husband passed away several years ago, and last year she began having trouble caring for herself and keeping up with her medications. Her granddaughter, who has been caring for her for the past 9 months, accompanies Ms. Long. You are the nurse responsible for performing her initial health history and assessment. During the history, the client timidly states that she feels very lucky to have someone caring for her at home so she does not have to go a nursing home. After this, she mentions that her granddaughter lost her job about 2 months ago but is still very busy and spends most of her days away from the house. You ask the client about her normal diet patterns, and she says that she typically has one meal a day in the evening when her granddaughter comes home and just snacks throughout the rest of the day. Upon examination, you realize that she is 5'1" and weighs 85 lbs. In addition, you notice that there appear to be several bruises at different stages of healing evident especially on her arms and legs. She also appears to have a stage II pressure ulcer on her coccyx.

As individuals continue to age, a variety of special and unique quality-of-life issues tend to occur. Some issues occur as the result of physical and cognitive changes of aging, both normal and pathological. Others develop with changing older adult roles. Regardless of the cause for these changes, they have the capacity to bring about great sadness and distress. Effective coping with these issues is often a deciding factor in the quality of life of older adults.

QUALITY OF LIFE (QOL)

Quality of life (QOL) is a concept that was relatively unexplored prior to the 1970s. Issues of cost-effectiveness and Medicare revisions stimulated exploration into the substantial amounts of money being spent to keep people alive for years on respirators and other life-sustaining equipment, only to have such people die or return to a life considered to be "not worth living." The first such article to appear in the *Journal of the American Geriatric Society* was a speech given by Senator Charles McMathias, Jr. (1979). He spoke of improving the QOL for the elderly amidst the controversy over the budget for health care and medical research. In 1983, gerontologists Pearlman and Speer wrote "Quality of Life Considerations in Geriatric Care," a document that contained their opinion on the definition of QOL for the elderly and the ramifications for decisions about euthanasia and terminating life support. They also explored related key concepts in the definition of QOL. Since then, the research on QOL considerations has expanded greatly. The discussion of QOL frequently surrounds the treatment choices to be made with older adults. In these cases, the process often compares "curing the disease" with the impact of that cure on QOL. This is sometimes referred to as the risk-benefit ratio.

The concept of QOL is consistently characterized by two attributes, multidimensionality and individuality. The multidimensional nature of

EVIDENCE-BASED PRACTICE

Title of Study: Medical Staff's Decision-Making Process in the Nursing Home
Authors: Cohen-Mansfield, J., Lipson, S.
Purpose: To describe the medical decision-making process at the time of status change events in a large suburban nursing home.
Methods: Questionnaires that described the medical decision-making process for 70 residents of a large nonprofit nursing home facility were completed by three female nurse practitioners and six male physicians.
Findings: The most frequently cited treatment considered and chosen was hospitalization, with family members involved in 39% of decisions and nurses involved in 34%. Quality of life was the most important consideration, and the effectiveness of treatment options and the specific characteristics of the resident and the family's wishes were other factors involved in the decision-making process.
Implications: Multiple considerations are involved in the decision-making process. They include: treatment options, the physician–patient relationship, family considerations, and quality of life.

Journal of Gerontology, Medical Sciences 2003, Vol. 58A, No. 3, 271—278.

the concept has been the focus of much scholarly work. Spitzer et al. (1981) were among the first to explore the multidimensional nature of QOL as activity, daily living, health, support, and outlook. Gurland and Katz (1991) performed an extensive review of QOL literature in an older adult population. Using content analysis, they developed a list of 15 domains in which QOL should be evaluated for older adults. These domains include:

- mobility
- activities of daily living
- organizational skills
- orientational skills
- receptive communication
- expressive communication
- health and perceived health
- mood and symptoms
- social and interpersonal relations
- autonomy
- financial management

- environmental fit
- gratification, future image
- general well-being
- effective coordination

Other researchers have attempted to define the concept broadly by identifying specific QOL domains. Ferrans (1990) reviewed the definitions of QOL and found them to fall into five broad categories:

- normal life
- happiness
- satisfaction
- achievement of personal goals
- social utility

In an attempt to describe individual QOL values, many researchers have evaluated the QOL specific to individuals from varied cultural backgrounds, age groups, and diseases. For a definition of QOL to evolve, it is necessary that the dimensions of life influenced by the individual and disease group be identified. Current models of QOL tend to focus on four specific areas of function and well-being: psychological, physiological, spiritual, and social (Ferrell, Grant, Padilla, Vemuri, & Rhiner, 1991). More recently, Bergland and Narum (2007) surveyed 282 elderly women and found that quality of life was defined by continuity, empowerment, and the quest for meaning.

In order to appropriately assess QOL for older adults receiving nursing care, it is important that this general model be used as a guideline. Issues surrounding the QOL of older adults are vast, but this chapter will explore four specific issues that have a great impact on the domains of QOL. While the issues have the capacity to affect all domains, elder mistreatment impacts the psychological domain of health for older adults; pain is the major physical issue; the spirituality of older adults will be the focus of the spiritual domain; and grandparenting will guide the discussion of the social domain.

CULTURAL FOCUS

In an attempt to describe individual QOL values, many researchers have evaluated the QOL specific to individuals from varied cultural backgrounds, age groups, and diseases. For a definition of QOL to evolve, it is necessary that the dimensions of life influenced by the individual and disease group be identified.

ELDER MISTREATMENT

It is estimated that approximately 1 million cases of elder mistreatment (EM) occur each year. However, this number is likely a severe underestimation, as elder abuse is frequently not reported for several reasons. Victims may fear retaliation, feel shame, or have a desire or need to protect the abuser (Cronin, 2007). Lack of mandatory universal reporting laws is another reason. Table 10.1 lists mandatory reporting elder abuse laws by state. The incidence of EM is likely to rise with the increasing older adult population.

Types of abuse include physical and psychological abuse and neglect, sexual abuse, and financial abuse. Physical abuse may involve intentionally causing pain or injuring older adults, while psychological abuse involves threatening, insulting, or socially isolating the older adult (Cronin, 2007). Physical and psychological neglect are often the most challenging forms of elder mistreatment to assess because of the associated decline in physical and cognitive functioning common in these victims. Active physical neglect arises from the purposeful withholding of necessities, whereas passive neglect results from the caregiver's inability to identify the older adult's needs or to perform the tasks essential to meet the older adult's needs. The term *neglect* implies a failure to perform an obligation and, therefore, raises questions regarding whether a family does have an obligation to provide care for an older adult. It is important to assess whether the caregiver is purposefully neglecting the older adult victim or is simply not physically or cognitively capable of caring for this person. Financial abuse may occur when the older adult's funds, property, or assets are used for wrongful purposes, and sexual abuse involves the sexual assault or rape of an older adult.

Characteristics that may place older adults at risk for abuse include (a) female gender, (b) advanced age, (c) functional dependence, (d) history of intergenerational conflict, (e) passive or stoic personality, (f) social isolation, (g) physical and/or cognitive deficits, and (h) history of abuse. Characteristics that increase risks for caregivers to abuse an older adult include (a) substance abuse, (b) mental illness, (c) lack of knowledge or experience with caregiving, (d) financial stressors, (e) history of abuse as a child, (f) lack of outside interests and involvement, (g) extreme life stressors, (h) aggressive and unsympathetic personality, and (i) unrealistic expectations of the situation (Fillit & Picariello, 1998).

Effective assessment of elder mistreatment is the responsibility of nurses and health care professionals in all settings. The greatest potential for reducing and/or preventing older adult mistreatment is early identification and intervention. The nurse should be alert to signs and symptoms of possible elder mistreatment, which may include: (a) patterns of unexplained injuries; (b) indication that the older adult is fearful of their

TABLE 10.1 American Bar Association Recommended Guidelines for State Courts Handling Cases Involving Elder Abuse, 1995

State	Health Professional	Human Services Professional	Clergy	Law Enforcement	Long-Term Care Facility Employee	Financial Professionals and Staff	Other	Any Person
Alabama	•							
Alaska	•			•	•			
Arizona	•	•	•	•	•			
Arkansas	•	•		•	•			
California	•	•	•	•		•		
Colorado								
Connecticut	•	•	•	•	•			
Delaware	•	•		•	•		•	•
District of Columbia				•	•			
Florida	•	•		•	•	•	•	
Georgia	•	•	•	•	•		•	
Hawaii	•	•		•	•		•	
Idaho				•	•		•	
Illinois								
Indiana	•	•		•	•			•
Iowa								
Kansas	•			•				
Kentucky							•	
Louisiana								
Maine	•			•				
Maryland	•	•		•				•
Massachusetts	•	•		•			•	•
Michigan	•	•		•			•	•

244

Minnesota
Mississippi
Missouri
Montana
Nebraska
Nevada
New Hampshire
New Jersey
New Mexico
New York
North Carolina
North Dakota
Ohio
Oklahoma
Oregon
Pennsylvania
Rhode Island
South Carolina
South Dakota
Tennessee
Texas
Utah
Vermont
Virginia
Washington
West Virginia
Wisconsin
Wyoming

Source: American Bar Association Recommended Guidelines for State Courts Handling Cases Involving Edler Abuse, 1995. Retrieved June 28, 2005, from http://www.abanet.org/media/factbooks/eldt1.html

caregiver; (c) anger or indifference by the caregiver toward the individual; (d) excessive concern by the caregiver regarding the individual's assets; (e) injuries or unexplained infections present in the client's genital region; (f) severe, unexplained dehydration or malnutrition, hypo- or hyperthermia related to environmental exposure; (g) poor hygiene of the client; or (h) unexplained management of medication. It is important to note and understand that victims may feel dependent upon the perpetrator and fear reprisal if they report the mistreatment (Cronin, 2007). In addition to the victims' reluctance to report the mistreatment, barriers to detection also are increased in that the signs and symptoms of abuse are commonly occurring clinical conditions among older adults. For example, changes in behavior may be a result of psychological abuse or an early sign of disease change or onset. (Cronin, 2007).

While interviewing the older adult, the nurse must try to remain nonjudgmental and begin with nonthreatening questions. It is important to interview the individual alone during this portion of the assessment and to be alert for any inconsistencies between history and physical findings.

If elder abuse or neglect is suspected, the health care provider must report it immediately to the local Adult Protective Services (Hogstel, 2001). However, these agencies are often understaffed and overburdened. Consequently, the ability to quickly assess and protect older adults against elder mistreatment is often compromised. However, an appropriate investigation must be conducted and intervention begun to ensure the older adult's safety. Statutes designed to safeguard older adults from elder mistreatment have been passed in all 50 states. In these statutes, elder mistreatment is

---

EVIDENCE-BASED PRACTICE

Title of Study: A Comparison of Three Measures of Elder Abuse

Author: Meeks-Sjostrom, D.

Purpose: To present and compare three measurements for assessing elder abuse.

Methods: Through a literature review, three measures for assessing elder abuse were identified, reviewed, and evaluated according to their characteristics and uses.

Findings: The three measures identified were: (1) The indicators of abuse (IOA), a 22-item tool for identifying abuse, completed by a health care professional following a home assessment; (2) The Elder Abuse and Neglect Assessment (EAI).

Implications: The data from this study strengthened support for the use of the measures to detect elder mistreatment in multiple environments of care.

Journal of Nursing Scholarship, Vol. 36, No. 3, 247–250.

---

defined in terms of acts of commission (intentional infliction of harm), or acts of omission (harm occurring through neglect) by a caregiver. The definition of a caregiver may vary among states, but it generally includes a relative or friend who is concerned and involved in some way with helping manage one's condition (Kassan, 2003).

PAIN

Pain is a major problem for older adults and those who care for them. Flaherty (2007) reports that 25% to 50% of community-dwelling older adults and 45% to 80% of nursing home residents experience untreated pain. Marcus (2004) reports that there are many poor consequences of pain. These include depression, decreased socialization, sleep disturbances, impaired functional ability, and increased health care utilization and costs.

Despite the great prevalence and impact of pain on older adults, there are many barriers that prevent success in this area. Some nurses believe that pain is a natural and expected part of aging, and this remains one of the most prevalent myths and a barrier to appropriate pain assessment and management. Other barriers include older adults' hesitancy to report pain, because they may believe that it is an expected part of aging and nothing can be done for it, or they simply may be afraid to bother their nurse.

Both normal and pathological changes of aging affect the presentation of pain in older adults. However, mixed findings have been found regarding whether or not the older adult's perception of pain decreases with age. Because objective biological markers of pain are not available, nurses must rely on the patient's self-report. There are many standardized tools for assessing pain in older adults, but the most frequently used measure of pain is a numeric rating scale where the client is asked to rank their pain on a scale from 1 to 10, with 1 being very little pain, and 10 being the worst pain imaginable. However, some research suggests that the abstract nature of these scales makes them difficult to use for some older adults, especially those with cognitive impairments. Another available tool is Visual Analogue Scales (VAS), which are straight horizontal 100 mm lines with verbal pain descriptors on the left and on the right sides. Older adults are asked to indicate a position on the scale that represents their pain. These tests also are not perfect. The "Faces Scale" depicts facial expressions on a scale from 0 to 6 with 0 for a smile, indicating no pain, and 6 for a crying grimace, indicating lots of pain. Determining the right tool for each patient is necessary to utilize these objective measures effectively.

For older adults with cognitive impairments, clients may not be able to verbalize pain appropriately. In these clients, yelling, wandering, and repetitive or aggressive behavior may be signs of pain. In caring for the cognitively impaired, the nurse needs to be aware of known painful conditions. Evaluation of behavior for the signs and symptoms of pain is essential for effective assessment and management (Horgas, 2007). The five-item Pain Assessment in Advanced Dementia Scale (PAINAD) has been effective for assessing pain in this population (Warden, Hurley, & Volicer, 2003).

Once the presence of pain is identified, it is important to look for the underlying cause of pain and determine whether it is acute or chronic. When possible, the cause of pain should be targeted for interventions and then the use of both pharmacological and nonpharmacological pain management strategies implemented. The most common pharmaceutical medications used to treat pain in older adults are acetaminophen, nonsteroidal and anti-inflammatory drugs (NSAIDs), and opioids. However, the frequent adverse drug reactions and analgesic sensitivity in this older adult population (see Chapter 6) underscore the need for the old cliché to "start low and go slow" (American Geriatric Society, 1998). For example, NSAIDs contribute to gastric ulceration and mask pain. Older adults have also been found to respond to morphine as if they were given a larger dose, suggesting the need to decrease morphine dosages in this population. It is important to note that pain medication for older adults should be given on a regular basis, not PRN, or as needed (American Geriatric Society, 1998). Collaborative pain medications, such as antidepressants, anticonvulsants, and anxiolytics, may also be helpful in pharmacologically reducing pain among older adults.

In addition to pharmacological pain management strategies, nonpharmacological pain interventions are receiving much attention for their effectiveness in reducing pain among older adults. Exercise, educational and cognitive therapy, massage, acupuncture, therapeutic touch, reiki, and reflexology are all currently being investigated as potential adjuncts to pain management. While the research is still forthcoming, early evidence suggests that these interventions are effective in reducing pain in multiple populations. The problem of pain in older adults is an ongoing concern in need of further clinical investigation. Pain management at the end of life will be discussed in Chapter 12.

GRANDPARENTING

The increase in lifespan has created a generation of grandparents that was nonexistent in the past. Previous generations did not live a sufficient length

CULTURAL FOCUS

It is estimated that 25% of Black and Hispanic grandmothers live in households with grandchildren compared to less than one-tenth of White grandmothers (Szinovacz, 1998). Nurses must be aware of these trends and their impact on the health of older adult grandparents.

of time for grandchildren to know their grandparents.While this is certainly a wonderful phenomenon, it is not universal. Due to the longer lifespan of women, it has been revealed that grandchildren are more likely to know their grandmothers than their grandfathers (Hogstel, 2001). Moreover, grandparenthood differs among cultures. For example, grandparenthood occurs at younger ages for Black and Hispanic women as compared to White women.

In addition to the rising availability of grandparents, a substantial increase has been seen in the number of grandparents raising grandchildren. It is estimated that 25% of Black and Hispanic grandmothers live in households with grandchildren compared to less than one-tenth of White grandmothers (Szinovacz, 1998). Reasons for this increase in grandparents raising grandchildren often stem from child mistreatment and neglect and may include: (a) impairment of the biological parents through substance abuse, (b) rise in rates of teen pregnancy, (c) presence of acquired immunodeficiency syndrome (AIDS), (d) incarceration, (e) mental illness, (f) emotional problems, and (g) premature parental death.

Grandparents who raise grandchildren are at higher risk for health problems than older adults who do not serve in this caregiving role. Moreover, grandparents raising grandchildren may also have financial problems and other caregiving responsibilities (e.g., Spouse). Grandparents caring for grandchildren are more likely to have (a) higher rates of chronic diseases, (b) female gender, (c) high rates of unemployment, and (d) less than a 12th-grade education (Hogstel, 2001). In caring for older adults, nurses must understand that grandparenting can be a stressful role and those grandparents caring for grandchildren may experience greater stress. Consequently, nursing interventions to maintain health, prevent stress-related illness, and increase social support for the grandparent should be implemented with these older adult clients.

SPIRITUALITY

The presence of spirituality in the lives of older adults once was not acknowledged. In fact, the original work of Rowe and Kahn (1997) on successful aging neglected to include the component of spirituality.

However, more recently, spirituality has been identified as an integral component of health and functioning. While the importance of spirituality is more readily acknowledged by society, expressions of spirituality are increasingly diverse. Some cultures express their spirituality through particularly religious practices, such as Buddhism or Taoism. Others have spiritual practices that are apart from formal religion. Spirituality represents a search for meaning in life, and this becomes especially important as older adults approach the end of life.

While the role of spirituality is strong through life for many adults, its role at the end of life is magnified. Older adults are more likely to explore the meaning of life and question the existence of an afterlife. End-of-life care has recently been the subject of a great deal of research, and the nursing role in promoting spiritual health at the end of life is becoming better articulated. This role will be discussed more fully in Chapter 12.

Spirituality is an inherent component of life for all people. It provides a framework within which people conduct the search for meaning and purpose in life. Koenig, McCullogh, and Larson (2001) define spirituality as "the personal quest for understanding answers to ultimate questions about life, about meaning, and about relationships that are sacred or transcendent" (p. 18). Spirituality differs from religion, which specifically concerns the spiritual beliefs and practices held by organized groups (e.g., Buddhist, Catholic, Protestant, Jewish). Religion is defined by Koenig et al. as "an organized system of beliefs, practices, rituals and symbols designed (a) to facilitate closeness to the sacred or transcendent (God, higher power, or ultimate truth/reality), and (b) to foster an understanding of one's relation and responsibility to others living together in a community" (p. 18). While many people pursue spirituality through a specific religion, participation in organized religion is not a prerequisite for spirituality. In fact, many older adults do not affiliate with an organized religion, yet possess a deep sense of spirituality.

CULTURAL FOCUS

While the importance of spirituality is more readily acknowledged by society, expressions of spirituality are increasingly diverse. Some cultures express their spirituality through particularly religious practices, such as Buddhism or Taoism. Others have spiritual practices that are apart from formal religion. Consequently, it is necessary to include spiritual assessment with older adults in order to identify deficits in the older adult's spiritual needs. Then interventions may be implemented to help the older adult improve spiritual connectedness.

It is of great importance that nurses understand that spirituality and the practice of religion vary greatly among older adults. While the process of aging often fosters a search for the meaning of life, not all older adults search in the same way. The nurse is likely to practice a religion different from the older adult, so it is important that the nurse does not impose their personal beliefs and religious views on their patients. The nurse must be open and understanding, allowing the older adult to pursue spirituality in their own unique way.

The presence of spirituality has been associated with relief from physical, mental, and addictive disorders and with enhanced quality of life and survival. Understanding the role of spirituality in the health and functioning of older adults underscores the need to plan care around this important life component. Consequently, it is imperative that nurses who care for older adults are well-prepared to assess and manage spiritual needs. Older adults who engage in religious and spiritual practice often cope better psychologically and have better physical health than those who don't (Koenig, 2007). Older adults residing in nursing homes are potentially more at risk for poor mental and physical health due to the many losses that go along with the aging process, loss of loved ones, loss of home and independence, and loss of function, of which they have little or no control.

It is necessary to include spiritual assessment when working with older adults. In conducting spiritual assessments, the nurse may ask about many topics: (1) the individual's beliefs and practices; (2) what spirituality means to the client; (3) whether the client is affiliated with specific religions and is actively involved; (4) whether spirituality is a source of support and strength; and (5) whether the client has any special religious traditions, rituals, or practices they like to follow. Spiritual assessment scales are available, including Stoll's Spiritual Assessment Guide and O'Brien's Spiritual Assessment Scale. These instruments may be helpful to the nurse conducting spiritual assessments of older adults.

Spiritual assessments may reveal deficits in the older adult's spiritual needs; interventions may need to be implemented to help the older adult improve their spiritual connectedness. This process requires the nurse to discuss with the client the role of spirituality and religion in the lives of older adults. The nurse should encourage religious and spiritual beliefs and practices in all environments of care, as allowed by institutional policy. It is important for the nurse to be aware of the availability of religious personnel within each facility and call upon these members of the interdisciplinary team to help the older adult whenever necessary. Spiritual counseling and praying with the patient are often great sources of comfort to the patient and family.

CRITICAL THINKING CASE STUDY

Mr. Hawkins is a 62-year-old man with severe peripheral vascular disease secondary to NIDDM. He lives at home with his wife who provides his daily care. Over the past 6 weeks, he has become more dependent in all activities of daily living and has ceased his social activities. When his family comes to visit, he responds to their concerns with grunts. He prefers to watch television instead of spending time with his children and grandchildren. His appetite has been poor, and he is having difficulty sleeping at night. On top of this, the circulation in his left foot has led to early necrosis. Because he is not a good candidate for surgery, he was asked to consider having an amputation.

1. How is Mr. Hawkins typical of older adults with chronic illness?
2. What risk factors may have contributed to Mr. Hawkins chronic conditions?
3. What effect do Mr. Hawkins's chronic conditions have on his ability to independently complete his activities of daily living?
4. What other health problems do you expect Mr. Hawkins to be at risk for, given his current conditions?
5. What nursing interventions could you put into place to increase Mr. Hawkins's health functioning and quality of life?

SUMMARY

As the population of older adults continues to rise, the number of special problems that affect the quality of life unique to this population will expand. Regardless of the trajectory of these quality of life issues among older adults, nurses are in a key position to assess older adults for the risk and existence of these commonly occurring issues and implement strategies to reduce their negative consequences. In so doing, nurses can promote a high quality of life for older adults in all care settings.

REFERENCES

American Geriatric Society Panel on Chronic Pain in Older Persons. (1998). The management of chronic pain in older persons. *Journal of the American Geriatrics Society, 46*, 635–651.

Bergland, A., & Narum, I. (2007). Quality of life demands comprehension and further exploration. *Journal of Aging & Health, 19*(1) 39–61.

Cronin, G. (2007). Elder abuse: the same old story? *Emergency Nurse, 15*(3), 11–13.

Ferrans, C. E. (1990). Quality of life: Conceptual issues. *Seminars in Oncology Nursing, 6*, 248–254.

Ferrell, B., Grant, M., Padilla, G., Vemuri, S., & Rhiner, M. (1991). The experience of pain and perceptions of quality of life: Validation of a conceptual model. *The Hospice Journal, 7*, 9–24.

Flaherty, E. (2007). *Try this: Pain assessment in older adults.* Issue 7. Retrieved July 14, 2007, from http://www.hartfordign.org/publications/trythis/issue07.pdf

Gurland, B. J., & Katz, S. (1991). Quality of life and mental disorders of elders. In H. Katschnig, H. Freeman, & N. Sartorius (Eds.), *Quality of life in mental disorders* (pp. 198–202). London: John Wiley and Sons.

Hogstel, M. O. (2001). *Gerontology: Nursing care of the older adult.* Albany, NY: Delmar Thomson Learning.

Horgas, A. (2007). *Try this: Assessing pain in older adults with dementia.* Issue D2. Retrieved July 14, 2007, from http://www.hartfordign.org/publications/trythis/assessingPain.pdf

Kassan, G. (2003). Compliance, caregivers, and the consumer. Presentation given at Direct to Consumer Public meeting. Retrieved July 14, 2007, from http://www.fda.gov/cder/ddmac/DTCmeeting2003_presentations.html

Koenig, H. G. (2007). Religion and remission of depression in medical inpatients with heart failure/pulmonary disease. *Journal of Nervous and Mental Disease, 195*(5), 389–395.

Koenig, H. G., McCullogh, M., & Larson, D. B. (2001). *Handbook of religion and health.* New York: Oxford University Press.

Marcus, D. (2004). Management of nonmalignant chronic pain in older patients. *Clinical Geriatrics, 12*(6), 26–32.

McMathias, C. (1979). Improving the quality of life for the elderly. *Journal of the American Geriatrics Society, 28*, 385–388.

Pearlman, R. A., & Speer, J. B. (1983). Quality of life considerations in geriatric care. *Journal of the American Geriatrics Society, 3*, 113–120.

Rowe, J. W., & Kahn, R. L (1997). Successful aging. *Aging, 10*, 142–144.

Szinovacz, M. (1998). Grandparents today: a demographic profile. *Gerontologist, 8*(1), 37–52.

Spitzer, W. O., Dobson, A. J., Hall, J., Chesterman, E., Levi, J., Shepard, R., et al. (1981). Measuring the quality of life for cancer patients: Concise QL-index for use by physicians. *Journal of Chronic Disease, 34*, 584–597.

Warden, V., Hurley, A. C., & Volicer, L. (2003). Development and psychometric evaluation of the pain assessment in advanced dementia (PAINAD) Scale. *Journal of the American Medical Directors Association, 4*(1), 9–15.

CHAPTER ELEVEN

Environments of Care

Learning Objectives

1. Identify the most common environments of care for older adults.
2. Discuss the effects of caregiving on older adults caring for loved ones.
3. Discuss strategies for reducing the risk of caregiving.
4. List positive and negative aspects to home care.
5. Identify supportive interventions in the community.
6. State the risks of acute care hospitalization for older adults.
7. Discuss aspects of skilled nursing facility admission and care.
8. Discuss risk factors and prevention strategies for urinary tract infections and pressure ulcers in skilled nursing facilities.
9. Identify housing alternatives for older adults.
10. Discuss problems associated with homeless older adults.

You are the home care nurse assigned to see an 83-year-old male patient who was recently discharged to his home from the hospital after a fracture of the right tibia resulting from a fall. He has no other known health problems. When you make your first visit to the client's home, you notice that there are several stairs that one must walk up prior to entering the home. You notice that the only other way to enter the house is by walking up several stairs in the back onto the deck and going in the back door. Concerned about the fact that this patient has a history of falls, you make a notation of this in the client's chart. When you enter the client's home, you assess his vital signs and then ask to listen to his lungs and heart and to look at the right leg. You determine that all of these assessments are within normal limits. As you ask the patient about his pain, he grimaces but says that he is fine. However, you spend some time explaining to him that it is okay to discuss pain with you, and he admits to still being bothered by pain. He feels like his pain medicine is not really helping, especially because the pain has been preventing him from eating or sleeping properly. You decide to call the doctor to try to get a more effective medication for pain. In addition, you work with the patient on some deep breathing and guided imagery techniques. Before you leave, you ask to take a quick look around the house to assess for safety. The client agrees and states, "You should be very pleased; my wife picked up all the rugs around the house and put one of those funny plastic mats in the shower for me." You cannot see any evidence of cords or other barriers to affect mobility around the house and tell the client that all seems to be in place. You do, however, advise the client to try to create an alternative way of getting in and out of the house to help protect the client from falling down the stairs. You also add that it may be wise for him to stay inside for a little while until he is feeling more comfortable with getting around.

As individuals age, the incidence of chronic and acute illnesses increases. In many cases these illnesses result in a subsequent decline in functional status. Functional decline accompanied by loss of spouse or significant other and changes in economic status caused by either death of the family provider or retirement often force older adults to make changes to their environment in order to obtain functional or financial assistance. Some changes that need to be made include adapting the home to a lower level of functioning, having a friend or family member move in to provide informal care, or leaving the current home for an assisted-care environment.

While most older adults prefer to stay in their own homes as long as possible, many others move to a variety of living environments within a continuum of care, which extend from acute care facilities to long-term care settings. Aging in place is a concept that refers to remaining in one setting throughout the majority of older adulthood. Assisted-living facilities, retirement homes, continuing-care retirement communities, and congregate housing are alternatives to the older adult's home that facilitate aging in place to some extent. Regardless of where care is provided, it is essential that cultural competence is achieved. The U.S. Department of Health and Human Services, Office of Minority Health provides recommended standards for cultural competence in health care settings (see Cultural Focus).

Aging in place is important, because moving is emotionally challenging and there may be negative effects of relocating. Translocation syndrome may occur when there is a change in the environment of older adults. This may manifest as impaired physical health, depression, and disruption of established behavior patterns and social relationships.

CULTURAL FOCUS

Recommended Standards for Cultural Competence

1. Promote and support the attitudes, behaviors, knowledge, and skills necessary for staff to work respectfully and effectively with patients and each other in a culturally diverse work environment.
2. Have a comprehensive management strategy to address culturally and linguistically appropriate services, including strategic goals, plans, policies, procedures, and designated staff responsible for implementation.
3. Utilize formal mechanisms for community and consumer involvement in the design and execution of service delivery, including planning, policy making, operations, evaluation, training, and, as appropriate, treatment planning.
4. Develop and implement a strategy to recruit, retain, and promote qualified, diverse, and culturally competent administrative, clinical, and support staff that are trained and qualified to address the needs of the racial and ethnic communities being served.
5. Require and arrange for ongoing education and training for administrative, clinical, and support staff in culturally and linguistically competent service delivery.
6. Provide all clients with limited English proficiency (LEP) access to bilingual staff or interpretation services.
7. Provide oral and written notices, including translated signage at key points of contact, to clients in their primary language informing them of their right to receive no-cost interpreter services.
8. Translate and make available signage and commonly used written patient educational material and other materials for members of the predominant language groups in service areas.
9. Ensure that interpreters and bilingual staff can demonstrate bilingual proficiency and receive training that includes the skills and ethics of interpreting and knowledge in both languages of the terms and concepts relevant to clinical or nonclinical encounters. Family or friends are not considered adequate substitutes, because they usually lack these abilities.
10. Ensure that the clients' primary spoken language and self-identified race/ethnicity are included in the health care organization's management information system as well as any patient records used by provider staff.
11. Use a variety of methods to collect and utilize accurate demographic, cultural, epidemiological, and clinical outcome data for racial and ethnic groups in the service area, and become informed about the ethnic/cultural needs, resources, and assets of the surrounding community.
12. Undertake ongoing organizational self-assessments of cultural and linguistic competence, and integrate measures of access, satisfac-

tion, quality, and outcomes for CLAS into other organizational internal audits and performance improvement programs.

13. Develop structures and procedures to address cross-cultural ethical and legal conflicts in health care delivery and complaints or grievances by patients and staff about unfair, culturally insensitive, or discriminatory treatment, or difficulty in accessing services, or denial of services.

14. Prepare an annual progress report documenting the organizations' progress with implementing CLAS standards, including information on programs, staffing, and resources.

©1999, HHS Office of Minority Health and Resources for Cross Cultural Health Care

---

HOME CARE

It is estimated that approximately 95% of older adults live in the community by themselves or with others. The remaining 5% live in nursing homes, assisted living, or continuing-care retirement homes. Of the 95% that live independently, the majority live with spouses or by themselves (Hogstel, 2001). The number of older adults living independently is expected to increase with the improving health of the aging population. Living in the same home environment through life has many advantages. The older adult may remain among neighbors who share memories and

---

EVIDENCE-BASED PRACTICE

Title of Study: Views of Community-Dwelling, Old-Old People on Barriers and Aids to Nutritional Health

Authors: Callen, B., Wells, T.

Purpose: An examination of both barriers and aids in the maintenance of the health of old–old community-dwelling residents from their perspective.

Methods: Interviews were conducted on 68 community-dwelling residents 80 years or older. Two open-ended questions were used related to barriers and aids to help nutritional health.

Findings: Despite reduced independence and increased physical limitations, the interviewees were positive about their lives and made great attempts to remain independent. Social connectiveness was noted as the main factor in remaining independent.

Implications: Knowledge of positive practices and negative barriers is helpful to older persons in maintaining health promotion.

Journal of Nursing Scholarship, Vol. 35, No. 3, 257–262.

now watch out for each other; sometimes older adults are surrogate parents or grandparents to new families who move into the neighborhood. But, there are also problems with remaining at home for a lifetime. Many homes require costly and difficult repairs and maintenance that older adults can no longer afford to manage. A decline in functional status, vision, and hearing often make adaptation to a home and socialization difficulty. There is no medical care or assistance with ADLs and IADLs built into the home, so the older adult either has to leave home to obtain care, or hire outside providers. The latter may be costly and expenses are not always covered by Medicare and private insurance.

Whether or not the older adult experiences a decline in health, an interdisciplinary approach to home care is essential to facilitate aging in place. Nursing, physical therapy, occupational therapy, speech-language pathology, assistance with personal care, and social work are all available to persons in the home setting. The interdisciplinary team works together to assist the client in regaining strength and returning to the pre-illness

---

EVIDENCE-BASED PRACTICE

Title of Study: Measuring Patient-Level Clinical Outcomes of Home Health Care

Authors: Keepnews, D., Capitman, J., Rosati, R.

Purpose: To examine the Outcomes Assessment and Information Set (OASIS) data to analyze patient-level outcomes of home health care.

Methods: Sixteen OASIS measures were compiled to construct an index. The measures were activities of daily living (ADLs) and instrumental activities of daily living (IADLs). Scores were taken at admission and at the time of discharge. Predictors of functional status at discharge were identified by regression analysis.

Findings: 78.1% of patients improved, 18.5% declined, and 2.8% showed no change. 57.2% variance in functional status at discharge was shown. The following were related negatively to functional outcomes of care: age, visual impairment, having Medicaid as a payer, urinary incontinence, cognitive impairment, and use of unplanned or emergency care. Treatment received for care of open wounds or lesions and cardiovascular or orthopedic conditions were positively associated with functional outcomes.

Implications: OASIS data is used to measure patient-level functional outcomes of short-term home health services. More research is needed to improve methods for determining patient outcomes and their predictors.

Journal of Nursing Scholarship, First Quarter 2004.

level of functioning. The team collaborates with the client and family, especially the caregiver.

Home care begins with an assessment on the initial visit, and this sets the stage for all subsequent visits. The initial assessment includes the assessment of the client's (a) assets, (b) social support, (c) environment, and (d) available community resources. The formal assessment of older adult Medicare recipients is called the Outcome and ASessment Information Set (OASIS). This is a group of data elements that forms the comprehensive assessment for an adult home care patient and provides the basis for measuring patient outcomes for purposes of outcome-based quality improvement (OBQI). The OASIS includes sociodemographic, environmental, support system, health status, and functional status attributes of the older adult. The purpose of this assessment is to provide the home health nurse with a picture of the client. Each home health agency uses its own assessment form. Older adults often have multiple diagnoses, chronic illnesses, and disabilities. Each part of the initial assessment is designed to aid the home health nurse to form a holistic view of the client and to then develop an appropriate plan of care that meets the client's individual needs. Reimbursement from Medicare and insurance depend on the assessment of the client and needs for skilled care as identified by the nurse.

Following the assessment, a plan of care is developed to help the client meet their goals. It is important to note that Medicare reimbursement for home care has become extremely limited over the past two decades. Thus, the nurse must utilize every available resource in order to help the client meet the goals in an efficient manner. Community resources are an important part of home health, and the home health nurse should identify community resources that may be useful (Hogstel, 2001). Community-based services include such programs as employment resources, senior center programs, senior housing, adult day care services, and alternative community-based living facilities. Many of these programs are funded through grants distributed through Area Agencies on Aging (AAA) or the federal government, and all can enhance the well-being of older adults and contribute to their ability to live independently, without financial distress and social isolation. Sometimes, the need for community resources does not arise until later visits or client discharge. Consequently, it is important to plan for resources from the start of visits to make sure the client has all necessary services at discharge (Hogstel, 2001).

Caregiving at Home

When older adults continue to reside at home, cognitive, health, and functional declines typically result in the need to have a caregiver live in the home as well. Moreover, it is reported that the caregiver burden is increasing. The Profile of Older Americans (AARP, 2007) reports that 53.6% (13.7 million) of older noninstitutionalized persons live with their elderly spouses, and it is estimated that family members provide approximately 80% of the care for older adults.

The caregiver often provides the majority of care when the older adult is recovering from an acute illness and continues until they can manage self-care activities. In some cases, however, the presence of chronic physical disease, such as stroke or diabetes, or cognitive problems, such as depression or dementia, require the caregiver to assist the dependent older adult with all ADLs. In many cases, the caregiver is also an older adult, most often a woman, with health problems of her own.

The experience of caregiving is very stressful and has been shown to result in the onset of depression, grief, fatigue, decreased socialization, and health problems of the caregiver (Sullivan, 2007). The Caregiver Strain Index (Robinson, 1983) may be helpful in identifying stressors of caregiving that can lead to greater problems throughout the caregiving period.

The caregiver's role and responsibilities may create stress that is situational, acute, or chronic in nature. Other variables associated with that stress are sociocultural issues. For example, caregiving is a more accepted part of the role in many cultural backgrounds, such as native Pacific Islanders. Thus, this role may receive more support and lead to less stress. In addition, family dynamics, attributes of the caregiver, and individual characteristics of the older adult influence caregiver stress. Unfortunately, approximately 50% of caregivers have been diagnosed with depression. "Caregivers may be prone to depression, grief, fatigue, and changes in social relationships. They may also experience physical health problems" (Sullivan, 2007, p. 1). Nurses must evaluate caregivers for signs of various diseases, including depression. Also, providing potential resources, such as respite programs, may help preserve the family member's mental health, which may enable the family member to continue caring for the loved one and delay nursing home placement.

It is important for home care nurses to assess clients at home for signs and symptoms of neglect. As discussed in Chapter 10, active physi-

---

CULTURAL FOCUS

Other variables associated with that stress are sociocultural issues. For example, caregiving is a more accepted part of the role in many cultural backgrounds, such as native Pacific Islanders. Thus, this role may receive more support and lead to less stress. In addition, family dynamics, attributes of the caregiver, and individual characteristics of the older adult influence caregiver stress.

---

cal neglect arises from the purposeful withholding of necessities, whereas passive neglect results from the caregiver's inability to identify the older adult's needs or to perform the tasks essential to meet the older adult's needs. The term *neglect* implies a failure to perform an obligation and, therefore, raises questions regarding whether a family has an obligation to provide care for an older adult. It is important to assess whether the caregiver is purposefully neglecting the older adult victim or is simply not physically or cognitively capable of caring for this person. Signs of neglect include pressure ulcers, malnutrition, dehydration, and poor hygiene. The nurse should also assess for signs and symptoms of physical abuse including, bruising, swelling, and depression. The identification of caregiver stress and early signs of abuse allow the nurse to intervene and prevent harm to the client.

Home care nurses are in a position to assess caregiver stress and provide interventions to relieve stress as necessary. Respite care for the older adult may be found for the older adult in a local skilled nursing facility so that the caregiver may vacation and rest. Other supportive services, such as home health aides, homemakers, chore services, or Meals on Wheels may also be obtained. The caregivers must be supported and encouraged to take care of themselves and pursue their own interests in activities. In this manner, the caregiver will remain in better health and be more actively engaged in society. This will ultimately assist the caregiver in the transition to noncaregiving status once the care recipient dies.

ACUTE CARE

Any older adult with acute or chronic illness will spend some time in a hospital or acute care facility. Fulmer (2001) reports that older adults generally spend twice the time in acute care facilities than their younger counterparts do. While older adults were historically excluded from surgery and other radical procedures because of a short projected lifespan, this is no longer the case. Approximately 60% of hospital admissions, depending on geographic area, are of older adults. However, despite the high prevalence of older adults in acute care facilities, this environment of care is poorly prepared to meet the commonly occurring problems of older adults. In fact, the potential to acquire delirium, nosocomial infections, and decubitus ulcers and to fall may make acute care settings very unsafe for older adults.

Over the past few decades, several intervention models have been introduced to make acute care facilities safer places for older adults. The Geriatric Nurse Resource Project at Yale University Medical Center (Fulmer, 1991a; 1991b) and New York University Medical Center enrolls interested nurses in geriatric care units into a program that provides training on the commonly occurring problems of aging and education on the best geriatric nursing practices. The nurse returns from the training program to act as a resource in their unit for the best care of older adults. This model has proven to be very effective at preventing many of the common problems that result from hospitalization of older adults and has served as a model for other hospitals to use.

The acute care environment offers an excellent opportunity to introduce health-promotion strategies to older adults, because they have the greatest need to adjust their lifestyle in order to return to a healthy status (see Chapter 5). When recovering from illness, older adults may be more amenable to learning information that they believe will prevent future hospital admissions and restore their health. Moreover, the acute care nurse is central in planning services for the older adult upon discharge. Referrals to alternative housing and home care are needed to help the older adult meet acute care goals in a shortened hospital stay environment. Supportive services at home will also assist in preventing hospital readmission for recurring or unresolved illnesses.

A thorough assessment of the environment to which the older adult is returning after acute care hospitalization helps to determine care needs after discharge. This may be done as part of an interdisciplinary care team in the acute care facility. While resolving the acute care illness, nurses caring for older adults may assist in scheduling visiting nurses or long-term care admissions. They can provide for follow-up care, transportation, home health aide and homemaking services, adult day care, or Meals on Wheels. These services will help older adults return to the home care environment more readily prepared to recover from the illness. In addition, helping older adults to locate health promotion programs, such as those that will aid in smoking-cessation, stress-management, weight-loss, or exercise, will allow them to enter these programs immediately after discharge, while they are still motivated to do so.

SKILLED NURSING FACILITIES

Skilled nursing facilities (SNFs) provide 24-hour nursing care to older adults who are unable to care for themselves. These facilities may be private or public, and they may receive reimbursement from Medicare, Medicaid, and private insurances, or the residents self-pay. Most SNFs provide medication administration, wound care, daily assessment, meals, and assistance with ADLs. Other available skilled services may be physical therapy, respiratory therapy, speech-language pathology services, and occupational therapy (Hogstel, 2001). Residents may stay in SNFs for short-term rehabilitation after surgery or medical illness, or they may reside in them throughout their lives.

The typical SNF resident is a female widow in her seventies or eighties who has two or more chronic health conditions requiring nursing care and assistance. However, there are more and more resident centenarians residing in nursing homes than ever before. Many residents of SNFs do not have close family members or regular visitors.

Upon admission to a nursing facility, the resident's private physician, or the facility physician, must perform a history and physical examination within 48 hours. The documentation specific to SNFs is known as the minimum data set (MDS). This is a core set of screening, clinical, and functional status elements, including common definitions and coding categories (See Figure 11.1). It forms the foundation of the comprehensive assessment for all residents of long-term care facilities certified to participate in Medicare or Medicaid and standardizes communication about resident problems and conditions within facilities, between facilities, and between facilities and outside agencies. This documentation must be completed on admission to the facility and in specified intervals throughout the SNF stay. Nursing facilities must provide information on the Resident Bill of Rights upon admission so that the resident and family understand the resident's rights and responsibilities within the SNF. The admission process should also involve a complete orientation and tour of the facility, as well as a discussion of programs and requirements for the resident and family, if possible. It is important that nurses provide an effective orientation and transition to the facility in the first few days to decrease the risk of negative health effects, which may be indicative of the translocation syndrome. The translocation syndrome, discussed earlier, is very likely to happen during admission to a nursing home or transfer to acute care from a nursing home environment, so great attention to the older adult is essential to minimize symptoms of translocation syndrome. Older adults must continually be assessed for alterations in function and cognition and be supported to participate in the environment at the highest possible level. Changes in function and cognition and how the move affects the individual must be diagnosed immediately and appropriate interventions implemented to ensure as safe a transition as possible.

Two commonly occurring problems in long-term care facilities include the frequent onset of urinary tract infections and pressure sores, or decubitus ulcers.

Urinary Tract Infections

Urinary tract infections (UTIs) are the most common infection among older adults and are caused by an accumulation of pathological bacteria in the urine. However, it is important to note that bacteria in the urine occurs commonly among older adults, especially women and those who dwell in long-term care faculties. Bacteriuria, which is the presence of

MINIMUM DATA SET (MDS) — *VERSION 2.0*
FOR NURSING HOME RESIDENT ASSESSMENT AND CARE SCREENING
BACKGROUND (FACE SHEET) INFORMATION AT ADMISSION

SECTION AB. DEMOGRAPHIC INFORMATION

1.	DATE OF ENTRY	Date the stay began. Note — Does not include readmission if record was closed at time of temporary discharge to hospital, etc. In such cases, use prior admission date

☐☐ – ☐☐ – ☐☐☐☐
Month   Day   Year

2.	ADMITTED FROM (AT ENTRY)	1. Private home/apt. with no home health services 2. Private home/apt. with home health services 3. Board and care/assisted living/group home 4. Nursing home 5. Acute care hospital 6. Psychiatric hospital, MR/DD facility 7. Rehabilitation hospital 8. Other
3.	LIVED ALONE (PRIOR TO ENTRY)	0. No 1. Yes 2. In other facility
4.	ZIP CODE OF PRIOR PRIMARY RESIDENCE	☐☐☐☐☐

5.	RESIDEN-TIAL HISTORY 5 YEARS PRIOR TO ENTRY	(*Check all settings* resident *lived in* during 5 years prior to date of entry given in item AB1 above)	
		Prior stay at this nursing home	a.
		Stay in other nursing home	b.
		Other residential facility—board and care home, assisted living, group home	c.
		MH/psychiatric setting	d.
		MR/DD setting	e.
		NONE OF ABOVE	f.

6.	LIFETIME OCCUPA-TION(S) [Put "/" between two occupations]	☐☐☐☐☐☐☐☐☐☐☐☐☐☐☐☐☐☐

7.	EDUCATION (*Highest Level Completed*)	1. No schooling 2. 8th grade/less 3. 9-11 grades 4. High school	5. Technical or trade school 6. Some college 7. Bachelor's degree 8. Graduate degree
8.	LANGUAGE	(*Code for correct response*) **a.** Primary Language 0. English 1. Spanish 2. French 3. Other **b. If other, specify**	
9.	MENTAL HEALTH HISTORY	Does resident's RECORD indicate any history of mental retardation, mental illness, or developmental disability problem? 0. No 1. Yes	

10.	CONDITIONS RELATED TO MR/DD STATUS	(*Check all conditions* that are related to MR/DD status that were manifested before age 22, and are likely to continue indefinitely)	
		Not applicable—no MR/DD (Skip to AB11)	a.
		MR/DD with organic condition	
		Down's syndrome	b.
		Autism	c.
		Epilepsy	d.
		Other organic condition related to MR/DD	e.
		MR/DD with no organic condition	f.

11.	DATE BACK-GROUND INFORMA-TION COMPLETED	☐☐ – ☐☐ – ☐☐☐☐ Month Day Year

SECTION AC. CUSTOMARY ROUTINE

1.	CUSTOMARY ROUTINE	(*Check all that apply.* If all information UNKNOWN, check last box only.)	
	(*In year prior to DATE OF ENTRY to this nursing home, or year last in community if now being admitted from another nursing home*)	**CYCLE OF DAILY EVENTS**	
		Stays up late at night (e.g., after 9 pm)	a.
		Naps regularly during day (at least 1 hour)	b.
		Goes out 1+ days a week	c.
		Stays busy with hobbies, reading, or fixed daily routine	d.
		Spends most of time alone or watching TV	e.
		Moves independently indoors (with appliances, if used)	f.
		Use of tobacco products at least daily	g.
		NONE OF ABOVE	h.
		EATING PATTERNS	
		Distinct food preferences	i.
		Eats between meals all or most days	j.
		Use of alcoholic beverage(s) at least weekly	k.
		NONE OF ABOVE	l.
		ADL PATTERNS	
		In bedclothes much of day	m.
		Wakens to toilet all or most nights	n.
		Has irregular bowel movement pattern	o.
		Showers for bathing	p.
		Bathing in PM	q.
		NONE OF ABOVE	r.
		INVOLVEMENT PATTERNS	
		Daily contact with relatives/close friends	s.
		Usually attends church, temple, synagogue (etc.)	t.
		Finds strength in faith	u.
		Daily animal companion/presence	v.
		Involved in group activities	w.
		NONE OF ABOVE	x.
		UNKNOWN—Resident/family unable to provide information	y.

SECTION AD. FACE SHEET SIGNATURES

SIGNATURES OF PERSONS COMPLETING FACE SHEET:

a. Signature of RN Assessment Coordinator	Date

I certify that the accompanying information accurately reflects resident assessment or tracking information for this resident and that I collected or coordinated collection of this information on the dates specified. To the best of my knowledge, this information was collected in accordance with applicable Medicare and Medicaid requirements. I understand that this information is used as a basis for ensuring that residents receive appropriate and quality care, and as a basis for payment from federal funds. I further understand that payment of such federal funds and continued participation in the government-funded health care programs is conditioned on the accuracy and truthfulness of this information, and that I may be personally subject to or may subject my organization to substantial criminal, civil, and/or administrative penalties for submitting false information. I also certify that I am authorized to submit this information by this facility on its behalf.

Signature and Title	Sections	Date
b.		
c.		
d.		
e.		
f.		
g.		

☐ = When box blank, must enter number or letter   ☐ a. = When letter in box, check if condition applies

MDS 2.0 September, 2000

FIGURE 11.1   Box 11-2 sample minimum data set documentation.

MINIMUM DATA SET (MDS) — VERSION 2.0
FOR NURSING HOME RESIDENT ASSESSMENT AND CARE SCREENING
FULL ASSESSMENT FORM
(Status in last 7 days, unless other time frame indicated)

SECTION A. IDENTIFICATION AND BACKGROUND INFORMATION

1. RESIDENT NAME
a. (First) b. (Middle Initial) c. (Last) d. (Jr/Sr)

2. ROOM NUMBER

3. ASSESSMENT REFERENCE DATE
a. Last day of MDS observation period
Month — Day — Year
b. Original (0) or corrected copy of form (enter number of correction)

4a. DATE OF REENTRY Date of reentry from most recent temporary discharge to a hospital in last 90 days (or since last assessment or admission if less than 90 days)
Month — Day — Year

5. MARITAL STATUS
1. Never married 3. Widowed 5. Divorced
2. Married 4. Separated

6. MEDICAL RECORD NO.

7. CURRENT PAYMENT SOURCES FOR N.H. STAY
(Billing Office to indicate; check all that apply in last 30 days)
Medicaid per diem	a.	VA per diem	f.
Medicare per diem	b.	Self or family pays for full per diem	g.
Medicare ancillary part A	c.	Medicaid resident liability or Medicare co-payment	h.
Medicare ancillary part B	d.	Private insurance per diem (including co-payment)	i.
CHAMPUS per diem	e.	Other per diem	j.

8. REASONS FOR ASSESSMENT
[Note—If this is a discharge or reentry assessment, only a limited subset of MDS items need be completed]
a. Primary reason for assessment
1. Admission assessment (required by day 14)
2. Annual assessment
3. Significant change in status assessment
4. Significant correction of prior full assessment
5. Quarterly review assessment
6. Discharged—return not anticipated
7. Discharged—return anticipated
8. Discharged prior to completing initial assessment
9. Reentry
10. Significant correction of prior quarterly assessment
0. NONE OF ABOVE
b. Codes for assessments required for Medicare PPS or the State
1. Medicare 5 day assessment
2. Medicare 30 day assessment
3. Medicare 60 day assessment
4. Medicare 90 day assessment
5. Medicare readmission/return assessment
6. Other state required assessment
7. Medicare 14 day assessment
8. Other Medicare required assessment

9. RESPONSIBILITY/ LEGAL GUARDIAN
(Check all that apply)
Legal guardian	a.	Durable power attorney/financial	d.
Other legal oversight	b.	Family member responsible	e.
Durable power of attorney/health care	c.	Patient responsible for self	f.
		NONE OF ABOVE	g.

10. ADVANCED DIRECTIVES
(For those items with supporting documentation in the medical record, check all that apply)
Living will	a.	Feeding restrictions	f.
Do not resuscitate	b.	Medication restrictions	g.
Do not hospitalize	c.	Other treatment restrictions	h.
Organ donation	d.	NONE OF ABOVE	i.
Autopsy request	e.		

SECTION B. COGNITIVE PATTERNS

1. COMATOSE (Persistent vegetative state/no discernible consciousness)
0. No 1. Yes (If yes, skip to Section G)

2. MEMORY (Recall of what was learned or known)
a. Short-term memory OK—seems/appears to recall after 5 minutes
0. Memory OK 1. Memory problem
b. Long-term memory OK—seems/appears to recall long past
0. Memory OK 1. Memory problem

---

3. MEMORY/ RECALL ABILITY
(Check all that resident was normally able to recall during last 7 days)
Current season	a.	That he/she is in a nursing home	d.
Location of own room	b.		
Staff names/faces	c.	NONE OF ABOVE are recalled	e.

4. COGNITIVE SKILLS FOR DAILY DECISION-MAKING
(Made decisions regarding tasks of daily life)
0. INDEPENDENT—decisions consistent/reasonable
1. MODIFIED INDEPENDENCE—some difficulty in new situations only
2. MODERATELY IMPAIRED—decisions poor; cues/supervision required
3. SEVERELY IMPAIRED—never/rarely made decisions

5. INDICATORS OF DELIRIUM— PERIODIC DISORDERED THINKING/ AWARENESS
(Code for behavior in the last 7 days) [Note: Accurate assessment requires conversations with staff and family who have direct knowledge of resident's behavior over this time].
0. Behavior not present
1. Behavior present, not of recent onset
2. Behavior present, over last 7 days appears different from resident's usual functioning (e.g., new onset or worsening)
a. EASILY DISTRACTED—(e.g., difficulty paying attention; gets sidetracked)
b. PERIODS OF ALTERED PERCEPTION OR AWARENESS OF SURROUNDINGS—(e.g., moves lips or talks to someone not present; believes he/she is somewhere else; confuses night and day)
c. EPISODES OF DISORGANIZED SPEECH—(e.g., speech is incoherent, nonsensical, irrelevant, or rambling from subject to subject; loses train of thought)
d. PERIODS OF RESTLESSNESS—(e.g., fidgeting or picking at skin, clothing, napkins, etc; frequent position changes; repetitive physical movements or calling out)
e. PERIODS OF LETHARGY—(e.g., sluggishness; staring into space; difficult to arouse; little body movement)
f. MENTAL FUNCTION VARIES OVER THE COURSE OF THE DAY—(e.g., sometimes better, sometimes worse; behaviors sometimes present, sometimes not)

6. CHANGE IN COGNITIVE STATUS
Resident's cognitive status, skills, or abilities have changed as compared to status of 90 days ago (or since last assessment if less than 90 days)
0. No change 1. Improved 2. Deteriorated

SECTION C. COMMUNICATION/HEARING PATTERNS

1. HEARING (With hearing appliance, if used)
0. HEARS ADEQUATELY—normal talk, TV, phone
1. MINIMAL DIFFICULTY when not in quiet setting
2. HEARS IN SPECIAL SITUATIONS ONLY—speaker has to adjust tonal quality and speak distinctly
3. HIGHLY IMPAIRED/absence of useful hearing

2. COMMUNICATION DEVICES/ TECHNIQUES
(Check all that apply during last 7 days)
Hearing aid, present and used	a.
Hearing aid, present and not used regularly	b.
Other receptive comm. techniques used (e.g., lip reading)	c.
NONE OF ABOVE	d.

3. MODES OF EXPRESSION
(Check all used by resident to make needs known)
Speech	a.	Signs/gestures/sounds	d.
Writing messages to express or clarify needs	b.	Communication board	e.
American sign language or Braille	c.	Other	f.
		NONE OF ABOVE	g.

4. MAKING SELF UNDERSTOOD
(Expressing information content—however able)
0. UNDERSTOOD
1. USUALLY UNDERSTOOD—difficulty finding words or finishing thoughts
2. SOMETIMES UNDERSTOOD—ability is limited to making concrete requests
3. RARELY/NEVER UNDERSTOOD

5. SPEECH CLARITY
(Code for speech in the last 7 days)
0. CLEAR SPEECH—distinct, intelligible words
1. UNCLEAR SPEECH—slurred, mumbled words
2. NO SPEECH—absence of spoken words

6. ABILITY TO UNDERSTAND OTHERS
(Understanding verbal information content—however able)
0. UNDERSTANDS
1. USUALLY UNDERSTANDS—may miss some part/intent of message
2. SOMETIMES UNDERSTANDS—responds adequately to simple, direct communication
3. RARELY/NEVER UNDERSTANDS

7. CHANGE IN COMMUNICATION/ HEARING
Resident's ability to express, understand, or hear information has changed as compared to status of 90 days ago (or since last assessment if less than 90 days)
0. No change 1. Improved 2. Deteriorated

□ = When box blank, must enter number or letter [a.] = When letter in box, check if condition applies

MDS 2.0 September, 2000

FIGURE 11.1 Box 11-2 sample minimum data set documentation (*continued*).

Resident _____   Numeric Identifier _____

SECTION D. VISION PATTERNS

1.	VISION	(Ability to see in adequate light and with glasses if used)
		0. ADEQUATE—sees fine detail, including regular print in newspapers/books
		1. IMPAIRED—sees large print, but not regular print in newspapers/books
		2. MODERATELY IMPAIRED—limited vision; not able to see newspaper headlines, but can identify objects
		3. HIGHLY IMPAIRED—object identification in question, but eyes appear to follow objects
		4. SEVERELY IMPAIRED—no vision or sees only light, colors, or shapes; eyes do not appear to follow objects
2.	VISUAL LIMITATIONS/ DIFFICULTIES	Side vision problems—decreased peripheral vision (e.g., leaves food on one side of tray, difficulty traveling, bumps into people and objects, misjudges placement of chair when seating self)	a.
		Experiences any of following: sees halos or rings around lights; sees flashes of light; sees "curtains" over eyes	b.
		NONE OF ABOVE	c.
3.	VISUAL APPLIANCES	Glasses; contact lenses; magnifying glass 0. No 1. Yes

SECTION E. MOOD AND BEHAVIOR PATTERNS

1.	INDICATORS OF DEPRES- SION, ANXIETY, SAD MOOD	(Code for indicators observed in last 30 days, irrespective of the assumed cause) 0. Indicator not exhibited in last 30 days 1. Indicator of this type exhibited up to five days a week 2. Indicator of this type exhibited daily or almost daily (6, 7 days a week)

VERBAL EXPRESSIONS OF DISTRESS

a. Resident made negative statements—e.g., "Nothing matters; Would rather be dead; What's the use; Regrets having lived so long; Let me die"

b. Repetitive questions—e.g., "Where do I go; What do I do?"

c. Repetitive verbalizations—e.g., calling out for help, ("God help me")

d. Persistent anger with self or others—e.g., easily annoyed, anger at placement in nursing home; anger at care received

e. Self deprecation—e.g., "I am nothing; I am of no use to anyone"

f. Expressions of what appear to be unrealistic fears—e.g., fear of being abandoned, left alone, being with others

g. Recurrent statements that something terrible is about to happen—e.g., believes he or she is about to die, have a heart attack

h. Repetitive health complaints—e.g., persistently seeks medical attention, obsessive concern with body functions

i. Repetitive anxious complaints/concerns (non-health related) e.g., persistently seeks attention/reassurance regarding schedules, meals, laundry, clothing, relationship issues

SLEEP-CYCLE ISSUES

j. Unpleasant mood in morning

k. Insomnia/change in usual sleep pattern

SAD, APATHETIC, ANXIOUS APPEARANCE

l. Sad, pained, worried facial expressions—e.g., furrowed brows

m. Crying, tearfulness

n. Repetitive physical movements—e.g., pacing, hand wringing, restlessness, fidgeting, picking

LOSS OF INTEREST

o. Withdrawal from activities of interest—e.g., no interest in long standing activities or being with family/friends

p. Reduced social interaction

2.	MOOD PERSIS- TENCE	One or more indicators of depressed, sad or anxious mood were not easily altered by attempts to "cheer up", console, or reassure the resident over last 7 days
		0. No mood indicators 1. Indicators present, easily altered 2. Indicators present, not easily altered
3.	CHANGE IN MOOD	Resident's mood status has changed as compared to status of 90 days ago (or since last assessment if less than 90 days) 0. No change 1. Improved 2. Deteriorated
4.	BEHAVIORAL SYMPTOMS	(A) Behavioral symptom frequency in last 7 days

(A) Behavioral symptom frequency in last 7 days
0. Behavior not exhibited in last 7 days
1. Behavior of this type occurred 1 to 3 days in last 7 days
2. Behavior of this type occurred 4 to 6 days, but less than daily
3. Behavior of this type occurred daily

(B) Behavioral symptom alterability in last 7 days
0. Behavior not present OR behavior was easily altered
1. Behavior was not easily altered

		(A)	(B)
a. WANDERING (moved with no rational purpose, seemingly oblivious to needs or safety)			
b. VERBALLY ABUSIVE BEHAVIORAL SYMPTOMS (others were threatened, screamed at, cursed at)			
c. PHYSICALLY ABUSIVE BEHAVIORAL SYMPTOMS (others were hit, shoved, scratched, sexually abused)			
d. SOCIALLY INAPPROPRIATE/DISRUPTIVE BEHAVIORAL SYMPTOMS (made disruptive sounds, noisiness, screaming, self-abusive acts, sexual behavior or disrobing in public, smeared/threw food/feces, hoarding, rummaged through others' belongings)			
e. RESISTS CARE (resisted taking medications/ injections, ADL assistance, or eating)			

5.	CHANGE IN BEHAVIORAL SYMPTOMS	Resident's behavior status has changed as compared to status of 90 days ago (or since last assessment if less than 90 days) 0. No change 1. Improved 2. Deteriorated

SECTION F. PSYCHOSOCIAL WELL-BEING

1.	SENSE OF INITIATIVE/ INVOLVE- MENT	At ease interacting with others	a.
		At ease doing planned or structured activities	b.
		At ease doing self-initiated activities (when information UNKNOWN, check last box only)	c.
		Establishes own goals	d.
		Pursues involvement in life of facility (e.g., makes/keeps friends; involved in group activities; responds positively to new activities; assists at religious services)	e.
		Accepts invitations into most group activities	f.
		NONE OF ABOVE	g.
2.	UNSETTLED RELATION- SHIPS	Covert/open conflict with or repeated criticism of staff	a.
		Unhappy with roommate	b.
		Unhappy with residents other than roommate	c.
		Openly expresses conflict/anger with family/friends	d.
		Absence of personal contact with family/friends	e.
		Recent loss of close family member/friend	f.
		Does not adjust easily to change in routines	g.
		NONE OF ABOVE	h.
3.	PAST ROLES	Strong identification with past roles and life status	a.
		Expresses sadness/anger/empty feeling over lost roles/status	b.
		Resident perceives that daily routine (customary routine, activities) is very different from prior pattern in the community	c.
		NONE OF ABOVE	d.

SECTION G. PHYSICAL FUNCTIONING AND STRUCTURAL PROBLEMS

1.	(A) ADL SELF-PERFORMANCE—(Code for resident's PERFORMANCE OVER ALL SHIFTS during last 7 days—Not including setup)

0. INDEPENDENT—No help or oversight —OR— Help/oversight provided only 1 or 2 times during last 7 days

1. SUPERVISION—Oversight, encouragement or cueing provided 3 or more times during last 7 days —OR— Supervision (3 or more times) plus physical assistance provided only 1 or 2 times during last 7 days

2. LIMITED ASSISTANCE—Resident highly involved in activity, received physical help in guided maneuvering of limbs or other nonweight bearing assistance 3 or more times — OR—More help provided only 1 or 2 times during last 7 days

3. EXTENSIVE ASSISTANCE—While resident performed part of activity, over last 7-day period, help of following type(s) provided 3 or more times:
—Weight-bearing support
—Full staff performance during part (but not all) of last 7 days

4. TOTAL DEPENDENCE—Full staff performance of activity during entire 7 days

8. ACTIVITY DID NOT OCCUR during entire 7 days

(B) ADL SUPPORT PROVIDED—(Code for MOST SUPPORT PROVIDED OVER ALL SHIFTS during last 7 days; code regardless of resident's self-performance classification)
0. No setup or physical help from staff
1. Setup help only
2. One person physical assist
3. Two+ persons physical assist
8. ADL activity itself did not occur during entire 7 days

		(A) SELF-PERF	(B) SUPPORT
a.	BED MOBILITY	How resident moves to and from lying position, turns side to side, and positions body while in bed	
b.	TRANSFER	How resident moves between surfaces—to/from: bed, chair, wheelchair, standing position (EXCLUDE to/from bath/toilet)	
c.	WALK IN ROOM	How resident walks between locations in his/her room	
d.	WALK IN CORRIDOR	How resident walks in corridor on unit	
e.	LOCOMO- TION ON UNIT	How resident moves between locations in his/her room and adjacent corridor on same floor. If in wheelchair, self-sufficiency once in chair	
f.	LOCOMO- TION OFF UNIT	How resident moves to and returns from off unit locations (e.g., areas set aside for dining, activities, or treatments). If facility has only one floor, how resident moves to and from distant areas on the floor. If in wheelchair, self-sufficiency once in chair	
g.	DRESSING	How resident puts on, fastens, and takes off all items of street clothing, including donning/removing prosthesis	
h.	EATING	How resident eats and drinks (regardless of skill). Includes intake of nourishment by other means (e.g., tube feeding, total parenteral nutrition)	
i.	TOILET USE	How resident uses the toilet room (or commode, bedpan, urinal); transfer on/off toilet, cleanses, changes pad, manages ostomy or catheter, adjusts clothes	
j.	PERSONAL HYGIENE	How resident maintains personal hygiene, including combing hair, brushing teeth, shaving, applying makeup, washing/drying face, hands, and perineum (EXCLUDE baths and showers)	

MDS 2.0 September, 2000

FIGURE 11.1 *(continued)*.

Resident _____ Numeric Identifier _____

2.	**BATHING**	How resident takes full-body bath/shower, sponge bath, and transfers in/out of tub/shower (EXCLUDE washing of back and hair.) *Code for most dependent in self-performance and support.* (A) BATHING SELF-PERFORMANCE codes appear below	(A)	(B)
		0. Independent—No help provided		
		1. Supervision—Oversight help only		
		2. Physical help limited to transfer only		
		3. Physical help in part of bathing activity		
		4. Total dependence		
		8. Activity itself did not occur during entire 7 days *(Bathing support codes are as defined in Item 1, code B above)*		
3.	**TEST FOR BALANCE** (see training manual)	*(Code for ability during test in the last 7 days)* 0. Maintained position as required in test 1. Unsteady, but able to rebalance self without physical support 2. Partial physical support during test; or stands (sits) but does not follow directions for test 3. Not able to attempt test without physical help		
		a. Balance while standing		
		b. Balance while sitting—position, trunk control		
4.	**FUNCTIONAL LIMITATION IN RANGE OF MOTION** (see training manual)	*(Code for limitations during last 7 days that interfered with daily functions or placed resident at risk of injury)* (A) RANGE OF MOTION (B) VOLUNTARY MOVEMENT 0. No limitation 0. No loss 1. Limitation on one side 1. Partial loss 2. Limitation on both sides 2. Full loss	(A)	(B)
		a. Neck		
		b. Arm—Including shoulder or elbow		
		c. Hand—Including wrist or fingers		
		d. Leg—Including hip or knee		
		e. Foot—Including ankle or toes		
		f. Other limitation or loss		
5.	**MODES OF LOCOMO-TION**	*(Check all that apply during last 7 days)*		
		Cane/walker/crutch **a.**	Wheelchair primary mode of locomotion **d.**	
		Wheeled self **b.**		
		Other person wheeled **c.**	NONE OF ABOVE **e.**	
6.	**MODES OF TRANSFER**	*(Check all that apply during last 7 days)*		
		Bedfast all or most of time **a.**	Lifted mechanically **d.**	
		Bed rails used for bed mobility or transfer **b.**	Transfer aid (e.g., slide board, trapeze, cane, walker, brace) **e.**	
		Lifted manually **c.**	NONE OF ABOVE **f.**	
7.	**TASK SEGMENTA-TION**	Some or all of ADL activities were broken into subtasks during last 7 days so that resident could perform them 0. No 1. Yes		
8.	**ADL FUNCTIONAL REHABILITA-TION POTENTIAL**	Resident believes he/she is capable of increased independence in at least some ADLs **a.**		
		Direct care staff believe resident is capable of increased independence in at least some ADLs **b.**		
		Resident able to perform tasks/activity but is very slow **c.**		
		Difference in ADL Self-Performance or ADL Support, comparing mornings to evenings **d.**		
		NONE OF ABOVE **e.**		
9.	**CHANGE IN ADL FUNCTION**	Resident's ADL self-performance status has changed as compared to status of 90 days ago (or since last assessment if less than 90 days) 0. No change 1. Improved 2. Deteriorated		

SECTION H. CONTINENCE IN LAST 14 DAYS

1.	CONTINENCE SELF-CONTROL CATEGORIES *(Code for resident's PERFORMANCE OVER ALL SHIFTS)*
	0. *CONTINENT*—Complete control [includes use of indwelling urinary catheter or ostomy device that does not leak urine or stool]
	1. *USUALLY CONTINENT*—BLADDER, incontinent episodes once a week or less; BOWEL, less than weekly
	2. *OCCASIONALLY INCONTINENT*—BLADDER, 2 or more times a week but not daily; BOWEL, once a week
	3. *FREQUENTLY INCONTINENT*—BLADDER, tended to be incontinent daily, but some control present (e.g., on day shift); BOWEL, 2-3 times a week
	4. *INCONTINENT*—Had inadequate control BLADDER, multiple daily episodes; BOWEL, all (or almost all) of the time

| **a.** | **BOWEL CONTI-NENCE** | Control of bowel movement, with appliance or bowel continence programs, if employed | |
| **b.** | **BLADDER CONTI-NENCE** | Control of urinary bladder function (if dribbles, volume insufficient to soak through underpants), with appliances (e.g., foley) or continence programs, if employed | |

2.	**BOWEL ELIMINATION PATTERN**	Bowel elimination pattern regular—at least one movement every three days **a.**	Diarrhea **c.**
		Constipation **b.**	Fecal impaction **d.**
			NONE OF ABOVE **e.**

MDS 2.0 September, 2000

3.	**APPLIANCES AND PROGRAMS**	Any scheduled toileting plan **a.**	Did not use toilet room/commode/urinal **f.**
		Bladder retraining program **b.**	Pads/briefs used **g.**
		External (condom) catheter **c.**	Enemas/irrigation **h.**
		Indwelling catheter **d.**	Ostomy present **i.**
		Intermittent catheter **e.**	NONE OF ABOVE **j.**
4.	**CHANGE IN URINARY CONTI-NENCE**	Resident's urinary continence has changed as compared to status of 90 days ago (or since last assessment if less than 90 days)	
		0. No change 1. Improved 2. Deteriorated	

SECTION I. DISEASE DIAGNOSES

Check only those diseases that have a relationship to current ADL status, cognitive status, mood and behavior status, medical treatments, nursing monitoring, or risk of death. (Do not list inactive diagnoses)

1.	DISEASES	*(If none apply, CHECK the NONE OF ABOVE box)*		
		ENDOCRINE/METABOLIC/NUTRITIONAL	Hemiplegia/Hemiparesis	**v.**
		Diabetes mellitus **a.**	Multiple sclerosis	**w.**
		Hyperthyroidism **b.**	Paraplegia	**x.**
		Hypothyroidism **c.**	Parkinson's disease	**y.**
		HEART/CIRCULATION	Quadriplegia	**z.**
		Arteriosclerotic heart disease (ASHD) **d.**	Seizure disorder	**aa.**
		Cardiac dysrhythmias **e.**	Transient ischemic attack (TIA)	**bb.**
		Congestive heart failure **f.**	Traumatic brain injury	**cc.**
		Deep vein thrombosis **g.**	**PSYCHIATRIC/MOOD**	
		Hypertension **h.**	Anxiety disorder	**dd.**
		Hypotension **i.**	Depression	**ee.**
		Peripheral vascular disease **j.**	Manic depression (bipolar disease)	**ff.**
		Other cardiovascular disease **k.**	Schizophrenia	**gg.**
		MUSCULOSKELETAL	**PULMONARY**	
		Arthritis **l.**	Asthma	**hh.**
		Hip fracture **m.**	Emphysema/COPD	**ii.**
		Missing limb (e.g., amputation) **n.**	**SENSORY**	
		Osteoporosis **o.**	Cataracts	**jj.**
		Pathological bone fracture **p.**	Diabetic retinopathy	**kk.**
		NEUROLOGICAL	Glaucoma	**ll.**
		Alzheimer's disease **q.**	Macular degeneration	**mm.**
		Aphasia **r.**	**OTHER**	
		Cerebral palsy **s.**	Allergies	**nn.**
		Cerebrovascular accident (stroke) **t.**	Anemia	**oo.**
			Cancer	**pp.**
		Dementia other than Alzheimer's disease **u.**	Renal failure	**qq.**
			NONE OF ABOVE	**rr.**
2.	INFECTIONS	*(If none apply, CHECK the NONE OF ABOVE box)*		
		Antibiotic resistant infection (e.g., Methicillin resistant staph) **a.**	Septicemia	**g.**
			Sexually transmitted diseases	**h.**
		Clostridium difficile (c. diff.) **b.**	Tuberculosis	**i.**
		Conjunctivitis **c.**	Urinary tract infection in last 30 days	**j.**
		HIV infection **d.**	Viral hepatitis	**k.**
		Pneumonia **e.**	Wound infection	**l.**
		Respiratory infection **f.**	NONE OF ABOVE	**m.**
3.	**OTHER CURRENT OR MORE DETAILED DIAGNOSES AND ICD-9 CODES**	**a.**	| | | • |
		b.	| | | • |
		c.	| | | • |
		d.	| | | • |

SECTION J. HEALTH CONDITIONS

1.	**PROBLEM CONDITIONS**	*(Check all problems present in last 7 days unless other time frame is indicated)*		
		INDICATORS OF FLUID STATUS	Dizziness/Vertigo	**f.**
		Weight gain or loss of 3 or more pounds within a 7 day period **a.**	Edema	**g.**
			Fever	**h.**
			Hallucinations	**i.**
		Inability to lie flat due to shortness of breath **b.**	Internal bleeding	**j.**
			Recurrent lung aspirations in last 90 days	**k.**
		Dehydrated; output exceeds input **c.**	Shortness of breath	**l.**
			Syncope (fainting)	**m.**
		Insufficient fluid; did NOT consume all/almost all liquids provided during last 3 days **d.**	Unsteady gait	**n.**
			Vomiting	**o.**
		OTHER	NONE OF ABOVE	**p.**
		Delusions **e.**		

FIGURE 11.1 Box 11-2 sample minimum data set documentation (*continued*).

SECTION M. SKIN CONDITION

				Number at Stage
1.	ULCERS (Due to any cause)	(Record the number of ulcers at each ulcer stage—regardless of cause. If none present at a stage, record "0" (zero). Code all that apply during last 7 days. Code 9 = 9 or more.) **[Requires full body exam.]**		
		a. Stage 1.	A persistent area of skin redness (without a break in the skin) that does not disappear when pressure is relieved.	
		b. Stage 2.	A partial thickness loss of skin layers that presents clinically as an abrasion, blister, or shallow crater.	
		c. Stage 3.	A full thickness of skin is lost, exposing the subcutaneous tissues - presents as a deep crater with or without undermining adjacent tissue.	
		d. Stage 4.	A full thickness of skin and subcutaneous tissue is lost, exposing muscle or bone.	
2.	TYPE OF ULCER	(For each type of ulcer, **code for the highest stage in the last 7 days** using scale in item M1—i.e., 0=none; stages 1, 2, 3, 4)		
		a. Pressure ulcer—any lesion caused by pressure resulting in damage of underlying tissue		
		b. Stasis ulcer—open lesion caused by poor circulation in the lower extremities		
3.	HISTORY OF RESOLVED ULCERS	Resident had an ulcer that was resolved or cured **in LAST 90 DAYS** 0. No 1. Yes		
4.	OTHER SKIN PROBLEMS OR LESIONS PRESENT	(Check all that apply during last 7 days)		
		Abrasions, bruises		a.
		Burns (second or third degree)		b.
		Open lesions other than ulcers, rashes, cuts (e.g., cancer lesions)		c.
		Rashes—e.g., intertrigo, eczema, drug rash, heat rash, herpes zoster		d.
		Skin desensitized to pain or pressure		e.
		Skin tears or cuts (other than surgery)		f.
		Surgical wounds		g.
		NONE OF ABOVE		h.
5.	SKIN TREAT-MENTS	(Check all that apply during last 7 days)		
		Pressure relieving device(s) for chair		a.
		Pressure relieving device(s) for bed		b.
		Turning/repositioning program		c.
		Nutrition or hydration intervention to manage skin problems		d.
		Ulcer care		e.
		Surgical wound care		f.
		Application of dressings (with or without topical medications) other than to feet		g.
		Application of ointments/medications (other than to feet)		h.
		Other preventative or protective skin care (other than to feet)		i.
		NONE OF ABOVE		j.
6.	FOOT PROBLEMS AND CARE	(Check all that apply during last 7 days)		
		Resident has one or more foot problems—e.g., corns, callouses, bunions, hammer toes, overlapping toes, pain, structural problems		a.
		Infection of the foot—e.g., cellulitis, purulent drainage		b.
		Open lesions on the foot		c.
		Nails/calluses trimmed during **last 90 days**		d.
		Received preventative or protective foot care (e.g., used special shoes, inserts, pads, toe separators)		e.
		Application of dressings (with or without topical medications)		f.
		NONE OF ABOVE		g.

SECTION N. ACTIVITY PURSUIT PATTERNS

1.	TIME AWAKE	(Check appropriate time periods over last 7 days)	
		Resident awake all or most of time (i.e., naps no more than one hour per time period) in the:	
		Morning a.	Evening c.
		Afternoon b.	NONE OF ABOVE d.

(If resident is comatose, skip to Section O)

2.	AVERAGE TIME INVOLVED IN ACTIVITIES	(When awake and not receiving treatments or ADL care) 0. Most—more than 2/3 of time 2. Little—less than 1/3 of time 1. Some—from 1/3 to 2/3 of time 3. None	
3.	PREFERRED ACTIVITY SETTINGS	(Check all settings in which activities are preferred)	
		Own room a.	
		Day/activity room b.	Outside facility d.
		Inside NH/off unit c.	NONE OF ABOVE e.
4.	GENERAL ACTIVITY PREFER-ENCES (adapted to resident's current abilities)	(Check all PREFERENCES whether or not activity is currently available to resident)	
		Cards/other games a.	Trips/shopping g.
		Crafts/arts b.	Walking/wheeling outdoors h.
		Exercise/sports c.	Watching TV i.
		Music d.	Gardening or plants j.
		Reading/writing e.	Talking or conversing k.
		Spiritual/religious activities f.	Helping others l.
			NONE OF ABOVE m.

2.	PAIN SYMPTOMS	(Code the **highest level of pain** present in the **last 7 days**)		
		a. **FREQUENCY** with which resident complains or shows evidence of pain	b. **INTENSITY** of pain	
		0. No pain (**skip to J4**)	1. Mild pain	
		1. Pain less than daily	2. Moderate pain	
		2. Pain daily	3. Times when pain is horrible or excruciating	
3.	PAIN SITE	(If pain present, **check all sites** that apply in **last 7 days**)		
		Back pain	a.	Incisional pain	f.
		Bone pain	b.	Joint pain (other than hip)	g.
		Chest pain while doing usual activities	c.	Soft tissue pain (e.g., lesion, muscle)	h.
		Headache	d.	Stomach pain	i.
		Hip pain	e.	Other	j.
4.	ACCIDENTS	(Check all that apply)		
		Fell in **past 30 days**	a.	Hip fracture in **last 180 days**	c.
		Fell in **past 31-180 days**	b.	Other fracture in **last 180 days**	d.
				NONE OF ABOVE	e.
5.	STABILITY OF CONDITIONS	Conditions/diseases make resident's cognitive, ADL, mood or behavior patterns unstable—(fluctuating, precarious, or deteriorating)		a.
		Resident experiencing an acute episode or a flare-up of a recurrent or chronic problem		b.
		End-stage disease, 6 or fewer months to live		c.
		NONE OF ABOVE		d.

SECTION K. ORAL/NUTRITIONAL STATUS

1.	ORAL PROBLEMS	Chewing problem	a.
		Swallowing problem	b.
		Mouth pain	c.
		NONE OF ABOVE	d.
2.	HEIGHT AND WEIGHT	Record (a.) **height in inches** and (b.) **weight in pounds**. Base weight on most recent measure in **last 30 days**; measure weight consistently in accord with standard facility practice—e.g., in a.m. after voiding, before meal, with shoes off, and in nightclothes	
		a. HT (in.) ☐☐ b. WT (lb.) ☐☐☐	
3.	WEIGHT CHANGE	a. Weight loss—5 % or more in **last 30 days**; or 10 % or more in **last 180 days** 0. No 1. Yes	
		b. Weight gain—5 % or more in **last 30 days**, or 10 % or more in **last 180 days** 0. No 1. Yes	
4.	NUTRI-TIONAL PROBLEMS	Complains about the taste of many foods a.	Leaves 25% or more of food uneaten at most meals c.
		Regular or repetitive complaints of hunger b.	NONE OF ABOVE d.
5.	NUTRI-TIONAL APPROACH-ES	(Check all that apply in last 7 days)	
		Parenteral/IV a.	Dietary supplement between meals f.
		Feeding tube b.	
		Mechanically altered diet c.	Plate guard, stabilized built-up utensil, etc. g.
		Syringe (oral feeding) d.	On a planned weight change program h.
		Therapeutic diet e.	NONE OF ABOVE i.
6.	PARENTERAL OR ENTERAL INTAKE	(Skip to Section L if neither 5a nor 5b is checked)	
		a. Code the proportion of **total calories** the resident received through parenteral or tube feedings in the **last 7 days** 0. None 3. 51% to 75% 1. 1% to 25% 4. 76% to 100% 2. 26% to 50%	
		b. Code the average **fluid intake** per day by IV or tube in **last 7 days** 0. None 3. 1001 to 1500 cc/day 1. 1 to 500 cc/day 4. 1501 to 2000 cc/day 2. 501 to 1000 cc/day 5. 2001 or more cc/day	

SECTION L. ORAL/DENTAL STATUS

1.	ORAL STATUS AND DISEASE PREVENTION	Debris (soft, easily movable substances) present in mouth prior to going to bed at night	a.
		Has dentures or removable bridge	b.
		Some/all natural teeth lost—does not have or does not use dentures (or partial plates)	c.
		Broken, loose, or carious teeth	d.
		Inflamed gums (gingiva); swollen or bleeding gums; oral abscesses; ulcers or rashes	e.
		Daily cleaning of teeth/dentures or daily mouth care—by resident or staff	f.
		NONE OF ABOVE	g.

FIGURE 11.1   (continued).

Resident _____   Numeric Identifier _____

5.	PREFERS CHANGE IN DAILY ROUTINE	Code for resident preferences in daily routines 0. No change 1. Slight change 2. Major change	
		a. Type of activities in which resident is currently involved	
		b. Extent of resident involvement in activities	

SECTION O. MEDICATIONS

1.	NUMBER OF MEDICA-TIONS	(Record the number of different medications used in the last 7 days; enter "0" if none used)	
2.	NEW MEDICA-TIONS	(Resident currently receiving medications that were initiated during the last 90 days) 0. No 1. Yes	
3.	INJECTIONS	(Record the number of DAYS injections of any type received during the last 7 days; enter "0" if none used)	
4.	DAYS RECEIVED THE FOLLOWING MEDICATION	(Record the number of DAYS during last 7 days; enter "0" if not used. Note—enter "1" for long-acting meds used less than weekly)	

a. Antipsychotic	d. Hypnotic
b. Antianxiety	e. Diuretic
c. Antidepressant	

SECTION P. SPECIAL TREATMENTS AND PROCEDURES

1.	SPECIAL TREAT-MENTS, PROCE-DURES, AND PROGRAMS	a. SPECIAL CARE—Check treatments or programs received during the last 14 days

TREATMENTS		PROGRAMS	
Chemotherapy	Ventilator or respirator	l.	
Dialysis	a. PROGRAMS		
IV medication	b. Alcohol/drug treatment program	m.	
Intake/output	c. Alzheimer's/dementia special care unit	n.	
Monitoring acute medical condition	d. Hospice care	o.	
Ostomy care	e. Pediatric unit	p.	
Oxygen therapy	f. Respite care	q.	
Radiation	g. Training in skills required to return to the community (e.g., taking medications, house work, shopping, transportation, ADLs)	r.	
Suctioning	h.		
Tracheostomy care	i.		
Transfusions	k. NONE OF ABOVE	s.	

b. THERAPIES - Record the number of days and total minutes each of the following therapies was administered (for at least 15 minutes a day) in the last 7 calendar days (Enter 0 if none or less than 15 min. daily) [Note—count only post admission therapies] (A) = # of days administered for 15 minutes or more (B) = total # of minutes provided in last 7 days	DAYS (A)	MIN (B)
a. Speech - language pathology and audiology services		
b. Occupational therapy		
c. Physical therapy		
d. Respiratory therapy		
e. Psychological therapy (by any licensed mental health professional)		

2.	INTERVEN-TION PROGRAMS FOR MOOD, BEHAVIOR, COGNITIVE LOSS	(Check all interventions or strategies used in last 7 days—no matter where received)	
		Special behavior symptom evaluation program	a.
		Evaluation by a licensed mental health specialist in last 90 days	b.
		Group therapy	c.
		Resident-specific deliberate changes in the environment to address mood/behavior patterns—e.g., providing bureau in which to rummage	d.
		Reorientation—e.g., cueing	e.
		NONE OF ABOVE	f.

3.	NURSING REHABILITA-TION/ RESTOR-ATIVE CARE	Record the NUMBER OF DAYS each of the following rehabilitation or restorative techniques or practices or provided to the resident for more than or equal to 15 minutes per day in the last 7 days (Enter 0 if none or less than 15 min. daily.)

a. Range of motion (passive)		f. Walking	
b. Range of motion (active)		g. Dressing or grooming	
c. Splint or brace assistance		h. Eating or swallowing	
TRAINING AND SKILL PRACTICE IN:		i. Amputation/prosthesis care	
d. Bed mobility		j. Communication	
e. Transfer		k. Other	

4.	DEVICES AND RESTRAINTS	(Use the following codes for last 7 days:) 0. Not used 1. Used less than daily 2. Used daily	
		Bed rails	
		a. — Full bed rails on all open sides of bed	
		b. — Other types of side rails used (e.g., half rail, one side)	
		c. Trunk restraint	
		d. Limb restraint	
		e. Chair prevents rising	
5.	HOSPITAL STAY(S)	Record number of times resident was admitted to hospital with an overnight stay in last 90 days (or since last assessment if less than 90 days). (Enter 0 if no hospital admissions)	
6.	EMERGENCY ROOM (ER) VISIT(S)	Record number of times resident visited ER without an overnight stay in last 90 days (or since last assessment if less than 90 days). (Enter 0 if no ER visits)	
7.	PHYSICIAN VISITS	In the LAST 14 DAYS (or since admission if less than 14 days in facility) how many days has the physician (or authorized assistant or practitioner) examined the resident? (Enter 0 if none)	
8.	PHYSICIAN ORDERS	In the LAST 14 DAYS (or since admission if less than 14 days in facility) how many days has the physician (or authorized assistant or practitioner) changed the resident's orders? Do not include order renewals without change. (Enter 0 if none)	
9.	ABNORMAL LAB VALUES	Has the resident had any abnormal lab values during the last 90 days (or since admission)? 0. No 1. Yes	

SECTION Q. DISCHARGE POTENTIAL AND OVERALL STATUS

1.	DISCHARGE POTENTIAL	a. Resident expresses/indicates preference to return to the community 0. No 1. Yes	
		b. Resident has a support person who is positive towards discharge 0. No 1. Yes	
		c. Stay projected to be of a short duration— discharge projected within 90 days (do not include expected discharge due to death) 0. No 2. Within 31-90 days 1. Within 30 days 3. Discharge status uncertain	
2.	OVERALL CHANGE IN CARE NEEDS	Resident's overall self sufficiency has changed significantly as compared to status of 90 days ago (or since last assessment if less than 90 days) 0. No change 1. Improved—receives fewer 2. Deteriorated—receives supports, needs less more support restrictive level of care	

SECTION R. ASSESSMENT INFORMATION

1.	PARTICIPA-TION IN ASSESS-MENT	a. Resident: 0. No 1. Yes	
		b. Family: 0. No 1. Yes 2. No family	
		c. Significant other: 0. No 1. Yes 2. None	

2. SIGNATURE OF PERSON COORDINATING THE ASSESSMENT:

a. Signature of RN Assessment Coordinator (sign on above line)

b. Date RN Assessment Coordinator signed as complete			
	Month	Day	Year

MDS 2.0 September, 2000

FIGURE 11.1   Box 11-2 sample minimum data set documentation (*continued*).

bacteria in the urine, is generally asymptomatic and does not appear to cause renal damage or affect morbidity or mortality of older adults. It is always present among clients with long-term indwelling catheters and has a great economic impact among the older population.

EVIDENCE-BASED PRACTICE

Title of Study: The Minimum Data Set Depression Quality Indicator: Does It Reflect Differences in Care Processes?

Authors: Simmons, S., Cadogan, M., Cabrera, G., Al-Samarrai, N., Jorge, J., Levy-Storms, L., Osterweil, D., Schnelle, J.

Purpose: To determine whether those nursing homes that score differently on prevalence of depression (according to the minimum data set [MDS] quality indicator), also provide different care for the depressed client.

Methods: A cross-sectional study of 396 long-term residents in 14 skilled nursing homes. Of those care facilities, 10 were in the lower quartile and 4 in the upper quartile on the MDS depression quality indicator. By the use of resident interviews, direct observation, and medical records reviews, measurement of depressive symptoms were assessed. The staff was assessed relating to their care process, by trained researchers.

Findings: The prevalence noted by independent assessments was significantly higher than prevalence based on the MDS quality indicator and comparable between those homes reporting low versus high rates of depression (46% and 41%, respectively).

Implications: The MDS quality indicator underestimates the prevalence of depression, particularly in those homes reporting low or nonexistent rates. Nursing homes need to enhance staff recognition of depressive symptoms. Those nursing homes that report low prevalence of depression should not be accredited for providing better care.

The Gerontologist, Vol. 44, No. 4, 554–564.

When bacteriuria becomes pathological, the symptoms are generally incontinence, increased confusion, and falls among older adults (Amella, 2004). Other common symptoms among older adults include urinary frequency, dysuria, suprapubic discomfort, fever, and/or costovertebral tenderness. Diagnosis generally involves the collection of a urine specimen for culture and sensitivity. Antibiotic treatment of should only occur in the presence of symptoms, and a short course of antibiotics is usually recommended. Treatment for longer periods of time may be necessary among the older population, however, due to decreased natural immune responses. As stated earlier in this text, indwelling catheters should be avoided when possible due to the increased risk of developing infections. If indwelling catheters are necessary, meticulous catheter care is essential to prevent the development of UTIs and the resulting complications.

Pressure (Decubitus) Ulcers

Decubitus ulcers occur commonly in long-term care settings. They are classified according to the severity of the wound, usually in four stages or types (Table 11.1). Early stage pressure ulcers appear as a mild pink discoloration of the skin in White individuals and a darkened area on those with darker-pigmented skin. Early stage ulcers disappear a few hours after pressure is relieved on the area. Later stage decubiti take the form of very deep wounds extending through all layers of skin and underlying muscle. They require extensive, time-consuming, and costly treatments and place the older adult at high risk for septicemia should the wound become infected.

The most effective nursing intervention for pressure ulcers is prevention. At an average cost of $1.3 billion a year, decubitus ulcers are a substantial drain on the health care system. They are also very preventable. The Braden scale for pressure ulcer risk assessment is an effective tool for assessing risk. Use of the assessment of risk factors contained in this instrument enables nurses to identify and implement preventative measures to avoid the development of these wounds. Preventative measures include the utilization of pressure relieving devices, such as mattresses, pads and footwear, as well as regular and consistent skin assessment by knowledgeable nursing professionals.

Nutrition is essential in preventing decubitus ulcers. A large study conducted among older adults aged 65 and older (n = 1113) found that diets were inadequate in 16.7% of the older participants. Normal changes of aging place the older adult at a higher risk for nutritional deficiencies.

TABLE 11.1   National Pressure Ulcer Advisory Panel Pressure Ulcer Classification

Stage I	Intact skin with nonblanchable redness of a localized area, usually over a bony prominence. Darkly pigmented skin may not have visible blanching; its color may differ from that of the surrounding area.
Stage II	Partial-thickness loss of dermis presenting as a shallow open ulcer with a red pink wound bed, without slough. May also present as an intact or open or ruptured serum-filled blister.
Stage III	Full-thickness tissue loss. Subcutaneous fat may be visible, but bone, tendon, or muscle are not exposed. Slough may be present but does not obscure the depth of tissue loss. May include undermining and tunneling.
Stage IV	Full-thickness tissue loss with exposed bone, tendon, or muscle. Slough or eschar may be present on some parts of the wound bed. Often include undermining and tunneling.

Retrieved August 8, 2007, from http://www.npuap.org/pr2.htm

In addition, a decrease in the smell, vision, and taste senses and the high frequency of dental problems makes it difficult for the older adult to maintain adequate daily nutrition. Lifelong eating habits, such as a diet high in fat and cholesterol, are other obstacles to maintaining optimal nutrition. The diminishing senses of taste and smell result in less desire to eat and may lead to malnutrition. Diminishing taste is also accompanied by a decline in salivary flow that accompanies aging. Chronic illness, depression, loneliness, isolation, limited funds to purchase food, and not knowing healthy food choices are also significant factors in malnutrition among older adults. Once the nurse identifies the nutritional concerns and risk factors, it is necessary to plan care surrounding nutrition in the older adult. Eliminating risk factors for malnutrition and appropriate meal planning are essential nursing interventions. Encouraging family to bring the older adult food that they enjoy or coordinating home-delivered meals may be helpful in promoting nutrition. Dietary supplements may also be essential in providing needed nutrition among chronically ill older adults.

Once pressure ulcers have developed, daily care with recommended products is implemented according to wound stage. Stage one ulcers are usually massaged around the area of the wound and reassessed daily. Stage two ulcers are generally treated with occlusive dressings and reevaluated at regular intervals. Normal saline dressings are the treatment strategy for stage three and four ulcerations. As nutrition is necessary for decubitus ulcer prevention, it is also needed to heal a decubitus ulcer once it forms. Nutritional management in conjunction with effective wound care is integral to healing pressure ulcers.

ASSISTED LIVING

Assisted-living facilities (ALFs) developed in the 1980s to provide supportive residential housing for the rapidly growing elderly population. Prior to this time, women cared for their aging mothers, sisters, and mothers-in-law at home. However, the rising number of women returning to the workplace reduced the number of caregivers available for the informal care of older adults. Most SNFs were not a desirable alternative because of high cost and a focus on functional dependence, so lower cost ALFs, with a greater emphasis on autonomy, became an appealing housing alternative to older adults with minor to moderate functional impairments.

"ALFs generally follow a nonmedical model, focusing on resident autonomy, privacy, independence, dignity and respect, in a housing environment as homelike as possible" (Wink & Holcomb, 2002, p. 251). Because there are no physicians and often no nurses in ALFs, the cost is usually lower than a traditional SNF. The nonmedical model also precludes reimbursement by Medicare, although Medicare reimbursement for these services may be provided by an outside home care agency. The average monthly cost of ALFs is $1,873 per person (National Center for Assisted Living, 1998).

Currently, the National Center for Assisted Living (1998) estimates that there are more than 32,886 assisted-living residences in the United States, providing housing to approximately 789,000 people. The average annual income of ALF residents is $28,000, with financial resources of approximately $192,000 (Marosy, 1997). The average age of residents in ALFs in 2000 was 80 years with a range of 66 to 94 years. The services offered at ALFs vary, but there is 24-hour supervision, three meals a day plus snacks provided in a dining room setting, and a range of personal, health care, and recreational services. These services may be included in the monthly rate, or they may be offered at additional costs.

Advertisements for ALFs featuring attractive facilities and health care have greatly influenced their successful occupancy in the past decade. However, the health care and nursing services available at ALFs vary widely throughout the country. Wallace (2003) reports that some facilities have adequate 24-hour coverage, while others do not have registered nurses on site. Furthermore, the disparity in state regulations has led to varied interpretations of what an ALF is and can do and the role of nurses within these facilities. Older adults and their families should research extensively the services within these facilities prior to selling their homes and relocating.

CONTINUING CARE RETIREMENT COMMUNITIES

Continuing care retirement communities (CCRCs) are defined as "full service communities offering long-term contracts that provide for a continuum of care, including retirement, assisted living and nursing services, all on one campus" (New Life Styles,2005). CCRCs are a housing alternative for older adults that arose in the 1980s, and they continue to house a small number of older adults today (Resnick, 2000). Their purpose is to facilitate aging in place. CCRCs provide several levels of care, including independent living, assisted living, and skilled nursing care. Theoretically, the older adult may remain in the community by merely changing the level of care received as changes occur in health, functional, or cognitive status.

CCRCs are very expensive and require an entrance fee ranging from $20,000 to $400,000, as well as a monthly payment ranging from $200 to $2,500. Residence in a CCRC requires commitment to a long-term contract that specifies the housing, services, and nursing care provided. AARP (2007) reports that there are three types of CCRC contracts:

- Extensive contracts include unlimited long-term nursing care at minimal or no increase in monthly fee.
- Modified contracts include a specified amount of long-term care. If chronic conditions require more care beyond that specified time, the older adult is responsible for payments.
- Fee-for-service contracts require the older adult to pay the full daily rates for long-term nursing care.

CCRCs originated from religious or social groups interested in caring for members of their communities. More recently, private investors have begun to purchase and operate these communities. Older adults generally pay a large entrance fee or purchase a home within the community and then pay a monthly fee. Skilled levels of care are reimbursable under Medicare. However, independent and assisted livings are privately paid. As with ALFs, periodic home care services may be reimbursable under Medicare by home care nurses. Services provided depend on the level of care and range from basic recreational services in independent living to full care and meals in a skilled nursing environment.

A study of older adults relocating to CCRCs showed that they experienced relocation stress that was consistent with the translocation syndrome. Assistance by a wellness nurse was needed to help manage the consequences of translocation within the first 6 months in the community (Resnick, 1989). Research exploring the health-promoting behaviors of CCRC residents found that it is essential for the older adults in these communities and their care providers to focus on health promotion behaviors and activities in order to keep costs down and quality of life high (Resnick, 2000).

HOMELESS OLDER ADULTS

While older adults often populate a variety of environments of care, it is essential to acknowledge that homelessness is a significant problem among this population. Little is known about the homeless older population. The lack of knowledge stems from defining homelessness among older adults. For example, is an older resident who was discharged from assisted living because of changes in functional status and has no home to return to considered homeless? In addition, because the older homeless population rarely seeks health services, they are difficult to access. The few available studies estimate that there are between 60,000–400,000 older homeless adults in the United States today, with an estimated doubling of this number by the year 2030 (Burt, 1996).

The typical older homeless person is a male. Despite the lack of health service use among older homeless adults, this population suffers

CRITICAL THINKING CASE STUDY

Mrs. Hobson is an 89-year-old woman who has lived in her house for the past 60 years. Her husband passed away 25 years ago, and she relies on her two sons and daughter for groceries and transportation to health appointments. She is independent in all her activities of daily living. She lives in an inner city area that has deteriorated greatly over her time there. Last night, Mrs. Hobson's home was burglarized. Mrs. Hobson startled the burglar, and she was hit in the head with the crowbar used to break the window and enter the house. She was treated in the emergency room and sent home.

1. What challenge does living on her own provide for Mrs. Hobson?
2. What other housing alternatives might Mrs. Hobson consider?
3. If Mrs. Hobson were to move to a more supportive environment, what effects might she experience during this transition?
4. If Mrs. Hobson were to stay in her own home, what interventions could be implemented to make her safer and enable her to function at the highest possible degree of independence?

from substantial physical and mental illness, as well as alcohol and drug abuse. This places older adults at high risk for increased morbidity and mortality, including decreased bone density, increased risk of hip fracture from falls, and increased motor vehicle accidents (Felson, Kiel, Anderson, & Kamel, 1988). It is important for nurses to consider the projected increase in homelessness among older adults and focus research attention at meeting the health needs of this challenging population.

SUMMARY

With the proportionate increase in the occurrence of chronic and acute illnesses among older adults, the subsequent decline in functional status, and the numerous losses sustained by older adults, changes in the living environments are likely. Many older adults continue to live independently at home or with a caregiver. Often changes in the environment are necessary for financial reasons. In other cases, older adults may move to obtain health care or a more functional supportive environment.

Moving from one environment to another is often stressful for older adults. Translocation syndrome describes the symptoms older adults may experience when they must change environments. Translocation can be very difficult and result in adverse physical and emotional outcomes. There are many environments in which older adults may receive health care and supportive care. These include acute care facilities, nursing homes, assisted-living facilities, and continuing care retirement communities. It is often the nurse's role to assist the older adult to find the environment where health and functional needs can be met, and to relocate to the most stress-free environment possible.

REFERENCES

Amella, E. (2004). Presentation of illness in older adults. *American Journal of Nursing, 104*, 40–52.

American Association of Retired Persons. (2007). *Continuing care retirement communities.* Retrieved July 14, 2007, from http://www.aarp.org/families/housing_choices/other_options/a2004-02-26-retirementcommunity.html

Burt, M. R. (1996). Homelessness: Definitions and counts. In J. Baumohl (Ed.), *Homeless in America* (pp. 15–23). Phoenix, AZ: Oryx Press.

Felson, D. T., Kiel, D. P., Anderson, J. J., & Kamel, W. B. (1988). Alcohol consumption and hip fractures: The Framingham study. *American Journal of Epidemiology, 128*(5), 1102–1110.

Fulmer, T. (1991a). The geriatric nurse specialist role: A new model. *Nursing Management, 22*(3), 91–93.

Fulmer, T. (1991b). Grow your own experts in hospital elder care. *Geriatric Nursing,* March/April, 64–66.

Fulmer, T. (2001). Acute care. In J. J. Fitzpatrick, T. Fulmer, M. Wallace, & E. Flaherty (Eds.), *Geriatric nursing research digest* (pp. 103–105). New York: Springer Publishing Company.

Hogstel, M. O. (2001). Gerontology: Nursing care of the older adult. Albany, NY: Delmar Thomson Learning.

Marosy, J. P. (1997). Assisted living: Opportunities for partnerships in caring. *Caring, 16*(10), 72–78.

National Center for Assisted Living. (2001). *Facts and trends: The assisted living sourcebook 2001.* Retrieved July 14, 2007, from http://www.ahca.org/research/alsourcebook2001.pdf

New Life Styles. (2005). Types of Senior Housing and Care. Retrieved on August 25, 2007 http://www.newlifestyles.com/resources/articles/Selecting_a_Continuing.aspx

Resnick, B. (1989). Care for life. . . . Even if a life care community is Utopia, the move can be a dramatic change. Here's how to smooth the transition. *Geriatric Nursing— American Journal of Care for the Aging, 10*(3), 130–132.

Resnick, B. (2000). Continuing care retirement communities. In J. J. Fitzpatrick, T. Fulmer, M. Wallace, & E. Flaherty (Eds.), *Geriatric nursing research digest* (pp. 138–141). New York: Springer Publishing Company.

Robinson, B. (1983). Validation of a caregiver strain index. *Journal of Gerontology, 38*, 344–348.

Sullivan, T. M. (2007). Caregiver strain index (CSI). In *Try this: Best practices in nursing care to older adults* (issue 14). New York: The Hartford Institute for Geriatric Nursing, New York University, Division of Nursing.

Wallace, M. (2003). Is there a nurse in the house? The role of nurses in assisted living: Past, present & future. *Geriatric Nursing, 24*(4), 218–221.

Wink, D, M., & Holcomb, L. O. (2002). Clinical practice. Assisted living facilities as a site for NP practice. *Journal of the American Academy of Nurse Practitioners, 14*, 251–256.

CHAPTER TWELVE

End-of-Life Care

Learning Objectives

1. Identify the role of nurses in promoting the use of advance directives among clients.
2. Discuss legal resources for end-of-life planning.
3. Describe assessment parameters important in palliative care.
4. Describe the nurse's role in supporting a multidisciplinary team approach to palliative and end-of-life care.
5. Identify the rationale for the team approach to care management.
6. Identify physical, social, psychological, and spiritual needs and nursing interventions at the end of life.
7. Provide care to enhance the grieving process of families.
8. Discuss challenges to widows and widowers.
9. Discuss the role of hospice in a "good death."

Ms. Wallace is a 65-year-old woman with multiple sclerosis who is currently ventilator and feeding tube dependent. Her two sons are attempting to have her code status changed to DNR/DN. However, her daughter is fighting to maintain her at full code status. Ms. Wallace had appointed her husband as her health care proxy 5 years ago, but unfortunately he passed away 6 months ago. The client now is incapable of communicating her wishes, although each family member states that they know what she would want in this situation.

You are a nurse in her nursing home, and you have been taking care of her regularly for the past month. You have established a relationship with each member of her family and have spoken to each of them regarding their feelings surrounding the situation. Several family meetings have been held, but as of yet no compromise has been made. Her physician comes to you to discuss how this issue may be resolved.

The story of Ms. Wallace is typical of today's older adult. In this society, there remains a marked difference between the way people want to die and the way they actually do. If asked to envision perfect death, most people would likely exclude the words "hospital," "tubes," "medication," and "pain." Yet, many older adults die in hospitals, with breathing and feeding tubes, urinary catheters, and, unfortunately, much pain. The goal of palliative care is to allow older adults to die in a manner that they would consider a "good death." The World Health Organization (2005) defines palliative care as "the active total care of patients whose disease is not responsive to curative treatment. Control of pain, other symptoms, and psychological, social, and spiritual problems is paramount." This definition clearly underscores the multidimensional nature of end-of-life care with biological, psychological, social, and spiritual components.

End-of-life care has recently undergone a great deal of research, and the nursing role at the end of life is becoming better articulated. As one approaches the end of life, they may explore the meaning of life and question the possibility of an afterlife. There are many aspects to end-of-life care, including communication, physical care, spiritual care, emotional and psychological care, as well as working with the family in promoting effective grieving.

ADVANCE DIRECTIVES

A major advancement in closing the gap between what a patient wants and what actually happens at the end of life is the development of advance directives. Norton and Talerico (2000) report that experienced health care providers who are comfortable with end-of-life issues are more likely to assess the readiness of older adults to make decisions about advance directives. Older adults must be encouraged to complete advanced directives in order to have their wishes followed at the end of life. Nurses have a unique opportunity to encourage the development of advance directives in all environments of care.

In 1990, the Patient Self-Determination Act was created to require every health care institution to develop policies and procedures for advanced directives available to all who receive services in that facility. Hogstel (2001) reports, "Failure to comply with the act may result in the facility's loss of Medicare and Medicaid payments" (p. 552). The act was instrumental in helping older adults to consider advanced directives should their decision-making capacity be altered while they are hospitalized. Advanced directives are a mechanism in which individuals can make decisions about their lives and health care prior to becoming ill. While it is not required that older adults make these decisions (and many do not), it is required that hospitals provide clients with the option to do so. The use of verbal statements, living wills, and durable powers of attorney are all considered legitimate advance directives for future health care treatment decisions (Hogstel, 2001). An important Web site that may be helpful to older adults and health care providers in developing these statements is *Aging With Dignity* and may be accessed at http://www.agingwithdignity.org.

At the end of life, great care must be paid to the client's nutrition and hydration to maintain comfort, and the ethical issues related to maintaining nutrition and hydration have received a lot of attention. In some cases, nutrition and hydration through nasogastric or gastric tubes provides the only life-sustaining measure in the older adult's life. Ethical issues surrounding the decision to remove these life-sustaining issues are prevalent. Families' decisions about continuing, or removing these life-sustaining treatments often conflict with health care providers. In these cases, it is most appropriate to determine the client's wishes. Moreover, cultural values influence the decision to sustain or withhold nutrition and hydration at the end of life. Caralis, Davis, Wright, and Marcial (1993) found that Whites were more likely to withhold nutrition and hydration

---

EVIDENCE-BASED PRACTICE

Title of Study: Role Strain and Ease in Decision Making to Withdraw or Withhold Life Support for Elderly Relatives

Authors: Hansen, L., Archbold, P., Stewart, B.

Purpose: To describe the strain and ease in decision making of family care providers when the decision must be made whether to withdraw or withhold life support for elderly relatives in various settings. To describe role satisfaction derived from caregiving to their elderly relatives.

Methods: Seventeen family caregivers were interviewed to gather descriptions of their experiences when faced with decisions pertaining to life support issues for their elderly relatives.

Findings: Role strain was related to issues before, during, and after decision making regarding life support. Role strain involved multifaceted, complex, and dynamic issues related to caring for elderly relatives. Role satisfaction did not coincide with the experienced role strain the family caregivers experienced and described.

Implications: Research is needed in the areas of role strain, ease in decision making, and role satisfaction related to family care providers experiences with caring for their elderly relatives.

Journal of Nursing Scholarship, Vol. 36, No. 3, 233–238.

CULTURAL FOCUS

Cultural values influence the decision to sustain or withhold nutrition and hydration at the end of life. Caralis, Davis, Wright, and Marcial (1993) found that Whites were more likely to withhold nutrition and hydration at the end of life than were other cultural groups.

at the end of life than were other cultural groups. This process is greatly aided by the use of advance directives. In the absence of advance directives, ethical decision-making frameworks (Chapter 10) can be helpful in guiding decision making regarding these issues.

Verbal statements regarding potential health care problems and possible treatment decisions may be made by older adults to health care providers and trusted friends and family. These verbal comments indicate a thoughtful approach to decisions that are consistent with ethical principles and with the older adult's past decisions. They may be used to make health care decisions when the older adult is no longer able to do so. If these statements are spoken to health care providers, documenting them in the patient record provides the best evidence of the patient's wishes.

Another way in which older adults may make their desires for care known in the event they are unable to make decision for themselves is through living wills. Hogstel (2001, p. 553) defines living wills as documents that provide a written statement about preferences for life-sustaining treatment. Because the living will is a written form generally filed with the older adult's medical record, its usefulness is dependent upon the health care providers to implement the older adult's wishes (Hogstel, 2001).

A durable power of attorney for health care or medical power of attorney has power extended to making health care decisions in the event that decision-making capacity of the older adult is impaired. Similar to a power of attorney for financial decisions, the older adult designates a trusted person to make health care decisions for them. The agent in this case may receive diagnostic information, analyze potential treatment options, act as an advocate for the client, and give consent to, or refusal of, care. This is a legal advance directive that offers greater flexibility than a living will. The document is not limited to life-sustaining measures but may apply to nursing home placement, surgery, or other forms of nonemergency treatment. One of the great barriers to implementing a durable power of attorney is finding someone to function as a substitute decision maker since older adults may have outlived their significant others (Hogstel, 2001). In this case, they may petition or hire a court-appointed power of attorney in order to benefit from the flexibility offered by a durable power of attorney for health care.

FINANCIAL PLANNING FOR END OF LIFE

There are many options that may be useful in planning for future financial needs of older adulthood. Some of the options have limitations. For example, a *trust* is limited to those who have significant financial assets. Trusts allow the older adult to maintain maximum control of financial assets while transferring the management of funds in a specified manner to an identified party, such as a bank or financial planner. A trust designates beneficiaries, individuals who will be in receipt of financial assets in the manner in which the older adult specifies (Hogstel, 2001). Another financial option is a *joint tenancy*, which is limited to those who have a trusted friend or family member. By opening an account or purchasing a property with another person, the older adult gives the trusted family member or friend unlimited access to the property or account. While both of these options have limitations, they are extremely helpful for many older adults who have or anticipate having the need for assistance with financial affairs. A *will* is a written document that gives instructions for the distribution of property, savings, and assets upon the death of the older adult. These are important documents to help the older adults determine the disposition of their assets upon death.

Regardless of the amount of financial assets, it is important for older adults to consider designating power of attorney to a trusted relative or friend, in the event that the older adult anticipates altered decision-making capacity. This situation may arise if the older adult were to experience a medical or surgical illness or procedure and needed to make sure financial needs and obligations would be met during that time. In this case, the power of attorney can manage the older adult's financial affairs, including filing taxes, paying bills, and banking during the older adult's recovery from a medical illness. When the older adult's decision-making capacity remains impaired, the designated individual manages the financial affairs for the duration of the older adult's life. This later case is known as a durable power or attorney. Delegation of power of attorney can be very specific and provide limited instructions such as "pay bills for two months" or more general, providing the agent with the power to manage all financial and personal matters.

DIMENSIONS OF END-OF-LIFE CARE

Nurses care for clients at the end of life in multiple care settings. There are many aspects to end-of-life nursing care including communication, physical care, spiritual care, emotional and psychological care, as well as working with the family in promoting effective grieving. Physical dimensions include management of common symptoms at the end of life, while psychological dimensions include the completion of developmental tasks as well as management of depression, anxiety, and agitation. Spiritual aspects of care focus on the need to find meaning in life and death. Social aspects of care revolve around completing roles that were essential to life. The dying person's bill of rights is found in Table 12.1.

Regardless of the aspect of nursing care delivery, culturally competent care is essential when working with older adults. Sherman (2001) reports that "Members of the palliative care team bring their own cultural perspectives and life experiences. Hospice/Palliative care nurses must be culturally

TABLE 12.1   Dying Person's Bill of Rights

- I have the right to be treated as a living human being until I die.
- I have the right to maintain a sense of hopefulness, however changing its focus may be.
- I have the right to be cared for by those who can maintain a sense of hopefulness, however challenging this might be.
- I have the right to express my feelings and emotions about my approaching death, in my own way.
- I have the right to participate in decisions concerning my care.
- I have the right to expect continuing medical and nursing attention even though "cure" goals must be changed to "comfort" goals.
- I have the right not to die alone.
- I have the right to be free from pain.
- I have the right to have my questions answered honestly.
- I have the right not to be deceived.
- I have the right to have help from and for my family accepting my death.
- I have the right to die in peace and dignity.
- I have the right to retain my individuality and not be judged for my decisions, which may be contrary to the beliefs of others.
- I have the right to discuss and enlarge my religious and/or spiritual experiences regardless of what they may mean to others.
- I have the right to expect that the sanctity of the human body will be respected after death.
- I have the right to be cared for by caring, sensitive, knowledgeable people who will attempt to understand my needs and will be able to gain some satisfaction in helping me face my death.

Reprinted with permission from Sorrentino, S. A. (1999). *Assisting with patient care.* St. Louis: Mosby, p. 843.

sensitive and responsive, providing care in a culturally competent manner" (p. 23). The views of death differ among cultures as seen in Table 12.2.

Physical Dimension

The physical dimension of end-of-life care for older adults focuses on ensuring that patients are pain-free while meeting other needs. This is not a time for nurses to be influenced by myths that underlie the undertreatment of pain in older adults (see Chapter 10). Clients must be assessed regularly for the presence of pain. This can be accomplished with a standardized pain assessment tool. Pharmacological and nonpharmacological interventions must then be implemented on a regular schedule (not PRN) to ensure a pain-free death. No older adult should ever die in pain. The physical dimension also focuses on the older adults' declining functional ability. The ability to perform ADLs should be assessed daily using a standardized functional assessment tool (see Chapter 4). While the older adult should be encouraged to maintain independence as long as possible, assistance may be needed when the older adult is no longer able to complete ADLs independently. Other physical symptoms common at the end of life include dyspnea, cough, anorexia, constipation, diarrhea, nausea, vomiting, and fatigue. These phys-

TABLE 12.2   Cultural Views of Death

Native Americans	African Americans	Asian Americans	Latin Americans
Death is viewed in a circular pattern rather than linear.	Prior bad memories of health care make older adults concerned about making end-of-life decisions.	End-of-life care decisions may be made by family members who consider it their role, even if the older adult is competent to make decisions. This may also involve the nondisclosure of terminal illness to protect the older adult. Autopsy and organ donation are not acceptable, so as not to disturb the body.	Reluctance to make decisions on end-of-life issues or complete advance directives, as well as endorse the withholding or withdrawal of life prolonging treatment, use of hospice services, support physician-assisted death, and organ donation is common. The well-being of the family may be considered over the well-being of the client.

TABLE 12.3   Physical Symptoms at the End of Life

Physical Symptom	Nursing Interventions
Dyspnea	• Assess respiratory rate and effort as well as pattern of dyspnea and triggering/relieving factors (i.e., activity). • Respiratory rates >20 breaths/minute labored respirations, use of accessory muscles and diminished or adventitious lung sounds require follow-up and possible intervention. • Administer morphine solution by mouth, sublingual, or via suppository Q2H, PRN. Diuretics (e.g., Lasix), bronchodilators, steroids, antibiotics, anticholinergics, and sedatives should also be considered. • Administer oxygen as appropriate to relieve symptoms, especially in those who do not respond to morphine. • Keep environment cool and position client for full chest expansion.
Cough	• Assess etiology of cough. • If from excess fluids, treat accordingly with diuretics (e.g., Lasix). • Reduce smoking and make sure environmental air is clear, cool, and humidified. • Elevate head of bed. • Ensure proper fluid administration. • Administer cough suppressants/depressants, opiates, bronchodilators, and local anesthetics.
Anorexia	• Understand that lack of hunger is normal at the end of life. Food and fluids at the end of life may create distress and, thus, anorexia does not necessarily need to be treated. • Good mouth care, using a soft toothbrush or spongy oral swab, is essential to prevent dryness, mouth sores, dental problems, and infections. • If the client can tolerate fluids, provide soups, tomato juice, and sport drinks to prevent electrolyte imbalances.
Constipation	• Recognize impact of morphine preparations on constipation among older adults and administer prophylactic treatment for constipation. • Assess client's self-report as well as physical symptoms of constipation such as bowel distension, nausea, vomiting, or rectal impaction. • Recommended medications include stool softeners, such as docusate sodium (Colace), and stimulant laxatives, such as senna (Sennakot-S).

(continued)

TABLE 12.3   *(Continued)*

Physical Symptom	Nursing Interventions
	• Bowel suppositories and enemas may also be used to relieve constipation. • Be alert for the progression of constipation to bowel obstruction. This may present as steady abdominal pain and is a medical emergency.
Diarrhea	• Assess presence and etiology of diarrhea and remove cause, if possible. • Ensure adequate fiber and bulk in diet and adequate fluids. • Determine times throughout the day when older adults are most often incontinent through a bowel diary. • Once the pattern of incontinent episodes is determined, the older adult may be encouraged and assisted to the toilet a half hour before diarrhea usually occurs. • Consider the administration of diphenoxylate (Lomotil) or loperamide (Imodium).
Nausea & Vomiting	• Assess client's self report of nausea, along with aggravating/relieving factors. The use of diary may be helpful. • Assess vomiting as well as aggravating/relieving factors. It is important to note that retching and gagging may occur even in unresponsive clients. • Administer antiemetics around the clock (not prn). Antiemetics that may be effective include prochlorperazine (Compazine) and metoclopramide (Reglan) administered as a rectal suppository, intravenously, or parenterally. • Consider the combination preparation [ABHR] of lorazepam (Ativan), diphenhydramine (Benadryl), haloperidol (Haldol), and metochlopramide (Reglan) if antiemetics alone are not effective at relieving symptoms.
Fatigue	• Fatigue must be recognized as a major source of distress among older adults at the end of life and has a great impact on quality of life. • Treatment of symptoms such as pain, nausea and vomiting, and dyspnea significantly impact fatigue. • Light exercise and activity, alternating with periods of rest and relaxation, are effective at relieving fatigue. • Music and guided imagery may also be helpful at inducing rest and providing stimulation during fatigued periods.

Adapted from Matzo, M. L., & Sherman, D. W. (Eds.). (2001). *Palliative care nursing.* New York: Springer Publishing Company.

ical symptoms are summarized in Table 12.3 along with nursing interventions to reduce symptoms and their impact on quality of life.

Psychological Dimension

In psychological terms, the older adult's success in meeting the developmental tasks of aging must be assessed. While end of life is often difficult, this time also provides an opportunity to complete important developmental tasks of aging. The psychological dimension focuses on how the older adult feels about their self and their relationships with others. Are there unresolved personal issues? Are there unfinished tasks that still need to be completed so that the older adult feels that responsibilities have been met? Discussing some of these issues with older adults who are approaching the end of life will help to identify uncompleted tasks. While it may appear to be too late, some older adults have completed academic degrees, contacted estranged family members, and even have been married on their death beds. The nurse may be the one to make the phone call or mediate the discussion between two people who have not spoken in years. Nurses can play an important role in helping older adults to complete these developmental tasks and experience a good rather than a bad death.

In addition to the developmental task of aging, the psychological experience of dying must be considered. End of life often involves the development of depression, anxiety, confusion, agitation, and delirium. These symptoms and suggested nursing interventions are described in Table 12.4.

Social Dimension

In the social dimension, it is important to identify the roles that older adults have occupied and whether or not they have disengaged from these roles. With the rising numbers of older adults caring for grandchildren, the aging grandmother may be concerned about who will care for her grandchildren when she passes away. Older adults may be employed and worry about how their job responsibilities will be met upon their death. They may also be caregivers to ill or cognitively impaired spouses or siblings; the loved one's future care is likely to be a concern.

Spiritual Dimension

The spiritual dimension allows the older adult to transcend from this life into another existence. If the older adult has explored the meaning of their life and has an expectation of an afterlife, death may be peaceful. However, older adults often continue to struggle with the meaning of life even at the end. As discussed in Chapter 10, spiritual assessment and coun-

TABLE 12.4   Psychological Symptoms at the End of Life

Psychological Symptom	Nursing Interventions
Depression	• Assess cause of depression—consider unrelieved pain and anticipatory grieving. • Openly discuss older adult's fears and concerns regarding end of life, in order to assist in the resolution of depression. • Refer for counseling. • Implement suicide precautions, if necessary. • Consider administration of antidepressants, including selective serotonin reuptake inhibitors (SSRIs), such as fluoxetine (Prozac), paroxetine (Paxil), and sertraline (Zoloft); tricyclic antidepressants, such as amitriptyline (Elavil), imipramine (Tofranil) and, nortriptyline (Pamelor); monoamine oxidase inhibitors (MAOIs), such as phenelzine (Nardil) and tranylcypromine (Parnate); and the other atypical antidepressants, such as trazadone (Desyrel) and bupropion (Buspar).
Anxiety & Agitation	• Assess cause of anxiety/agitation—consider unrelieved pain, urinary retention, constipation, or nausea as source and treat appropriately. • Openly discuss older adults' fears and concerns regarding end of life, in order to assist in the resolution of anxiety-producing issues. • Administer anxiolytics, such as lorazepam (Ativan), diazepam (Valium), or clonazepam (Klonopin). However, remember that these medications may result in delirium among older adults. • If anxiolytic medications fail to relieve anxiety, consider the use of barbiturates, such as Phenobarbital, or neuroleptics, such as haloperidol (Haldol).
Delirium and Acute Confusion	• Assess delirium using standardized instrument, such as confusion assessment method (see Chapter 9). • Delirium is a frequent occurrence at end of life as a result of life-threatening conditions and treatment strategies. • Immediate detection and removal of the cause of delirium will enhance the patient's recovery. • While the delirium is resolving, it is important to keep the older adult safe through the use of detection systems to alert caregivers of wandering behavior and implementing fall prevention strategies. • A calm, soft-spoken approach to care is necessary, and the delirious older adult should not be forced to participate in caregiving activities that cause anxiety or agitation.

CRITICAL THINKING CASE STUDY

Mr. Casey, age 79, was admitted to the medical surgical unit for testing because of vague abdominal discomfort. He was admitted during your shift and was pleasant and respectful during the admission interview. He stated that he was a devout Catholic and attended church every Sunday. He also stated that he was sure the tests would show nothing, and he thought his physician was overreacting by admitting him to the hospital. However, over the course of several days, it was determined that Mr. Casey had end-stage abdominal cancer. Because he lived alone, he and his only relative, a sister, determined that he should remain in the hospital for the rest of his short life. He was only expected to live for a few more weeks.

1. What questions might be appropriate to ask Mr. Casey to determine the role of spirituality in his life and death?
2. What interventions might the nurse use to facilitate Mr. Casey's spirituality in the hospital environment?
3. Beyond spirituality, what other dimensions should be considered in planning care for Mr. Casey? Provide examples of open-ended questions that could be asked to facilitate each dimension.
4. Beyond the patient and family, what other health care providers may the nurses communicate with in order to facilitate the best possible end-of-life care for Mr. Casey?

seling are integral to the promotion of peaceful death. The nurse must explore spiritual concerns with the older adult in a respectful manner.

COMMUNICATION

Several steps are necessary to help older adults achieve "good deaths." One of the hallmarks of palliative care is communication between caregivers, families, and patients. Nurses can be instrumental in bringing together interdisciplinary teams to plan care for dying older adults and assess effectiveness in meeting multidimensional palliative care needs. This team approach provides clients comfort and the reassurance that they will not be abandoned. Nurses are responsible for consistently evaluating the needs of dying patients and calling the team together if those needs are not met. It is important that both the client and family are encouraged to participate in care planning and evaluation.

Nurses communicate with the physician, who plays an important role in effective symptom management. Consequently, regular pain assessments and responses to treatment will be communicated to the physician who can adjust medications to keep the client free of pain. In addition, communication with physical and occupational therapists ensures that physical function is maintained as long as possible and assistance is obtained when needed.

After assessing psychological and social issues, nurses consult with psychologists or counselors, who can help older adults complete developmental tasks of aging, and with social workers, who help to resolve social issues facing the older adult at the end of life. Nurses also work with pastoral care to assist the dying older adult to transcend life peacefully.

GRIEVING

Nurses' work with older adults at the end of life does not end when the older client passes away. Nurses are responsible for helping the family through the grieving process. Grieving begins before the older adult dies and proceeds differently for each family. Kubler-Ross (1964) describes several stages of grieving that must be experienced for successful resolution of the loss. These stages include denial, anger, bargaining, acceptance, and grieving. Progression through these stages is unpredictable, but necessary. Families who have lost an older relative never just "get over it."

A grief assessment helps to determine the type of grief, a family's reactions, the stages and tasks to be completed, and additional factors influencing the grief process. Once the nurse gathers information on the family's grief, an active listening approach assists with resolution. Utilizing principles of therapeutic communication, nurses identify problems with the grieving process and allow the family to talk through their situation, sharing experiences is appropriate so that the family knows they are not alone. Nurses may identify support systems, such as bereavement specialists and support groups, and they should encourage the family to conduct activities and attend rituals surrounding the older adult's death, even when this may be difficult, because these ceremonies put closure to the older adult's life. It is important to note that grief work is never completely finished, but the pain becomes less over time.

WIDOWHOOD

It is well understood that the life expectancy of women is longer than that of men. Moreover, societal trends have revealed that on average, women marry older men. These two factors often combine to produce a substantial number of older widows. The Federal Interagency Forum on Aging-Related Statistics (2004) reports that women are three times more likely to be widowed than men. There remains a paucity of research on the experience of widowhood. The research literature that is available focuses on the health effects of widowhood, with bleak outcomes. This literature reveals that widows and widowers demonstrate health-related effects as a result of their change in marital status (Dupre & Meadows, 2007). Moreover, it has been a common assumption for many years that widows are susceptible to reduced health status, increased depression, and addictions to both prescribed and easily available habit-forming substances.

Often, the combination of major caregiving duties that suddenly end when the spouse passes and the grief associated with this loss increases the risk of health problems and reduces functional status among older adults. Nurses may effectively work with widows to assist in the grieving process and provide support by consistently assessing for health risks, implementing interventions to prevent health problems, and promoting health and healing and effective communication. Support groups, spiritual intervention, and enhancement of socialization may aide in the bereavement process.

HOSPICE CARE

Hospice care at the end of life is an extremely valuable, yet underused, resource. Approximately 620,000 clients had hospice services in the United States in 2000. Although hospices have provided end-of-life and palliative care for individuals in the United States for over 20 years, it is a highly underutilized service (Hogstel, 2001). One-third of all hospice patients received hospice care for less than 7 weeks, illustrating the lack of use of this beneficial service. The majority of hospice patients were 65 years of age or older (Hoffman, 2005).

EVIDENCE-BASED PRACTICE

Title of Study: Nurses' Attitudes and Practice Related to Hospice Care
Authors: Cramer, L., McCorkle, R., Cherlin, E., Johnson-Hurzeler, R., Bradley, E.
Purpose: To describe nurses' characteristics, communications, and attitudes related to hospice and terminally ill care.
Methods: A self-administered questionnaire was completed by nurses to assess hospice-related training, knowledge, attitudes, demographics, and personal experiences.
Findings: Characteristics associated with hospice care included: religiousness, having an immediate family member or close friend who had used hospice care, and satisfaction with hospice caregivers. A greater self-knowledge was related to discussion with hospice patients.
Implications: The perceived benefit of hospice care by the nurses was related to the nurses' discussion of hospice with terminally ill persons.

Journal of Nursing Scholarship, Vol. 35, No. 3, 249–255.

Approximately 3,200 hospice programs currently exist in the United States, the District of Columbia, and Puerto Rico. Hospice originated as a home care program established in Connecticut, which became the first inpatient hospice facility in the United States when it added inpatient beds to its facility. This original program grew into the current U.S. model of hospice care (Hoffman, 2005). Hospice care focuses on the value of life and revolves around the belief that dying is a natural extension of the living process. Consequently, hospice clients are empowered to live with dignity, alert and free of pain. The goal of hospice care is to facilitate a "good death" for clients. Families and loved ones are involved in giving care to the dying while maintaining the highest possible quality of life. The environment aims to promote physical, psychological, social, and spiritual aspects of life within the context of differing cultural and spiritual values and beliefs. Nurses in all settings are in pivotal positions to identify patient appropriateness for hospice and to communicate with the client, family, and team about this resource at the end of life.

SUMMARY

End-of-life care has recently become recognized as an important part of the lives of older adults. The manner in which death is expressed differs among people, but the search for the meaning of life often takes place during older adulthood. Nurses play an important role in helping older adults to manage multiple dimensions of end of life such as physical and psychological symptoms, completion of roles and developmental tasks, and obtaining resources to determine the meaning of life.

Client's needs at the end of life are great and diverse. As nurses help the older adult cope with end of life, they must also care for the many needs of the older adults' family. Excellent communication with members of the health care team and the family is important. Equally important is meeting the physical, spiritual, emotional, and psychological needs of older adults to help them achieve a "good death."

CULTURAL FOCUS

The experience of dying differs for each older adult and is bound by both cultural and spiritual values and beliefs. In order to provide high quality hospice care, nurses must understand the individual values of the dying person and work toward meeting personal goals and needs.

REFERENCES

Caralis, P. V., Davis, B., Wright, K., & Marcial, E. (1993). The influence of ethnicity and race on attitudes towards advance directives, life prolonging treatments, and euthanasia. *Journal of Clinical Ethics, 4,* 155–165.

Dupre, M. E., & Meadows, S. O. (2007), Role strain and ease in decision making to withdraw or withhold life support for elderly relatives. *Journal of Family Issues, 28*(5), 623–652.

Federal Interagency Forum on Aging-Related Statistics. (2004). *Older Americans 2004: Key indicators of well-being.* Washington, DC: U.S. Government Printing Office.

Hogstel, M. O. (2001). *Gerontology: Nursing Care of the older adult.* Albany, NY: Delmar Thomson Learning.

Kubler-Ross, E. (1964). *On death and dying.* New York: Macmillan.

Hoffman, R. L. (2005). The evolution of hospice in America: Nursing's role in the movement. *Journal of Gerontological Nursing, 31*(7), 26–35.

Norton, S. A., & Talerico, K. A. (2000). Facilitating end-of-life decision-making: Strategies for communicating and assessing. *Journal of Gerontological Nursing, 26*(9), 6–13.

Sherman, D. W. (2001). Spirituality and culturally competent palliative care. In M. L. Matzo & D. Sherman (Eds.), *Palliative care nursing* (pp. 3–47). New York: Springer Publishing Company.

World Health Organization. (2005). *Definition of palliative care.* Retrieved June 6, 2005, from http://www.who.int/cancer/palliative/definition/en/

CHAPTER THIRTEEN

Future Trends and Needs

Learning Objectives

1. Project future demographics of older adulthood.
2. Discuss changes in the health care delivery system necessary to respond to an increased population of older adults.
3. Identify anticipated developments in normal, pathological, physical, and cognitive aging changes over the next century.
4. State the role of health promotion in increasing the population of older adults.
5. Discuss projected developments in geriatric assessment over the next century.
6. Report on advances in the development of environments of care for older adulthood.
7. Discuss future methods in which nurses may assist clients to have a "good death."

Mr. Hyer is a 65-year-old male with a diagnosis of AIDS. Recently, he has developed pneumocystis carinii pneumonia (PCP), and his death is now imminent. He is very weak and cannot perform care on his own. Mr. Hyer and his partner decide that it would be best for him to go to a hospice where they can help him to care for himself until his passing. They get a referral from the doctor, and Mr. Hyer is admitted to the hospice where you work. You have heard from the staff how strong Mr. Hyer is and how well he is dealing with this aspect of his life. One evening, you are with Mr. Hyer rubbing his back to help him get to sleep and he breaks down. "I don't want to die," he states. He tells you that he is not ready because he still has so much that he wants to do in his life. His niece is expecting a baby in a couple months, and he wants to be a part of that. He tells you how afraid of death he is and how he knows that everyone thinks that he is so strong but that really he is just as sad and afraid as everyone else, he just does not let anyone see that. "I am terrified to learn what lies in store for me in the near future," he explains. He says that he realizes that there is nothing that can be done for him at this point, but he just does not want to die. He also informs you how much he will miss his family and friends and hopes that they know how much they are loved and how much they mean to him. He also hopes that they realize that he did not want to have to leave them and that they are able to go on without him, especially his mother, sister, and partner.

The science of geriatric nursing has grown exponentially over the past several decades, and it continues to expand today. Geriatric nurse scientists have dedicated their research and careers to investigating how to assess, prevent, and manage the common and pathological changes of aging. As a result, the lifespan and quality of life for older adults have become better. Throughout this book, the current available research on the care of older adults has been presented. In this chapter, however, the future of the science of geriatric nursing will be envisioned. This vision is supported by the funding priorities of Table 13.1.

This chapter presents an exciting opportunity in which to visualize how and what older adulthood will be in the future. The increasing lifespan of older adults means that older adults will become the majority of the population. This, in turn, will produce changing roles and environments and necessary alterations in the health care delivery system. As nurses increase their understanding of normal and pathological changes of aging, nurse researchers and scientists will discover new ways to prevent these changes through advanced assessment, health promotion, medication, and various medical and surgical procedures. It is hoped that the reader will savor these exciting advances in the care of older adults and decide that they would like to participate in the care of this unprecedented number of older adults.

AMERICA CONTINUES TO GRAY

Believe it or not, by the year 2050, there will be more older adults than children aged 0 to 14. Stop and think about that for a minute. Think of the number of children running around on the beach during your summer vacation, or crying in the stores while you try to shop; and then think to yourself that next to every child will be at least one older adult. But don't stop your vision yet! In your head, you likely have a picture of a gray-haired, slightly sickly, and unfit elderly person or couple standing

TABLE 13.1 Research Priorities of the National Institute of Aging

PA Number	Institute	Date Open	Date Closed	Grant Type	Sponsors
PA-05-117	NIA	06/03/2005	09/02/2008	T35	Ruth L. Kirschstein National Research Service Award Short-Term Institutional Research Training Grants (T35)
PAR-05-061	NIA	03/02/2005	03/16/2008	R36	Aging Research Dissertation Awards to Increase Diversity
PAR-05-055	NIA	02/18/2005	05/11/2007	T32	Jointly Sponsored Ruth L. Kirschstein National Research Service Award Institutional Pre-doctoral Training Program in the Neurosciences
PA-05-036	NIA	12/29/2004	11/02/2007	P01, R01, R03, R21	Retirement Economics
PAS-05-022	NIA	11/24/2004	11/02/2007	R21	R21 Grants for Alzheimer's Disease Drug Discovery
PAR-05-021	NIA	11/23/2004	11/02/2007	R01	Alzheimer's Disease Pilot Clinical Trials
PA-04-158	NIA	09/20/2004	11/01/2007	RO1, RO3, R21	Ancillary Studies to the Ad Neuroimaging Initiative
PA-04-123	NIA	07/07/2004	11/02/2007	R03	Sociobehavioral Data Analysis and Archiving in Aging
PA-04-064	NIA	02/20/2004	04/01/2007	R41, R42, R43, R44	Technology and Aging: NIA SBIR/STTR Program Initiative

(continued)

TABLE 13.1 **Research Priorities of the National Institute of Aging** (*Continued*)

PA Number	Institute	Date Open	Date Closed	Grant Type	Sponsors
PA-04-026	NIA	11/21/2003	12/01/2006	R01	Acute Coronary Syndromes in Old Age
PA-03-167	NIA	09/04/2003	11/02/2006	R21	Aging Musculoskeletal and Skin Extracellular Matrix
PA-03-147	NIA	07/07/2003	07/30/2006	R01	Age-Related Changes in Tissue Function: Underlying Biological Mechanisms
PAS-03-128	NIA	05/23/2003	05/25/2006	R01	Genetics, Behavior, and Aging
PAS-03-122	NIA	05/13/2003	05/22/2006	R01, R21	Frailty in Old Age: Pathophysiology and Interventions
PA-03-069	NIA	02/10/2003	03/01/2006	R01	The Biological Basis of Hutchinson-Gilford Syndrome (HGS): Relationship to Mutations in the Lamin A/C Gene (LMNA) and to Other Known Laminopathies
PA-02-169	NIA	09/24/2002	09/25/2005	R01	Integrating Aging and Cancer Research
PA-02-116	NIA	06/25/2002	07/15/2005	R01, R21	Age-Related Prostate Growth: Biologic Mechanisms (R01 and R21)

Retrieved June 28, 2005, from http://grants1.nih.gov/grants/guide/pa-files/index.html?sort=office&year=active

next to your envisioned child. This is typical of what is seen in the older adult population today. However, the older adults who constitute the large elderly population of 2050 may very well have a full head of blond, red, or dark hair and be as physically fit as the 20-year-old athlete of today.

In fact, it is now well understood that individuals currently aged 65 years can be expected to live an average of 18 more years than they did 100 years ago, for a total of 83 years. Those aged 75 years can be expected to live an average of 11 more years, for a total of 86 years. The centenarians who are rare will be so commonplace that the White House will likely abandon sending them birthday cards. People continue to live longer primarily because of the advances in health care. Older adults are living improved lifestyles primarily due to advances in medications to treat diseases, immunizations to prevent disease, new diagnostic techniques to assist in the early detection and treatment of disease, and new medical and surgical procedures to treat acute and chronic diseases. As readers adjust the mental pictures of older adults on the beach or in the store, prepare to visualize this large population as both fit and healthy.

The cultural backgrounds of older adults are changing along with the vast increase in the population. Scommegna (2007) reports that there is an unprecedented shift in the cultural backgrounds of the U.S. population; the White population of adults over 65 is expected to decrease from approximately 87% to 75% of all older adults in the years 1990–2030. In turn, the percentage of African American older adults is expected to

---

CRITICAL THINKING CASE STUDY

Imagine you are a nurse in the year 2050. You are employed at a 120-bed acute-care teaching hospital in a major metropolitan area. Your specialty area is oncology and your unit has 6 beds.

1. What changes do you anticipate in the health care delivery system that make it possible for a major teaching hospital in a metropolitan area to remain viable with only 120 beds?
2. What changes do you anticipate in care of cancer patients that make it possible for an oncology unit to meet the needs of the environment of interest with only 6 beds?
3. What changes in the presentation of disease, assessment, and management of disease do you anticipate among the elderly in the year 2050?
4. What technological advances are likely to enhance health care delivery in the year 2050?

CULTURAL FOCUS

The next decades will bring an unprecedented shift in the cultural back-grounds of the U.S. population; and the White population of adults over 65 is expected to decrease from approximately 87% to 75% of all older adults in the years 1990–2030. In turn, the percentage of African American older adults is expected to rise from 8% to 9%; the percentage of Asian older adults is expected to increase from 1.4% to 5%; and the percentage of Hispanic older adults is expected to increase from 3.7% to 10.9%. These statistics are important, because they predict a change in the manner in which traditional Western medicine is accepted in this country.

rise from 8% to 9%; the percentage of Asian older adults is expected to increase from 1.4% to 5%; and the percentage of Hispanic older adults is expected to increase from 3.7% to 10.9%. These statistics are important, because they predict a change in the manner in which traditional Western medicine is accepted in this country.

With these improvements in health care and increased lifespan comes the challenge to overcome ageism among society. *Ageism* is defined as a negative attitude or bias toward older adults, or the belief that older people cannot or should not participate in societal activities or be given equal opportunities afforded to others. Today's nurses are well-positioned to fight ageism and dispel the many myths of aging. If the next generation can make this change, older adults of the future will be free to age without bias and restrictions on health care. Even though ageism will likely still exist among some, most people will have the opportunity to enjoy encounters with older adults more frequently and in better settings than is currently possible.

An additional research area that is likely to remain robust is the focus on theories of aging. As introduced in Chapter 1, there are several theoretical viewpoints that have been developed to describe why people age. These theories are sociological, psychological, moral or spiritual, and biological in nature. These theories provide insight into the common problems of aging, and they provide the framework for advances in pre-vention, assessment, and management of these problems. In time, greater insights are likely to be gained.

CHANGES IN THE HEALTH CARE DELIVERY SYSTEM

Everyone in the United States who reads the newspaper or watches the news on TV is aware of the problem of how to pay for health care for the ever-increasing older population. In fact, the U.S. health care delivery

RESEARCH FOCUS

Title of Study: Stereotypes of the Elderly in U.S. Television Commercials From the 1950s to the 1990s.

Authors: Miller, D. W., Leyell, T. S., Mazachek, J.

Purpose: To investigate the prevalence of negative stereotyping of older adults within the U.S. advertising industry.

Methods: The authors viewed U.S. television commercials between the years 1950 and 1990 in search of ageism trends.

Findings: Surprisingly, the researchers found little negative stereotyping of older adults within the television commercials examined. The study did not support that television advertising propagated negative ageism stereotypes as originally hypothesized. In fact, trends toward positive stereotyping of older adults were noted.

Implications: While the results did not reveal support for negative stereotyping of older adults, the possibility was hypothesized. Nurses should continue to be cautious of negative stereotyping in the media and the implications of negative perceptions on the health care of older adults.

International Journal of Aging & Human Development, August 2004, Vol. 58, No. 4, pp. 315–326.

---

system has undergone enormous changes over the past several decades in attempts to find a way to pay for the health care of older adults. As discussed in Chapter 2, it is commonly understood that as people continue to age, they tend to develop more health problems. These health problems require increased use of the health care system. With a larger number of older adults and greater use of the system, Medicare, the primary health insurance of older adults, is in great danger of being unable to fund needed health care services. While several attempts have been made to curtail Medicare spending (see managed care discussion, Chapter 2), these attempts have been unsuccessful, and the problem of how to pay for the health care needs of older adults remains.

Currently, major discussion about the health care delivery system centers on the payment for medications for older adults. While this is one facet of the problem, future solutions to the cost-effective delivery of health care to older adults must address the health care delivery system itself. The attitude that everyone must make use of everything available to restore and promote health has resulted in heavy medication and medical system usage. In a society where so much is available, it is currently unthinkable to withhold medications or services, even if the effectiveness is questionable and can be problematic for older adults. This is an ethical problem, the discussion of which will likely continue for decades to come. Regardless of the ethical issues raised by the current health care delivery system, revisions can be expected in the methods of reimbursement, the amount of care delivered, and the role of the gatekeeper.

Two more cost-cutting strategies will be likely to generate research in the coming decades. First, it is well-known that healthier older adults require fewer health care services. Yet, the current health care delivery system does not often support the use of preventative services for older adults. It is hoped that, in the future, reimbursement will be provided for more wellness visits, exercise, smoking cessation, and health promotion programs.

In addition, nursing medication errors account for millions of dollars spent on health care every year. An Institute of Medicine (IOM) expert panel identified four environmental factors that consistently contribute to the quality of care delivered and the patient outcomes seen (Kohn, Corrigan, & Donaldson, 2000)): management, workforce, work processes, and organizational culture factors. The IOM panel also proposed recommendations to prevent these errors from occurring in the future, including: (a) developing governing boards that focus on safety, (b) introducing evidence-based management of organizational structures and processes, (c) assuring high levels of leadership ability, (d) providing sufficient staffing, (e) promoting ongoing learning and decision support at the point of care, (f) encouraging interdisciplinary collaboration, (g) creating work designs that promote safety, and (h) achieving an organizational culture that continuously addresses patient safety (pp. 16–17). The next decades will likely see system changes in terms of quality assurance programs instituted in all facilities to reduce these costly errors.

In addition to the need for sufficient funds to pay for affordable and accessible care, more health care providers will be needed to care for the older adult population. Health care providers, including, physicians, nurses, therapists, and support personnel, must be educated on the special needs of older adults, including the topics in this book. While medical and nursing schools are beginning to offer courses in gerontology within the curriculum, many programs still do not have a required course in gerontology. Federal and private support has been increasingly available to educate providers regarding gerontology. It is hoped that this funding trend continues and the workforce to care for the rising older population is prepared to accomplish this task.

ETHICAL, LEGAL, AND FINANCIAL ISSUES FOR OLDER ADULTS

With all that is known about the increasing lifespan of older adults, advance directives and financial planning have undoubtedly become household words. Upon admission to any hospital, nursing home, or home care agency, a discussion regarding advance directives is supposed to ensue. The desired outcome is a decision about what the client would like done if certain changes in their health were to occur. However, the reality is that few people are able to make that decision when it is needed. Many health care professionals find themselves caring for older adults at the end of life, without advance directives, health care proxies, and the other well-documented legal methods designed to remove health care professionals from the decision-making process. Thus, ethical decision making on the part of nurses, physicians, and other health care providers is part of everyday practice.

While ethical decision-making principles are not likely to change in the future, it is anticipated that use of the legal system will enable older adults to formulate advance directives. Because these legal mechanisms for making health care decisions are fairly new, it is only logical to conclude that over time they will become easier to use and be used more frequently with older adults entering the health care system. Closer relationships between attorneys and health care providers are likely to follow. In addition, more attorneys may pursue this area of law in order to assist older adults in making these difficult decisions prior to a crisis.

In addition to the need for legal documents to guide the health care decision-making process, it is also necessary for older adults to plan financially for their extended lives. Just as the Medicare system anticipated reimbursing the health care system for a much shorter period of time for each older adult, so too, the Social Security system did not anticipate paying older adults a monthly stipend until their eighth, ninth, and tenth decades of life. Yet, that is exactly what they are doing and will be doing increasingly in the future. Current discussion about the future of the Social Security system concerns the privatization of funds, which are paid into the system by members of the current workforce. In other words, money paid into the Social Security system from currently employed citizens would be invested in the stock market. The strength of this would likely be a good return on the investments and a boost to the economy. The downside of this plan lies in its risk of losing some, if not all, Social Security funds.

Regardless of how the Social Security issue resolves, older adults should consider doing some financial planning of their own. While it is not always possible for lower wage workers to put away money from their weekly paychecks, retirement funds are a good solution to financing post-retirement years as a supplement to (or in place of) Social Security. Many private companies have seen the need and opportunity for financial planning services for older adults and offer these services as needed. Of course, all investments should be well researched prior to committing any capital. Older adults may also consider postponing retirement so that they have a shorter period of time without income.

NORMAL CHANGES OF AGING

Groups of health care professionals that gather each year at the Geronto-logical Society of America (GSA) and American Geriatric Society (AGS) can frequently be found debating the issue of whether normal changes of aging are actually *normal changes of aging*. Perhaps they are so highly influenced by the health and environment of older adults that they are not normal at all, just common. If the latter is true, the improved health and environment of older adults are likely to minimize the frequency of these so-called normal changes of aging.

What this means is that the current picture of older adults may no longer be accurate. With preventative exercise, diets, medications, and restorative procedures, geriatric hearts and lungs may be as strong as those of 20-year-olds. Cultural backgrounds also play an important role in how a person ages. For example, people with darker skin possess more natural protection against the sun and, thus, may wrinkle less than older adults with lighter skin. It is generally agreed that biological aging changes begin to appear commonly in the third decade of life, with subsequent linear decline until death, but it is important in the future for nurses to refrain from making assumptions about normal aging. The assistance of talented hair stylists will make the hair of older adults blond, red, or bru-nette; Botox, collagen injections, and highly skilled plastic surgeons will leave older skin as smooth as a baby's. Older adults will have 32 teeth and will be eating nachos, dripping with spicy salsa. Oral erectile agents such as Viagra™ and related products will continue to revolutionize the sexuality of older adults. Gone will be the hearing aides and eyeglasses, as the need for these are eliminated with hearing implants, laser Lasik™ treatments, and cataract removal.

Indeed these age-defying procedures are currently available and used frequently enough to expect their continued popularity. Yet, there are costs associated with these procedures, and availability does not mean that they will be used or desired by all. The normal changes of aging may

---

CULTURAL FOCUS

Cultural backgrounds also play an important role in how a person ages. For example, people with darker skin possess more natural protection against the sun and, thus, may wrinkle less than older adults with lighter skin. It is generally agreed that biological aging changes begin to appear commonly in the third decade of life, with subsequent linear decline until death. Therefore, it is important for nurses to refrain from making assumptions about normal aging.

---

be more difficult to predict in the future; however, the advances that have produced greater variability in the aging process have also contributed to the excitement of working with this population.

WELLNESS, HEALTH PROMOTION, AND HEALTH EDUCATION

There are many modern scientific advances that may claim partial responsibility for the increased longevity of older adults. However, the adoption of healthier lifestyles undoubtedly plays a big part in improved health and the longer life of older adults. Moreover, as originally discussed in Chapter 5, older adults are never "too old" to improve their nutritional level, start exercising, get a better night's sleep, and improve their overall safety. These health-promotion strategies, supported by Healthy People 2010, will continue during the twenty-first century to affect the lives of all people beginning in childhood.

Barriers to healthy lifestyles for the young and old still remain, and are a focus for further study by nurse researchers. Lack of motivation to improve health will remain a barrier for years to come, and nurses must continue to research the best ways to educate clients about the importance of good nutrition, exercise, smoking cessation, moderation in alcohol intake, and safety practices so that they can help individuals adopt these behaviors.

Further research on health promotion will likely examine ways to reduce additional barriers to healthy lifestyles. In the low-income population, for example, lack of money for healthy food and transportation and a lack of safe places to exercise will continue to be barriers to health. In the current decades of post-welfare reform, sometimes simply being able to find and afford food prevails over the need to eat a healthy diet. Also, the need for two jobs precludes extra time at the gym or on a volleyball team. Research that continues to uncover the benefits of health-promoting practices will build the evidence for change to a healthier lifestyle, but the means and methods to adopt these lifestyles also require further investigation.

MEDICATION MANAGEMENT

There is no doubt that the pharmaceutical industry is prospering in the current economy. For almost every disease that has been diagnosed over the past 200 years, a medication has developed to prevent or treat that disease. While not all the medications are effective at *curing* the disease, they may be effective at reducing the symptoms, prolonging life, or providing the psychological support that something is being done. Based upon the current growth in the pharmaceutical industry, it is expected that the development of new medications will continue for years to come.

It is well known that the more medications older adults are taking, the higher the risk for adverse reactions. Medications to prevent and manage disease and symptoms are needed, but more prudent use of medications in the older adult population is essential. Cautious medication usage in older adults is needed, and so too is the need to contain medication costs, which may or may not be reimbursable under Medicare in the future. Ethical considerations must be addressed when looking at the short- and long-term outcomes of medication usage in older individuals.

Excessive and inappropriate prescription and OTC drug use will likely be a major concern of professionals caring for older adults. However, on the other end of the continuum, older adults are disproportionately undermedicated in the areas of immunizations and pain medication. With older adulthood comes declining immunity. Reimmunization of vaccine-preventable diseases is necessary to both decrease the risk of carrying the disease and of developing it. In addition, the higher incidence of acute and chronic diseases in older adults puts them at an increased risk for pain. Even though pain is very prevalent among older adults, many barriers prevent effective pain reduction in this population. Besides finding ways to reduce excessive medication use in older adults, there is also a need for improved immunization and pain management. Furthermore, the prevalence of illegal drug use among older adults will continue to be an important area for research among gerontological investigators. The shift in cultural backgrounds in the United States also predicts a change in the manner in which traditional Western medicine is accepted in this country. Consequently, culturally competent care is essential among nurses caring for older adults, and improved understanding regarding complementary and alternative therapy will be necessary.

Cultural Focus

The shift in cultural backgrounds in the United States also predicts a change in the manner in which traditional Western medicine is accepted in this country. Consequently, culturally competent care is essential among nurses caring for older adults, and improved understanding regarding complementary and alternative therapy will be necessary.

GERIATRIC ASSESSMENT

Geriatric nurses have made incredible strides in the assessment of older adults over the past decade. One needs to look at the large number of publications provided by nursing researchers to understand how far nurses have come in attempts to more effectively assess the common problems associated with aging.

While assessment instruments are widely available, more needs to be done to effectively disseminate current assessment tools and develop new ones. For example, the Mini Mental State Examination and the Geriatric Depression Scale are in common use. However, the Pittsburgh Sleep Quality Index and the Beers Criteria for inappropriate medications are lesser known and underutilized. Further research into assessing older adults should focus on how to best disseminate these assessment instruments to nurses caring for older adults.

In addition, there are many common problems of aging for which no assessment instrument is currently available, or for which the currently available instrument is not as effective as it could be. Currently, no tools exist to assess the risk for translocation syndrome, or to alert health care providers to hazardous herbal medications. Although there are numerous pain assessment scales, assessing pain in cognitively impaired older adults remains problematic. Furthermore, many of the excellent tools available lack reliability and validity studies to support their use in further research and practice. In the twenty-first century, it is expected that these instruments will be further developed, refined, and tested to enhance the quality of geriatric nursing practice.

ADVANCES IN ACUTE ILLNESSES AND CHRONIC DISEASE MANAGEMENT

The next five decades will bring about unprecedented advances in the diagnosis, treatment, and cure of diseases that have plagued the population for centuries. Drawing from the Human Genome Project, advances have already begun in the genetic marking of diseases early in adulthood or childhood. Identified diseases can be managed with medication or surgical treatment to prevent onset. Genetic marking is commonly seen in daughters or sisters of women who have breast cancer and now struggle with the decision of whether to have a breast removed in the absence of clinical disease. Genetic markings are also currently available for other forms of cancer and heart disease and are used to help prevent the onset of clinical disease later in life.

Acute heart diseases, such as congestive heart failure (CHF) angina and myocardial infarction (MI), are likely to diminish in numbers as a result of preventative health promotion strategies and medications. When these acute conditions occur, they are likely to cause less morbidity and mortality in the future than they have in the past, because more effective treatments are available.

The coming decades will possibly see the emergence of vaccines to prevent many of the common diseases associated with aging, such as HIV and Alzheimer's disease. With better utilization of currently available vaccines to prevent influenza, viral pneumonia, and common childhood diseases, the United States could theoretically find these vaccine-preventable diseases eradicated. Of course, full eradication would require 100% immunization of the population concurrent with the absence of clinical disease. Even though this is theoretically possible, it is not likely to happen in the near or distant future. Most would agree that a high percentage of the population could benefit from the reduction of communicable diseases. Thus, continued development and dissemination of vaccines are worthy goals.

Many other acute conditions are seen in older adults: urinary tract infections (UTIs), sexually transmitted diseases (STDs), Lyme disease, decubitus ulcers, osteoarthritis, osteoporosis, stroke, obstructive pulmonary disease (COPD), Parkinson's disease, diabetes, and so on. The coming years are likely to see substantial improvements in early diagnosis, medications, and surgical interventions. While acute diseases such as UTIs, STDs, and Lyme are curable, these diseases will likely be detected earlier and cured faster, with fewer negative consequences in older adults. The advances in the prevention of decubitus ulcers and the improved overall health of older adults will likely contribute to a marked reduction in the number of these painful and costly sores among chronically ill older adults. New medications and surgical treatments for arthritis and new methods of screening and preventing osteoporosis and treating fractures will reduce the morbidity and mortality of these chronic illnesses. With safer work conditions and a decline in the number of smokers in the United States, a decline will also be seen in the number of older adults with COPD. A cure for Parkinson's disease is on the horizon. Improved prevention and management of diabetes is actively being investigated.

Regardless of the trajectory of acute and chronic diseases in the future, nursing will assume a leading role in reducing the consequences of diseases in older adults. The life-threatening complications of acute and chronic illnesses in older adults, such as changes in mental status, dehydration, septicemia, and pneumonia, will be greatly reduced by advanced research and improved clinical practice in geriatric nursing.

SPECIAL ISSUES OF AGING

Older adults experience a number of problems related to physical and cognitive difficulties and the normal and pathological changes of aging. These problems often impact both the independence of older adults and their quality of life. One specific problem resulting from many of the pathological diseases is pain. Much research has focused on the experience of pain among older adults during the past several decades, and improved understanding of the pain experience, more effective assessment tools for detecting pain in normal and cognitively impaired adults, and enhanced pain management have resulted. Pain has become the fifth vital sign, and ways in which to reduce pain will continue to be examined.

A recent news item highlighted the issue of driving among older adults. An elderly man attempting to depress the brake in his car accidentally hit the accelerator, crashed into an open-air market, and killed several adults and children. As the population of older adults increases, so too does the number of older drivers. Legislation is being proposed, and in some cases has been adopted, to regulate the driving privileges of older adults so that this type of accident does not happen again. Advocates for older adults fear the impact of such legislation on the independence and quality of life of this population. Modifications to highways, roads, and automobiles can enhance the ability of older adults to drive safely. These are better alternatives than regulating the driving privileges of older adults.

Other issues among older adults that will continue to be studied in the future center around quality of life. More effective assessments in this area will ease the difficulty associated with ethical treatment decisions and end-of-life care. Issues of elder mistreatment will foster the development of improved detection and increased availability of resources to prevent this abuse. More emphasis will be placed on resources to support older grandparents and enhance the quality of their lives as well.

PSYCHOLOGICAL AND COGNITIVE ISSUES IN AGING

Advances in the prevention, assessment, treatment, and management of the three Ds (depression, dementia, and delirium) have been steadily forthcoming over the last half of the twentieth century. Undoubtedly, they will continue to receive much attention and investigation as gerontological nursing progresses. Because many older adults live for decades with unrecognized and untreated depression, enhanced assessment tools administered in the form of a single question can now help identify older adults at risk. This allows for earlier and more effective treatment. In addition, the development of new SSRI antidepressant medications with low side-effect profiles has led to more effective treatment of this prevalent disorder. Future research will undoubtedly seek to discover more effective assessment and medication management, as well as the development of traditional and alternative therapies for depression management.

There are over 60 diseases in older adults that present with signs and symptoms of dementia. The loss of mental function is a major fear of those approaching older adulthood, as well as those caring for them. How to prevent dementias will continue to be a topic of study, particularly the prevention of Alzheimer's disease, the most common dementia, will receive a substantial amount of research.

Currently, the investigation of an Alzheimer's vaccine is underway. Stimulation of antibodies to beta-amyloid (the substance that makes up most of the amyloid plaques consistent with Alzheimer's disease) is thought to prevent disease development. Further research is also investigating the role of lithium in blocking the development of neurological plaques and tangles. Newer research suggests that the reduction of estrogen use in older women is a possible cause of Alzheimer's disease. In addition to research on prevention, studies will explore ways to better manage this disease with medication, improved nursing interventions, and environments for optimal care.

Like dementia, delirium is receiving research attention. The suggested causes of delirium are (a) a decreased ability to manage change, (b) several environmental assaults, (c) impaired sensory function, (d) acute and chronic disease, (e) medications, and (f) urinary catheterization. With increased knowledge of the contributors to delirium, prevention will become a benchmark of quality nursing care.

ENVIRONMENTS OF CARE

The future will undoubtedly find more older adults living at home and fewer living in long-term care facilities. This shift in housing, fueled by both the improved health of older adults and the poor reputation of nursing homes, has already begun. The vacancy rate in nursing homes approaches 50% in some states and is projected to rise. But, with the increased number of older adults living at home, there is a greater need for more community resources. Transportation, home-delivered meals, assistance with ADLs, and social activities are among the many needs of older adults living at home. It is likely that the future will see an expansion of these services to allow older adults to live safely at home.

Although the growth of assisted-living facilities and continuing-care retirement communities will continue as an alternative to living at home, these facilities will remain an alternative for wealthier older adults. The improved health status of older adults will likely stabilize the number of acute-care hospital admissions that have grown with the graying of America. However, there is a need for acute-care nurses to develop a better knowledge base and greater expertise for assessing and managing hospitalized older adults in order to prevent the iatrogenesis common during these hospital admissions.

SPIRITUALITY AND END-OF-LIFE CARE

Unquestionably, the role of nurses in end-of-life care has gained importance during the past several decades. The end-of-life nursing care knowledge base is stronger than it has ever been, but there is more to know. There is growing evidence of the role of managing physical, psychological, social, and spiritual needs at the end of life. This research will likely continue. Nurses in all care settings must be aware of the necessary care for older adults at the end of life in order to implement the best nursing practices.

Along the same lines, the need to assist older adults in having a peaceful "good death" has never been stronger. Recent attempts at promoting end-of-life education in nursing have helped to bring this issue to the forefront, but many older adults continue to die daily in a less-than-desirable manner. It is the goal of all gerontological nurses that older adults die on their own terms. Consequently, additional research is needed. Integration of end-of-life care into nursing curricula must be promoted. While hospice is an excellent resource for end-of-life care, it is underutilized. Over the next decades, it is hoped that nurses will gain greater knowledge and have expanded resources to address the issues of end-of-life care.

CONCLUSION

The aging of America is extremely exciting! Gerontological research has brought forth improvements in every area of older adult care. Moreover, these advances have already succeeded in extending the lifespan, and they will continue to produce unprecedented changes in the care of the older adult population. From a vaccine to prevent cognitive impairment to the development of a revised Medicare plan, the twenty-first century is full of possibilities. Gerontological nurses will undoubtedly play a major role in these innovations. However, the most gratifying result will be the improved health and quality of life of the elderly.

REFERENCES

Kohn, L. T., Corrigan, J. M., & Donaldson M. S. (2000). *To err is human: Building a safer health system*. Washington, DC: Institute of Medicine.

Scommegna, P. (2007). U.S. growing bigger, older and more diverse. *Population Reference Bureau*. Retrieved July 12, 2007, from http://www.prb.org/Articles/2004/US GrowingBiggerOlderandMoreDiverse.aspx

Web Resources

Hartford Institute of Geriatric Nursing: http://www.hartfordign.org
Alliance for Aging Research: http://www.agingresearch.org
Geronurseonline: http://www.geronurseonline.org/
American Association of Retired Persons: http://www.aarp.org/
National Institute of Aging: http://www.nia.nih.gov/
American Cancer Society: http://www.cancer.org/
Stanford Geriatric Education Center: http://sgec.stanford.edu/
Administration on Aging: http://www.aoa.gov/

Index

Page numbers ending in *t* (e.g. 101*t*) indicate a table on referenced page